The Clinical Neurobiology
of Fibromyalgia
and Myofascial Pain:
Therapeutic Implications

The Clinical Neurobiology of Fibromyalgia and Myofascial Pain: Therapeutic Implications has been co-published simultaneously as *Journal of Musculoskeletal Pain*, Volume 10, Numbers 1/2 2002.

The *Journal of Musculoskeletal Pain* Monographic "Separates"

Below is a list of "separates," which in serials librarianship means a special issue simultaneously published as a special journal issue or double-issue *and* as a "separate" hardbound monograph. [This is a format which we also call a "DocuSerial."]

"Separates" are published because specialized libraries or professionals may wish to purchase a specific thematic issue by itself in a format which can be separately cataloged and shelved, as opposed to purchasing the journal on an on-going basis. Faculty members may also more easily consider a "separate" for classroom adoption.

"Separates" are carefully classified separately with the major book jobbers so that the journal tie-in can be noted on new book order slips to avoid duplicate purchasing.

You may wish to visit Haworth's website at . . .

http://www.HaworthPress.com

. . . to search our online catalog for complete tables of contents of these separates and related publications.

You may also call 1-800-HAWORTH [outside US/Canada: 607-722-5857], or Fax 1-800-895-0582 [outside US/Canada: 607-771-0012], or e-mail at:

getinfo@haworthpressinc.com

The Clinical Neurobiology of Fibromyalgia and Myofascial Pain: Therapeutic Implications, edited by Robert M. Bennett, MD (Vol. 10, No. 1/2, 2002). *Covers the latest developments in pain research: examines the results of a wide scope of basic and applied research on soft-tissue pain.*

International MYOPAIN Society–MYOPAIN '01: Abstracts from the 5th World Congress on Myofascial Pain and Fibromyalgia, Portland, Oregon, USA, September 9-September 13, 2001 (Vol. 9, Suppl. #5, 2001)

Muscle Pain, Myofascial Pain, and Fibromyalgia: Recent Advances, edited by Leonardo Vecchiet, MD, and Maria Adele Giamberardino, MD (Vol. 7, No. 1/2, 1999). *Covers the latest developments in musculoskeletal pain that were presented at the MYOPAIN '98 Congress in Silvi Marina, Italy.*

MYOPAIN '98: Abstracts from the 4th World Congress on Myofascial Pain and Fibromyalgia, Silvi Marina [TE], ITALY, August 24-August 27, 1998, edited by Leonardo Vecchiet, MD, and Maria Adele Giamberardino, MD (Vol. 6, Supp. #2, 1998).

The Neuroscience and Endocrinology of Fibromyalgia, edited by Stanley R. Pillemer, MD (Vol. 6, No. 3, 1998). *"I recommend this book to all health care providers who want to offer the most up-to-date therapy for their patients with fibromyalgia." [David Borestein, MD, Clinical Professor of Medicine, The George Washington University Medical Center, Arthritis and Rheumatism]*

Muscle Pain Syndromes and Fibromyalgia: Pressure Algometry for Quantification of Diagnosis and Treatment Outcome, edited by Andrew A. Fischer, MD, PhD (Vol. 6, No. 1, 1998). *"Should help researchers in developing new and expanded studies for the appropriate role of pressure algometry." [Martin Grabois, MD, Professor and Chairman, Physical Medicine and Rehabilitation, Baylor College of Medicine, Houston, Texas]*

Musculoskeletal Pain Emanating from the Head and Neck: Current Concepts in Diagnosis, Management, and Cost Containment, edited by Murray E. Allen, MD (Vol. 4, No. 4, 1996). *"Exciting because it contains a distillation of recent research that is of value to all who treat and serve those with whiplash-related injuries." [National Association of Rehabilitation Professionals in the Private Sector]*

Clinical Overview and Pathogenesis of the Fibromyalgia Syndrome, Myofascial Pain Syndrome, and Other Pain Syndromes, edited by I. Jon Russell, MD, PhD (Vol. 4, No. 1/2, 1996). *The featured speakers at the MYOPAIN '95 Third World Congress are here distilled into an anthology that represents a state of the art in fibromyalgia syndrome and myofascial pain syndrome from that conference.*

The Clinical Neurobiology of Fibromyalgia and Myofascial Pain: Therapeutic Implications

Robert M. Bennett, MD
Editor

The Clinical Neurobiology of Fibromyalgia and Myofascial Pain: Therapeutic Implications has been co-published simultaneously as *Journal of Musculoskeletal Pain*, Volume 10, Numbers 1/2 2002.

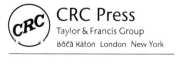

CRC Press
Taylor & Francis Group
Boca Raton London New York

CRC Press is an imprint of the
Taylor & Francis Group, an **informa** business

CRC Press
Taylor & Francis Group
6000 Broken Sound Parkway NW, Suite 300
Boca Raton, FL 33487-2742

© 2002 by Taylor & Francis Group, LLC
CRC Press is an imprint of Taylor & Francis Group, an Informa business

No claim to original U.S. Government works

Visit the Taylor & Francis Web site at
http://www.taylorandfrancis.com

and the CRC Press Web site at
http://www.crcpress.com

Indexing, Abstracting & Website/Internet Coverage

This section provides you with a list of major indexing & abstracting services. That is to say, each service began covering this periodical during the year noted in the right column. Most Websites which are listed below have indicated that they will either post, disseminate, compile, archive, cite, or alert their own Website users with research-based content from this work. [This list is as current as the copyright date of this publication.]

[continued]

[continued]

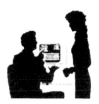

The Clinical Neurobiology of Fibromyalgia and Myofascial Pain: Therapeutic Implications

CONTENTS

ABOUT THE EDITOR

Robert M. Bennett, MD, FRCP, FACP, is Professor of Medicine at Oregon Health Sciences University in Portland, where he served as Chairman of the Division of Arthritis and Rheumatic Diseases from 1976 to 2000. Dr. Bennett is currently President of the International MYOPAIN Society. His clinical research interests have included fibromyalgia, systemic lupus erythematosus, and overlap syndromes. An accomplished leader in the field of soft tissue pain, he was the first to report adult growth hormone deficiency in a subset of fibromyalgia patients in 1992 and has subsequently documented the benefits of growth hormone replacement. Dr. Bennett has published over 300 articles and book chapters. He has served on the editorial boards of *Pain, Arthritis & Rheumatism, Geriatrics*, the *Journal of Musculoskeletal Pain*, and the *Journal of Functional Syndromes*. He is a past president of the American College of Rheumatology-Western Region and is cited in *Best Doctors in America, Who's Who in America, Who's Who in Science and Engineering*, and *Who's Who in the World*.

Preface:
MYOPAIN 2001

The long-awaited Fifth World Congress [MYOPAIN 2001] on Myofascial Pain [MPS] and Fibromyalgia [FMS] was held in beautiful Portland, Oregon, USA from September 9 to 13, 2001.

The dramatic events of September 11, 2001 caught the attention of those attending the conference from a total of 30 countries. There was a palpable sense of outrage at the terrorist attack upon the World Trade Towers containing thousands of innocent civilians. From the international community represented at the meeting, there was a sincere outpouring of empathy for the families who lost loved ones in this senseless tragedy. At one point during the meeting, the activities of the day were officially stopped for a few moments of silent reflection to honor the memory of those who had died or were suffering a loss.

While the cultural flavor of each MYOPAIN meeting has been unique to its location country, the clinical and scientific objectives have always been the same. Briefly stated, the goals have been: to present the results of basic and applied research regarding soft-tissue pain, to facilitate communication between clinicians and investigators, and to gain renewed momentum for three more years of productivity.

The history of the triennial MYOPAIN meetings has been described in editorials which preface publications regarding each of the four prior proceedings (1-4). A new development at MYOPAIN 1998 was the official inauguration of The International MYOPAIN Society [IMS]. A mandate to form such an organization was voted by the attendees at MYOPAIN 1995. After about two years of development, during which I was privileged to serve as Founding President, the organizational

[Haworth co-indexing entry note]: "Preface: MYOPAIN 2001." Russell, I. Jon. Co-published simultaneously in *Journal of Musculoskeletal Pain* [The Haworth Medical Press, an imprint of The Haworth Press, Inc.] Vol. 10, No. 1/2, 2002, pp. xv-xviii; and: *The Clinical Neurobiology of Fibromyalgia and Myofascial Pain: Therapeutic Implications* [ed: Robert M. Bennett] The Haworth Medical Press, an imprint of The Haworth Press, Inc., 2002, pp. xv-xviii. Single or multiple copies of this article are available for a fee from The Haworth Document Delivery Service [1-800-HAWORTH, 9:00 a.m. - 5:00 p.m. [EST]. E-mail address: getinfo@ haworthpressinc.com].

xv

structure of IMS took shape. It was officially incorporated as a non-profit, tax-exempt organization in the state of Texas and in Washington, DC. This status was officially approved by the Interim IMS Board of Directors in September, 1997. Those actions of the Interim Board of Directors and the new IMS officers were approved by the IMS members in business session on August 27, 1998 during the MYOPAIN meeting. Since its inception, the membership of IMS has grown to over 400 health care professionals interested in soft tissue pain conditions. The MYOPAIN 2001 meeting was the first of the triennial meetings to be fully organized and sponsored by IMS.

Since Dr. Robert M. Bennett was the host of MYOPAIN 2001 and served as guest editor of this proceedings, it is appropriate to profile him in this preface to the MYOPAIN 2001 Proceedings.

Robert M. Bennett, MD, FRCP, FACP. Dr. Bennett is Professor of Medicine at Oregon Health Sciences University in Portland, Oregon. He was Chairman of the Division of Arthritis and Rheumatic Diseases at Oregon Health Science University for 24 years [1976-2000]. Dr. Bennett is currently the President of the International MYOPAIN Society. From 1998 to 2001, he served as Vice President for the International MYOPAIN Society and Program Chairman for the MYOPAIN 2001 meeting in Portland, Oregon, USA. He was born and educated in England, and did his basic rheumatology training with Professor Eric Bywaters at the Royal Postgraduate Medical School in London. He has lived in the USA since 1972 and did additional training with Professor Daniel McCarty at the University of Chicago. His clinical research interests have included fibromyalgia, systemic lupus erythematosus, and overlap syndromes. He is an accomplished leader in the field of soft tissue pain. He was first to report adult growth hormone deficiency in a subset of fibromyalgia patients in 1992 and has subsequently documented the benefits of growth hormone replacement. He holds the use-patents for the utilization of growth hormone in fibromyalgia, chronic fatigue syndrome, rheumatoid arthritis, and polymyalgia rheumatica. His bench research involves the molecular characterization of cell surface deoxyribonucleic acid receptors, which he first described in 1983. He has published over 300 articles and book chapters. He is/has been on the editorial boards of *Pain, Arthritis and Rheumatism, Geriatrics*, the *Journal of Musculoskeletal Pain*, and the *Journal of Functional Syndromes*. He is a past president of the American College of Rheumatology Western Region. He is cited in *Best Doctors in America, Who's Who in America, Who's Who in Science and Engineering*, and *Who's Who in the World*.

The scientific program organized by Dr. Bennett and the IMS 2001 Program Committee offered a strong focus on the role of the central nervous system in the pathogenesis of soft tissue pain syndromes. Topical balance at the MYOPAIN 2001 meeting was ensured by a mixture of invited plenary lectures. In addition, 113 original abstracts, covering a wide range of topics, were presented at the meeting and are available in published form (5). In his Introduction to the proceedings, Dr. Bennett will be describing the meeting in more detail.

This current double issue of the *Journal of Musculoskeletal Pain* provides a synopsis of the plenary presentations at MYOPAIN 2001. It is fair to say that the extended summaries provided in these pages represent the "state of the art" for FMS and MPS as of September 2001. They also provide the basis upon which all who read these pages can regroup for the next assault. There is much to be done if we [collectively] are to be ready to present new information and findings at the MYOPAIN 2004 meeting in Munich, Germany.

The current officers of IMS are: Robert M. Bennet, MD, [USA], President; Dieter Pongratz, MD, [Germany], Vice President and Program Chairman for MYOPAIN 2004 in Munich, Germany; and Robert Gerwin, MD, Secretary/Treasurer. Dr. Gerwin will be the program chairman for the MYOPAIN 2007 meeting to be held in Washington, DC. The IMS Board is composed of Leonardo Vecchiet, MD [Italy], Chairman; Bente Danneskiold-Samsøe, MD, [Denmark], Member; James Fricton, DDS, [USA], Member; I. Jon Russell, MD, PhD [USA], Member; and Jack Scott, BA [USA], Member. The IMS Staff roster now includes: Barbara Runnels, MEd, and Rachel Brewer, BS. Continuing medical education accreditation was accomplished with the Accreditation Council for Continuing Medical Education through the Office of Continuing Medical Education under the direction of Susan Duncan, MEd at The University of Texas Health Science Center at San Antonio, This team of medical education professionals provided the administrative support for both the MYOPAIN 1995 and MYOPAIN 2001 meetings, so we are pleased that they have also agreed to assist with the planning of MYOPAIN 2004 in Munich as well.

The first responsibility of IMS is to maintain the high quality MYOPAIN meeting system, but it will also facilitate scholarly regional meetings between triennial international meetings, serve as a resource for expert opinion in the growing field of soft-tissue pain, facilitate interaction between members, and offer training/research scholarships to students at several levels of training. Membership in IMS is open to a wide variety of health care professionals and support staff. The first IMS Special Interest Group [Myofascial Pain Study Group], headed by Dr. Gerwin, is already making plans for a 2003 Focus on Pain meeting in cooperation with IMS.

Now the IMS needs you, the health care providers of the world who are interested in the care of persons suffering from soft tissue pain conditions. Needed are your energy, your ideas, your vision of the future, and your ability to lead IMS into the new century. Your membership and your commitment will make the difference. It takes many to make a united whole.

I. Jon Russell, MD, PhD

REFERENCES

1. Fricton JR, Awad EA, (editors): Myofascial Pain and Fibromyalgia. Adv Pain Res Ther 17:1-346,1990.

2. Russell IJ: MYOPAIN '92. J Musculoske Pain 1(3/4):xv-xvi,1993.

3. Russell IJ: MYOPAIN '95. J Musculoske Pain 4(1/2):xi-xiii, 1996.

4. Russell IJ: Preface: MYOPAIN '98. J Musculoske Pain 7(1/2):xix-xxi,1999.

5. Russell IJ editor: Abstracts from the 5th World Congress on Myofascial Pain and Fibromyalgia, Portland, Oregon, USA, September 9-September 13, 2001. J Musculoske Pain 9(Suppl #5):1-113, 2001.

Introduction:
The Fifth World Congress on Myofascial Pain and Fibromyalgia, MYOPAIN 2001, Portland, Oregon, USA, September 9-13, 2001

Soft tissue pain is the primary symptom that the myofascial pain syndrome [MPS] patient and the fibromyalgia syndrome [FMS] patient have in common. It is apparent, from the accounts of physicians around the world, that these syndromes are very common and, for most physicians, difficult to treat. There is, therefore, an acknowledged need for a more complete understanding of pain generation and processing in these disorders and a desire to provide a more rational approach to their management. Thus, it was appropriate that the theme of this fifth World Congress of MYOPAIN should focus on the neurobiology of pain.

MYOPAIN 2001 was attended by participants from 30 countries, providing about 150 podium and poster presentations relating to soft tissue pain disorders. The fields of endeavor included physicians from a variety of medical and surgical specialties, dental practitioners, basic science investigators, nurses, physical therapists, and a number of other paramedical disciplines. Mealtimes provided opportunities for direct interactions between investigators and clinicians, between doctors in training and experienced therapists, to meet and share vital conversations about problems experienced and potential solutions. A number of relevant exhibitors provided viewpoints and resources that would have been missed without them.

[Haworth co-indexing entry note]: "Introduction: The Fifth World Congress on Myofascial Pain and Fibromyalgia, MYOPAIN 2001, Portland, Oregon, USA, September 9-13, 2001." Bennett, Robert M. Co-published simultaneously in *Journal of Musculoskeletal Pain* [The Haworth Medical Press, an imprint of The Haworth Press, Inc.] Vol. 10, No. 1/2, 2002, pp. 1-3; and: *The Clinical Neurobiology of Fibromyalgia and Myofascial Pain: Therapeutic Implications* [ed: Robert M. Bennett] The Haworth Medical Press, an imprint of The Haworth Press, Inc., 2002, pp. 1-3. Single or multiple copies of this article are available for a fee from The Haworth Document Delivery Service [1-800-HAWORTH, 9:00 a.m. - 5:00 p.m. [EST] E-mail address: getinfo@haworthpressinc.com].

In this age of increasingly large meetings, with their multiple concurrent sessions, the challenge for the avid learner is to decide which sessions to attend and which to write off. It often represents an impossible quandary. The MYOPAIN series of meetings takes a different approach. It assumes that the attendees are better served by providing high quality material on a wide range of topics, in an all plenary program. In this style of meeting, it is possible to take in everything that is provided and miss nothing over an intensive three and one half day period. The three morning sessions were composed of didactic presentations of the basic sciences relevant to the neurobiology of pain, followed by clinical and therapeutic descriptions of regional pain syndromes, and concluding with the diagnosis and management of chronic widespread pain. During the noon hours and early evenings, time was specifically allocated to the viewing original new research presented by the investigators at their posters. The afternoon sessions provided opportunity for podium presentations of the best of the poster abstracts from that day. These sessions allowed review of what was learned from the poster presentations and an opportunity to see how the larger audience related to the new information. Finally, on the last day of the meeting, special workshops were provided on selected key topics to help new clinicians and investigators to get up to speed on fibromyalgia, myofascial pain syndrome, and on how to write for the medical literature. A new feature of this meeting was the provision of thematic symposia on two important topics: 1. Novel Approaches to the Management of Fibromyalgia, and 2. Torture and Myofascial Pain Syndrome.

A full listing of the scheduled topics was made available to Congress attendees in the form of a program booklet. For those not in attendance, the manuscripts of the invited morning session speakers are provided. These proceedings will also be available from the publisher [see below] to nonsubscribers in bookform. The abstracts, presented during the poster sessions, have already been published (1) and are available to *Journal* subscribers and others from The Haworth Press at 1-800-HAWORTH or on line at *<http://www.haworthpressinc.com>*.

It is my hope that this volume of the proceedings will provide a comprehensive update on the latest developments in soft tissue pain and a valuable point of reference for both clinicians and scientists in the field.

Robert M. Bennett, MD, FRCP, FACP
Professor of Medicine
Division of Arthritis and Rheumatic Diseases
Oregon Health and Science University
Portland, Oregon, USA

REFERENCE

1. Russell IJ, editor: Abstracts from the 5th World Congress on Myofascial Pain and Fibromyalgia, Portland, Oregon, USA, September 9-September 13, 2001. J Musculoske Pain 9(Suppl #5):1-113, 2001.

PRESIDENTIAL ADDRESS

Muscle Pain and Aging

Leonardo Vecchiet

SUMMARY. Objectives: Pain complaints at the musculoskeletal level, especially in their chronic manifestations, increase with age. The objectives of this review article are to discuss the physiologic and pathologic factors that may contribute to changes in sensitivity towards muscle pain with aging.

Findings: Very few psychophysical studies have explored the physiologic changes in muscle sensitivity with age. The largest population study so far conducted would indicate a decrease in pain threshold [pressure and electrical stimuli], particularly in elderly men. The profile of this hypersensitivity runs parallel to that of an increased oxidative damage to muscle fibers documented with the aging process. The global prevalence of pathologic events potentially painful for the muscle in-

Leonardo Vecchiet, MD, is affiliated with the Department of Medicine and Science of Aging, "G. D'Annunzio" University of Chieti, Italy.

Address correspondence to: Leonardo Vecchiet, MD, Semeiotica Medica, Policlinico "SS. Annunziata," via dei Vestini s.n., 66013 Chieti Scalo [CH], Italy [E-mail: vecchiet@unich.it].

[Haworth co-indexing entry note]: "Muscle Pain and Aging." Vecchiet, Leonardo. Co-published simultaneously in *Journal of Musculoskeletal Pain* [The Haworth Medical Press, an imprint of The Haworth Press, Inc.] Vol. 10, No. 1/2, 2002, pp. 5-22; and: *The Clinical Neurobiology of Fibromyalgia and Myofascial Pain: Therapeutic Implications* [ed: Robert M. Bennett] The Haworth Medical Press, an imprint of The Haworth Press, Inc., 2002, pp. 5-22. Single or multiple copies of this article are available for a fee from The Haworth Document Delivery Service [1-800-HAWORTH, 9:00 a.m. - 5:00 p.m. [EST]. E-mail address: getinfo@haworthpressinc.com].

creases with age. The increase, however, mostly regards primary muscle pain, e.g., myofascial pain due to trigger points from microtraumatic events, or muscle pain secondary to deep somatic structure involvement, e.g., referred muscle pain/hyperalgesia from osteoarthritic joints. In contrast, the same phenomenon is not observed for muscle pain secondary to visceral pathology–especially in its acute form–which, instead decreases with age. The extent of the pain symptom due to pathologic conditions does not increase proportionally to that of the underlying pathologic process, probably due to reduced reactivity of the elderly tissues towards inflammatory events [lesser capacity of producing algogenic substances].

Conclusions: The increased complaints of musculoskeletal pain with aging appear the result of a complex interaction between the physiologic process of aging, which seems to promote muscle damage and muscle hypersensitivity especially in the male sex, and the increased prevalence with age of most potentially painful pathologic conditions of the muscle itself or of other deep somatic structures. Future clinical and research efforts should aim at better understanding the pathophysiology of the increased pain in muscles in the elderly to help prevent not only the suffering to the patient but also the disabling consequences of the pain symptom at this level. *[Article copies available for a fee from The Haworth Document Delivery Service: 1-800-HAWORTH. E-mail address: <getinfo@haworthpressinc.com> Website: <http://www.HaworthPress.com> © 2002 by The Haworth Press, Inc. All rights reserved.]*

KEYWORDS. Muscle pain threshold, oxidative damage, elderly, primary and secondary muscle pain/hyperalgesia

INTRODUCTION

Pain in the musculoskeletal domain is one of the most frequent forms of pain in humans, in relation to a high number of conditions that may cause the symptom, both physiologic–such as physical exercise–and pathologic (1-3). Though muscle pain is dominant in every stage of life, it has been shown to increase with the aging process, so that complaints of the symptom–especially forms of chronic musculoskeletal pain–are more frequent in the elderly than in the younger population (4,5).

The aim of the present report is to discuss the factors that may contribute to changes in sensitivity towards muscle pain with aging. An indispensable premise to this discussion is an analysis of the general elements that may alter pain perception in relation to senescence.

PAIN IN THE ELDERLY

In the past few decades, there has been an exponential rise in the average individual life expectancy, which has led to a significant percentage increase in the elderly population. Pain in the elderly has therefore become a topical subject, destined to play an increasingly important role in the field of pain research and management in the forthcoming years (6).

When analyzing the problem of pain manifestations in older people, two fundamental elements need to be considered: 1. the impact of the physiologic process of aging on the system involved in perception, transmission, and elaboration of the painful signal; 2. the prevalence and incidence of potentially painful pathologies in old age.

While numerous epidemiologic investigations have been carried out to explore the frequency of the pathologic algogenic conditions of various body districts in the elderly (4), very few studies have so far examined the possible changes in pain perception as a function of age *per se*, i.e., in the absence of any pathology (5). In addition, the design and results of these studies are often controversial (4). It therefore seemed important to pay particular attention to the problem of the relationship between the physiologic aging process and the transmission/elaboration of the painful signal.

Physiologic Changes in Pain Perception in the Elderly

The progression of age, even in excellent health, in itself implies a decline in the functionality of the various body systems, which appears to be more marked the higher the level of "specialization" of the systems. Typical examples are the progressive reduction of visual and auditory capacities–producing the classic situations termed "presbyopia" and "presbycusis"–or reduction of the ability to discriminate tactile stimuli. It has been shown that the age-related changes in vision, audition, and skin senses are mainly determined by changes in transduction processes and receptor function (7). On this basis, it has been hypothesized that also the system involved in reception, transmission, and elaboration of the pain signals may undergo a similar, physiologic deterioration ultimately leading to a reduction of the capacity to perceive pain, thus producing a situation of "presbyalgia" in the elderly (6).

According to Harkins (5), the possible occurrence of "presbyalgia" could hypothetically be attributed to one or more of the five following conditions: a. age-dependent loss of receptors for pain [nociceptors];

b. changes in primary nociceptive afferents; c. changes in more central mechanisms subserving pain sensation and perception; d. changes in descending pain control mechanisms; e. birth cohort differences in social and cultural history that influence the meaning of pain. To date, no clear evidence exists that the aging process *per se* induces anatomofunctional changes in nociceptors [e.g., changes in density of nociceptors) and primary nociceptive afferents. The studies performed in the field–almost exclusively experimental psychophysical investigations to analyze thresholds of pain perception and tolerance–have, in fact, shown controversial results, which are sometimes difficult to interpret. Regarding thermal stimuli applied to the skin–radiant heat or contact heat, for instance–some researchers reported no variations of sensory thresholds as a function of age (8-11) while others found higher values in the elderly (12-14).

Regarding cold thermal stimuli–cold pressor test–Walsh found a different effect of the aging process in the two sexes, i.e., a decrease and a minimal increase in pain tolerance thresholds with age, in men and women, respectively (15).

Pressure stimuli applied on the Achilles tendon have shown lower levels of tolerance thresholds in the elderly (16).

As for electrical stimuli applied to the skin, in old compared to young subjects, some researchers found lower values of perception and tolerance thresholds (17), some reported higher values of sensory thresholds (18), and other groups did not find any significant change with age (19). Likewise, also electrical stimulation of the tooth pulp produced different results in the various studies, sometimes showing a reduced discrimination accuracy of the painful sensation (20) and sometimes the absolute absence of perception changes in old age (21).

It is thus difficult to draw definite conclusions on the fibroreceptor nociceptive function in the elderly on the basis of the mentioned studies, also considering that most of these studies were conducted in the "young-old" [65-75 years], while only a few of them examined the "old-old" [76-90 years] and practically never the category of the "oldest-old" [> 90 years].

A further reason for doubt on the validity of studies of this type is the "cross-sectional" experimental design in which a group of elderly people are directly compared with a group of young people. A "longitudinal" design would be far more appropriate, as progressive changes of the measured parameters are examined in different decades of age from youth to old age. According to Harkins et al. (6), the "cross-sectional" design only allows speculation on *differences between ages* and not on *changes due to aging.*

Relatively recent psychophysical studies by Harkins himself (5,22), conducted using a longitudinal design, in fact appear more reliable, showing at least one specific change of the nociceptive system in the elderly: a different reactivity towards the 1st and 2nd pain evoked in the hairy skin. As well known, thermal stimuli applied to hairy skin, for instance at limb level, normally produce two distinct painful sensations in succession. The first pain is described as sharp, pricking, very well localized, and seldom outlasting the duration of the stimulus. This sensation is attributed to the activation of A-delta type II mechano-heat afferents, small and lightly myelinated, whose conduction velocity ranges from 10 to 30 meters per second; these afferents have an anatomic distribution mainly in hairy skin. The first pain is followed by a painless period of up to 1 second, after which the second pain occurs. This is a burning sensation, diffuse and scarcely localized, whose duration frequently outlasts that of the stimulus. The sensation is produced by the activation of C fibers, i.e., unmyelinated fibers, whose conduction velocity ranges from 0.5 to 2 meters per second. The results of the above-mentioned recent studies suggest that elderly people preferentially employ the information transmitted by C-fibers rather than those mediated by A-delta type II fibers. In fact, although the intensity of perceived pain in response to a nociceptive thermal stimulus applied to hairy skin does not substantially differ among the various age groups, a change in the quality of the perceived sensation takes place with the aging process. In other words, the elderly do not describe brief thermal stimuli as sharp or pricking as frequently as younger subjects do; rather, they tend to describe the sensations as burning.

Furthermore, differences due to age also exist in the response times to 1st and 2nd pain, i.e., the elderly with respect to the young present longer reaction times to sensation onset to 1st but not 2nd pain (22). On the whole, these findings would suggest an age-dependent change in the conduction properties of the A-delta type II nociceptive fibers, in line with the hypothesis of an age-related small-fiber peripheral neuropathy (5). According to the same author, however, the clinical impact of this change on the global capacity of pain perception in the old would be minimal, if not insignificant.

Regarding the central mechanisms underlying perception and control of the pain sensation, no studies exist to date documenting possible differences between young and old people in relation to the aging process *per se*, i.e., in the absence of any pathology. In the case of elderly people affected with pathologic processes of the central nervous system, such as Alzheimer's disease, altered reactions towards painful events are often observed in the clinical setting, e.g., apathy, hyporeactivity, which suggests that this type of pathology may in some way influence the central mechanisms underlying both sensitivity and responsiveness to pain (6). Also in this case, however, there is an almost complete lack of controlled studies which would allow the drawing of definite conclusions with this respect.

Lastly, the role exerted by sociocultural factors on the pain experience is also controversial. In some cases, in fact, the elderly could tend to minimize the pain experience because "culturally" conditioned to consider suffering an unavoidable consequence of the aging process. In other circumstances, in contrast, they might emphasize their symptoms in an unconscious desire to attract the attention of others, particularly family members, especially if they feel lonely and neglected (4-6).

Pathologic Painful Conditions in the Elderly

It is well established that the elderly are subject to potentially painful conditions in various body structures much more frequently than younger people. Demonstrative examples are osteoarthritis, osteoporosis, or atherosclerosis [and therefore tendency to ischemia in various districts] which, on the whole, produce an age-related increase in both the incidence and prevalence of numerous forms of pain (4).

While there is a significant increase in the number of pathologies with algogenic components as age progresses, however, the same cannot be said for the intensity of the symptom. In fact, numerous studies show that in spite of the progressive worsening of the osteoarticular findings at x-rays, the pain complaint by the patient does not increase in parallel; in contrast, it sometimes diminishes (4,6).

Some studies, including research by our group, have clearly evidenced that the progressive increase in the atherosclerosis process at coronary level observed with age does not involve a parallel increase in the painful symptomatology at precordial or sternal level (23). It is well known, in fact, that the highest number of painless myocardial infarctions occur in the elderly. The problem of the relationship between the extent of the pathologic process and the degree of the perceived pain needs to be considered, regarding not only the anatomopathologic alterations but also the tissue reactive capacities of the subject, which may diminish as age progresses, thus determining a reduction of the capacity to produce algogenic substances in the course of inflammatory or ischemic processes (23).

MUSCLE PAIN IN THE ELDERLY

In line with the considerations already made for pain in general, pain at muscle level in the elderly is also likely to be the result of two main factors, 1. the impact of the physiologic aging process on muscle sensitivity to pain; 2. the prevalence and incidence of the pathologies with algogenic potential at muscle level in old age.

Physiologic Changes in Muscle Pain Perception in the Elderly

As already reported in the previous sections, while there are a number of studies that have examined the possible changes in pain sensitivity as a function of aging in physiologic conditions at skin level, research on muscle sensitivity is extremely scarce and often controversial. A study by Jensen at al. (24), in which pressure stimuli were applied to muscles of the cephalic region, showed increased sensory thresholds in subjects of over 65 years of age with respect to younger people. A recent, vast epidemiologic study by our group showed, however, results in the opposite direction. In this study, pain thresholds to pressure stimulation were measured in healthy individuals of seven different decades of age, from 20 years to > 80 years. Forty subjects [20 women and 20 men] were considered for each decade. Thresholds were measured systematically at the sites of the classic fibromyalgic tender spots and in at least three points along each of the following muscles: deltoid, trapezius, quadriceps, gastrocnemius [on both sides]. At the age of 20-30 years, thresholds at all sites were significantly lower in women than in men. Subsequently, in women thresholds tended to remain stable throughout the various decades of age, while in men they declined progressively, equaling women's values at the age of 80, with no significant difference between the two sexes at this stage. Preliminary results using another sensory modality, i.e., electrical stimulation selectively applied to muscles, also confirmed the same trend observed with the pressure stimulation. Thus, the results here of the sensory evaluation in normal muscles in humans not only failed to evidence a trend towards an increase–which would have supported the hypothesis of "presbyalgia"– but showed, in contrast, at least in the male sex, a net trend towards increased pain sensitivity (Vecchiet et al., unpublished data).

The question arises as to whether there is a correlate of this sensory asset at anatomofunctional level. What is the pattern of anatomo-functional changes in the skeletal muscle in the absence of any pathology, simply as a function of the aging process?

Bioptic studies have been performed by several groups, including ours, to examine this issue (25). Regarding our studies, these have been conducted on 800 specimens from muscle biopsies of normal subjects of different decades of age, from youth to old age, and are part of a complex collaborative inter-university project, called NEURIGEN Project [coordinator: Leonardo Vecchiet]. This project has involved the work of researchers from several Italian Universities, namely the "G. D'Annunzio" University of Chieti, and the Universities of Perugia, Rome, Pavia, and Bari. The studies performed in the ambit of the NEURIGEN project have addressed multiple aspects of muscle morpho-functionality but a number of them have concentrated particularly on the role of oxidative stress. The following sections report the most significant outcomes of the studies performed.

The Effects of Age on Skeletal Muscle

A number of specific changes, particularly biochemical changes, have been shown to occur in muscles with the aging process. The effects of aging on skeletal muscle manifest in three main ways. Firstly, muscle mass and strength both undergo a general decline [age-related changes in muscle mass = sarcopenia] (25). Secondly, mitochondrial abnormalities become evident, reflecting underlying physiological changes that occur with aging. Thirdly, and perhaps as a consequence of the two previous phenomena, the susceptibility to certain neuromuscular diseases increases (26).

Morphometric examination of muscles has shown that atrophy with aging is caused mainly by loss of fibers and to a lesser extent by reduction of fiber size, mostly of type II fibers (27,28). An age-related reduction of the total number of fibers could involve loss of a specific type of fiber, which, in turn, may alter the fiber type proportion. Lexell and Downham (29), however, showed that the proportion of the different types of fibers appears to be unaffected by increasing age, while type II fibers are significantly smaller in old muscles. This suggests that the loss of fibers that occurs with increasing age generally affects both fiber types to the same extent, while the size of the remaining type II fibers generally decreases. Morphological elementary lesions also observed in aged muscles are: severe multinuclear atrophy, anomalous splitting, nemaline myopathy, presence of ragged-red fibers, and central nuclei (30). In particular, it has been found that skeletal muscle specimens from aged subjects are characterized by the presence of cytochrome c oxidase negative/ragged red fibers, that is fibers lacking cytochrome c oxidase activity and with subsarcolemmal mitochondrial proliferation (31).

Muscle tissue, being the largest with a low protein turnover, reflects aging changes more markedly than other tissues. The decrement in muscle mass and functionality is associated with a generalized physiological decline that is common to all aging organisms (25).

The age-dependent accumulation of lipids that are more prone to peroxidation may also, following peroxidation, increase. Aging affects the metabolic capacity of the skeletal muscle, in particular the glycolytic and respiratory capacity (32), in relation to the loss of water that occurs with age and the resulting rigidity of the mitochondrial membrane. Temporary or sustained loss of mitochondrial function and adenosine 5'-triphosphate production can have a major impact on the reliability of cellular defenses and repair processes. This may result in increased mutational load, increased accumulation of dysfunctional cellular macromolecules, and a decreased capacity to mount an appropriate stress response when challenged. As it will be discussed in more detail in the next section [*Muscle Oxidative Damage and the Aging Process*], probable age-associated loss of function in mitochondria is suggested by the evidence of increased mitochondrial deoxyribonucleic acid [mtDNA] deletions (33,34) and point mutations (35,36), increased oxidative damage to mtDNA (37) and increased levels of aberrant forms of mtDNA (38). The potential for lipid peroxidation in the inner mitochondrial membrane increases (39), making the mitochondria more susceptible to damage by oxidants. The type of deletions and point mutations in mtDNA that cause inherited myopathies are also observed to increase with age (38).

It is plausible that the accumulation of all mtDNA defects accounts for the age-related deficits in mitochondrial bioenergetic capacity and function. Studies that have examined the content of cytochrome oxidase in mitochondria show a progressive and random loss in this enzyme closely correlating with age-associated decline in mitochondrial ribonucleic acid synthesis (40). A study of human diaphragm muscle indicated that cytochrome c oxidase decreases markedly beyond the seventh decade of life. The mtDNA deletions are hypothesized to create tissue bioenergy mosaics that may account for losses in bioenergetic capacity (40). The loss of functional mitochondria with age appears to be partially compensated by the increased workload of the remaining intact population of mitochondria.

The activity of various marker enzymes has also been measured in skeletal muscle from individuals of different ages to quantify the effect of aging on the metabolic capacity of the muscle. A decrease in the activity of cytochrome oxidase appears to be involved in the age-related increases in the production of mitochondria-derived oxidants (38). A functional consequence of oxidant damage is increased membrane rigidity, which can lead to a decline in receptor-mediated signaling.

Several studies have reported age-related reductions of skeletal muscle mitochondrial enzyme activity, and high-energy phosphate metabolism, which are associated with the decline in skeletal muscle strength and endurance capacity that occurs with aging (41). A recent study by Pastoris et al. [unpublished data] was carried out as part of the NEURIGEN project onto muscle biopsies from 700 sedentary subjects whose age ranged from 17 to 91 years. It explored the changes in the metabolic capacity of human skeletal muscles with the aging process. In specimens from one of the three following muscles: vastus lateralis, rectus abdominis, and gluteus maximus, the authors measured the activities of various marker enzymes related to glycolysis, Krebs' cycle, and the electron transfer chain. The results showed an impairment of the glycolytic pathway, which led the authors to conclude that aging significantly compromises the glycolytic capacity.

There is currently no evidence that most of the above reported age-related changes in muscle structure and function might account for changes in muscle pain sensitivity/complaint occurring with age. In our opinion, however, the aspect of the oxidative stress/damage to muscle tissue, which will be addressed in detail in the following section, might have some implication in the process of pain perception.

Muscle Oxidative Damage and the Aging Process

A role for oxidative damage in normal aging is supported by studies in experimental animals, but there has always been limited evidence in man (42). In recent years, a number of studies by this group, in the context of the NEURIGEN project, have instead been devoted to detection of oxidative damage to skeletal muscles in humans.

In 1999, Mecocci et al. (43) examined markers of oxidative damage to DNA, lipids, and proteins in 66 muscle biopsy specimens from humans aged 25 to 93 years. Age-dependent increases were found in 8-hydroxy-2-deoxyguanosine [OH^8dG], a marker of oxidative damage to DNA, in malondialdehyde [MDA], a marker of lipid peroxidation, and to a lesser extent in protein carbonyl groups, a marker of protein oxidation. The increases in OH^8dG were significantly correlated to increases in MDA. These results provide evidence for a role of oxidative damage in human aging which may contribute to age-dependent losses of muscle strength and stamina.

In the same year, another study was conducted by Pansarasa et al. (28) to explore the role of reactive oxygen species [ROS] in human skeletal muscle aging. Human muscle samples were obtained from patients hospitalized for reasons other than muscle problems in an open study with matched pairs of individuals of different ages. The subjects ranged in age from 17 to 91 years; they were grouped as follows: 17-25, 26-35, 36-45, 46-55, 56-65, 66-75, 76-85, and 86-91-year-old groups. To investigate the relationship between muscle aging and oxidative damage, the following were measured: total and Mn-dependent superoxide dismutase [total SOD, MnSOD], glutathione peroxidase [GSHPx], and catalase [CAT] activities; total, reduced, and oxidized glutathione [GSHtot, GSH, and GSSG] levels; lipid peroxidation [LPO], and protein carbonyl content [PrC]. Total SOD activity decreased significantly with age in the 66-75-year-old group, although MnSOD activity increased significantly in the 76-85-year-old group. The activity of the two hydrogen peroxide detoxifying enzymes [GSHPx and CAT] did not change with age, nor did GSHtot and GSH levels. The GSSG levels increased significantly [76-85 and 86-91-year-old groups] with age, as did GSHtot and GSH levels. A significant increase was observed in LPO levels [66-75 and 76-85-year-old groups], although the PrC content showed a trend towards an increase without gaining the statistical significance. These results support the idea that ROS play an important role in the human skeletal muscle aging process.

Another study by Cormio et al. (44) investigated the MtDNA deletions in aging. According to the "mitochondrial theory of aging," the age-related increase in ROS is responsible for the bioenergetic decay of mitochondria in aging through a mutagenic effect on mitochondrial DNA [mtDNA]. Theoretically, such an effect should be more relevant in the nervous tissue and skeletal muscle, which are postmitotic tissues that are highly dependent on oxidative metabolism. A wide search for mtDNA deletions [$mtDNA^{4977}$, $mtDNA^{7436}$, $mtDNA^{10422}$, and others] was performed in the skeletal muscle in five age-classes of healthy individuals [135 subjects]. The results showed that healthy individuals have an age-related increase in the number of mtDNA deleted species and in the average level of $mtDNA^{4977}$. The data of this study thus support the idea of a quantitative and qualitative increase of mtDNA deletions in aging.

Another recent study (45) addressed specifically the issue of the age and sex differences in human skeletal muscle with regard to the role of ROS. As already reported above, previous studies conducted in experimental animals, have indicated that ROS are involved in the aging process. Based on these premises, the objective of the study by Pansarasa et al. (45) was to evaluate the relationship between oxidative damage and human skeletal muscle aging, measuring the activity of the main antioxidant enzymes superoxide dismutase [total and MnSOD], glutathione peroxidase [GPx] and catalase in the skeletal muscle of men and women in the age groups: young [17-40 years], adult [41-65 years] and aged [66-91 years]. The authors also measured GSH and glutathione disulfide [GSSG] levels and the redox index; LPO and PrC. Total SOD activity was lower in the 66-91-year-old vs. the 17-40-year-old men; MnSOD activity was significantly greater in 66-91-year-old vs. 17-40-year-old women. The GPx activity remained unchanged. The activity of catalase was lower in adults than in young men but higher in the aged. The following were also observed: no changes in GSH levels, significantly higher GSSG levels only in aged men vs. adult men, and a significant decrease in aged women vs. aged men. The PrC increased significantly in the 41-65 and 66-91-year-old vs. the 17-40-year-old men. Finally, young women showed lower LPO levels than young men. Significantly higher LPO levels were observed in aged men vs. both young and adult men, and the same trend was found in women. The authors concluded that oxidative damage may play a crucial role in the decline of functional activity in human skeletal muscle with normal aging in both sexes; and that *men appear to be more subject to oxidative stress than women.*

The global outcome of the studies performed thus point to an evident increase in the oxidative damage to muscle with aging. It is of course difficult to precisely relate this increase to the changes in muscle sensitivity that have been observed in the elderly. However, it is not unlikely that these two parameters are somehow linked for basically two reasons. First, the changes in both pain sensitivity and oxidative damage appear to have similar profiles with age: an increase which preferentially affects men rather than women. Second, a similar concomitance of the two parameters, i.e., increased muscle pain sensitivity [decreased pressure/electrical pain threshold] and increased oxidative damage is present in a pathology that has been depicted as a condition of "early muscle aging," namely chronic fatigue syndrome [CFS].

Chronic Fatigue Syndrome: An Early Process of Muscle Aging?

Patients with CFS mainly complain of symptoms in the musculo-skeletal domain, namely fatigue and often myalgias. Previous studies have shown that these patients present diffuse and selective muscle hyperalgesia, i.e., the musculoskeletal tissue is hypersensitive to painful stimuli at every body site, while the overlying subcutaneous and skin tissues [unlike patients with fibromyalgia syndrome] are instead normosensitive (46,47). In addition to diffuse muscle hyperalgesia, CFS patients present a number of abnormalities at muscle biopsy, i.e., morphostructural alterations of the sarcomere, fatty degeneration and fibrous regeneration, inversion of the cytochrome oxidase/succinate dehydrogenase ratio, pleio/polymorphism and monstrosity of mito-chondria, reduction of some mitochondrial enzymatic activities and increments of common deletion 4977 bp of mitochondrial DNA 150-3,000 times the normal values. The global picture of these alterations in CFS patients suggests a degenerative status of muscle tissue, index of a decreased functional capacity, which is very similar to the picture observed in elderly normal subjects. In addition to these findings, CFS patients also present specific indices of muscle oxidative damage, here again very similar to those observed in elderly people (47). A recent study by Fulle et al. (48), has indeed documented specific oxidative alterations in the vastus lateralis muscle of patients with CFS. In this study, the authors detected oxidative damage to DNA and lipids in muscle specimens of CFS patients as compared to age-matched controls, as well as increased activity of the antioxidant enzymes catalase, GPx and transferase, and increases in GSHtot plasma levels. From this outcome, the authors hypothesized that in CFS there is oxidative stress in muscle, which results in an increase in antioxidant defenses. Furthermore, in muscle membranes, fluidity and fatty acid composition were significantly different in specimens from CFS patients as compared to controls and to patients suffering from fibromyalgia. These data support an organic origin of CFS, in which muscle suffers oxidative damage and is, at the same time, the site of selective hyperalgesia.

On the basis of what has been reported about the similar profile of oxidative damage and muscle hypersensitivity in conditions of physiologic and "early" [CFS] aging processes, one could speculate that the increased oxidative damage to muscle with the aging process somehow interferes with nociceptor function, although the exact mechanism through which this process would take place of course still needs to be identified.

Pathologic Muscle Pain Conditions in the Elderly

Most epidemiological studies report that the overall complaints of pain at musculoskeletal level increase with age (5,6). In other words, the elderly would suffer from musculoskeletal pain more frequently than younger people. However, the problem of pathologic muscle pain and aging is very complex and does not appear to have been satisfactorily addressed in the population studies performed so far.

A first important distinction must be made between primary and secondary forms of muscle pain, while a second fundamental distinction regards acute and chronic muscle pain.

Pain arising primarily in muscle structures, e.g., due to myofascial trigger points from microtraumatic events, would seem to increase with age, in relation to a raised percentage of risk factors [e.g., increased susceptibility of muscle tissue to trauma, increase in skeletal deformations leading to an abnormal load on muscles, increased percentage of abnormal postural attitudes, etc.]. Some forms of secondary muscle pain can also increase, for instance referred muscle pain and hyperalgesia from joints in relation to an increased incidence of joint pathology—especially osteoarthritis—with age (49). In contrast, the most typical form of secondary muscle pain, i.e., referred muscle pain from visceral structures, definitely declines. In fact, pain from internal organs is markedly less frequent in the elderly than in the young, especially in its acute manifestations (4). Thus the elderly appear on the whole more prone to complain from primary muscle pain or muscle pain secondary to algogenic foci in the joint, but less affected with muscle pain/hyperalgesia as a consequence of painful conditions of viscera. The reasons for these differences are far from being elucidated and will need to be addressed in future studies where the incidence of the single painful muscle conditions are explored in relation to the progression of age.

CONCLUSIONS

Painful manifestations in the elderly appear to result from the complex interaction between the "physiologic" changes in the function of the nociceptive system and the different incidence of pathologies with algogenic potential at the level of the different body structures occurring with age. While the physiologic reactivity towards painful stimuli appears to be slightly decreased in skin, the opposite phenomenon would be observed at muscle level. Senescent muscles would in fact be more sensitive towards painful stimuli than young muscles, especially in the male sex, a finding excluding a possible condition of "presbyalgia" due to age at muscle level. Though a cause-effect relationship is still difficult to establish to date, it is interesting to note that this muscle hypersensitivity to painful stimuli preferentially affecting elderly male subjects runs parallel to the profile of the oxidative damage to muscle tissue, which also increases with age, in a more pronounced fashion in the male than female sex.

Regarding potentially painful pathologic conditions, there is an overall exponential increase in their number with age and this is particularly true for conditions affecting the musculoskeletal domain either primarily [e.g., repeated microtraumas leading to trigger point formation] or secondarily [joint pathology giving rise to referred muscle involvement]. This leads to an overall increase in pain complaints due to pathologic events, though often the extent of the perceived pain does not increase in parallel with that of the underlying pathology, probably due to a lesser capacity of the elderly tissues to produce algogenic substances in response to pathologic events.

The result of the interaction of both physiologic and pathologic factors, however, point to a general increase in the pain complaints/susceptibility of the skeletal muscle in the elderly. In spite of this situation–of greater muscle suffering with age–the studies specifically devoted to the evaluation of muscle pain in the elderly still remain very limited in number. This situation is partly due to the objectively higher difficulty of assessing the symptom in standardized conditions in the elderly, especially if they present with cognitive impairment (5). However, it is also due, in large part, to a diffuse "sociocultural" attitude, according to which suffering should be accepted as an unavoidable component of the aging process.

It is extremely important for this attitude to change and for an increasing number of research studies in the field of pain to be carried out in the elderly. A thorough knowledge of the factors that intervene in pain expression in old age is indispensable to set up adequate therapeutic protocols, also considering that the responsiveness towards analgesics is modified with age and that for many compounds the interval between the effective dose and the dose provoking toxicity is progressively reduced (5,6). Research in the field of muscle pain is all the more important since the symptom at this level is not only the cause of considerable suffering to the patient but also often involves, for the specific function of the structure, a marked degree of disability which becomes a crucial problem for an old person (4).

From what has been synthetically reported, it is evident that the problem of pain, particularly muscle pain, in the elderly represents the challenge of the future for the pain clinician and researcher, the challenge of relieving the burden on an increasing portion of the general population. Since senescence represents a disease *per se*, every possible effort should be made to eliminate or decrease at least the algogenic component that so often accompanies old age.

REFERENCES

1. Vecchiet L, Giamberardino MA, Marini I: Immediate muscular pain from physical activity. Adv Pain Res Ther 10: 193-206,1987.

2. Vecchiet L, Dragani L, de Bigontina P, Obletter G, Giamberardino MA: Experimental referred pain and hyperalgesia from muscles in humans, New Trends in Referred Pain and Hyperalgesia, Pain Research and Clinical Management. Edited by L Vecchiet, D Albe-Fessard, U Lindblom, MA Giamberardino. Elsevier, Amsterdam, 1993, pp. 239-249.

3. Vecchiet L, Vecchiet J, Bellomo R, Giamberardino MA: Muscle pain from physical exercise. J Musculoske Pain 7(1&2): 43-53,1999.

4. Helme RD, Gibson SJ: Pain in older people, epidemiology of pain. Edited by IK Crombie, IASP Press, Seattle, 1999, pp. 103-112.

5. Harkins SW: Aging and Pain. The management of pain, 3rd ed. of the JJ Bonica manual. Edited by J Loeser. Lea & Febiger, Philadelphia, 2000, pp. 813-823.

6. Harkins SW, Kwentus J, Price DD: Pain and suffering in the elderly, The management of pain, 2nd ed. Edited by JJ Bonica. Lea & Febiger, Philadelphia, 1990, pp. 552-559.

7. Hinchliffe R: Aging and sensory threshold. J Gerontol 17: 45-49, 1962.

8. Birren JE, Shapiro HB, Miller JH: The effect of salicylate upon pain sensitivity. J Pharmacol Exp Ther 100: 67-71, 1959.

9. Hardy JD, Wolff HG, Goodell H: The pain threshold in man. Am J Psychiat 99: 744-751,1943.

10. Kenshalo DR Sr: Somesthetic sensitivity in young and elderly humans. J Gerontol 41: 732-742, 1986.

11. Schumacher GA, Goodell H, Hardy JD: Uniformity of the pain threshold in man. Science 92: 110-112, 1940.

12. Chapman WP, Jones CM: Variations in cutaneous and visceral pain sensitivity in normal subjects. J Clin Invest 23: 81-91,1941.

13. Procacci P, Della Corte M, Zoppi M: Pain threshold measurement in man, Recent advances on pain: pathophysiology and clinical aspects. Edited by JJ Bonica, P Procacci, C Pagni, Charles C Thomas, Springfield, IL, 1974, pp. 105-147.

14. Sherman ED, Robillard E: Sensitivity to pain in relationship to age. J Am Geriatr Soc 12: 1037-1044, 1964.

15. Walsh NE, Schoenfeld L, Ramamurthy S: Normative model for cold pressor test. Am J Phys Med Rehabil 68: 6-11, 1989.

16. Woodrow KM, Friedman GD, Siegelaub AB: Pain tolerance: differences according to age, sex and race. Psychosom Med 34: 548-556, 1972.

17. Collins G, Stone LA: Pain sensitivity, age and activity level in chronic schizophrenics and in normals. Br J Psychiat 12: 33-35, 1966.

18. Tucker MA, Andrew MF, Ogle SJ, Davison JG: Age associated change in pain threshold measured by transcutaneous neuronal electrical sitmulation. Age Ageing 18: 241-246, 1989.

19. Evans ER, Rendall MS, Bartek JP: Current perception threshold in ageing. Age Ageing 18: 241-246, 1989.

20. Harkins SW, Chapman CR: The perception of induced dental pain in young and elderly women. J Gerontol 32: 428-435, 1977.

21. Mumford JM: Pain perception in man on electrically stimulating the teeth, Pain. Edited by A Soulairac, J Cahan, J Charpentier. Academic Press, London, 1968, pp. 224-229.

22. Harkins S: Geriatric pain: pain perception in the old. Clin Geriatr Med 12: 435-445, 1996.

23. Buzzelli G, Vecchiet L, Matassi L: Rilievi sul comportamento del dolore precordiale in rapporto all'età. Rivista Critica di Clinica Medica 6: 873-886, 1968.

24. Jensen R, Rasmussen B, Pedersen B, Lous I, Olesen J: Cephalic muscle tenderness and pressure pain threshold in a general population. Pain 48: 197-203, 1992.

25. Navarro A, López-Cepero JM, Sánchez del Pino MJ: Skeletal muscle and aging. Front Biosci 6: 26-44, 2001.

26. Flanigan KM, Lauria G, Griffin JW, Kund RW: Age-related biology and diseases of muscle and nerve. Neurologic Clinics 16: 659-669, 1998.

27. Lexell J, Taylor CC, Sjostrom M: What is the cause of the ageing atrophy? Total number, size and proportion of different fiber types studied in whole vastus lateralis muscle from 15- to 83-year-old men. J Neurol Sci 84: 275-294, 1988.

28. Pansarasa O, Bertorelli L, Vecchiet J, Felzani G, Marzatico F: Age-dependent changes of antioxidant activities and markers of free radical damage in human skeletal muscle. Free Radical Biol & Med 27: 617-622, 1999.

29. Lexell J, Downham D: What is the effect of ageing on type II muscle fibers? J Neurol Sci 107: 250-251, 1992.

30. Ribacchi R, Ribacchi F, Prosperini AP, Marchetti G, Montanari G, Vecchiet L: Morphological and morphometric variability of skeletal muscle in relation to aging, Fourth World Congress on Myofascial Pain and Fibromyalgia, Silvi Marina, August 24-27, 1998, Abstract Book (Plenary Sessions). Edited by MGA, Rome, 1998, p. 52.

31. Moraes CT, Ricci E, Petruzzella V, Shanske S, Di Mauro S, Schon EA, Bonilla E: Molecular analysis of the muscle pathology associated with mitochondrial DNA deletions. Nat Genet 1: 359-367, 1992.

32. Cooper JM, Mann VM, Schapira AH: Analyses of mitochondrial respiratory chain function and mitochondrial DNA deletion in human skeletal muscle: effect of ageing. J Neurol Sci 113: 91-98, 1992.

33. Cortopassi GA, Arnheim N: Detection of a specific mitochondrial DNA deletion in tissue of older humans. Nucleic Acids Res 18: 6927-6933, 1990.

34. Linnane AW, Baumer A, Maxwell RJ, Preston H, Zhang CF, Marzuki S: Mitochondrial gene mutation: the ageing process and degenerative diseases. Biochem Int 22: 1067-1076, 1990.

35. Munscher C, Rieger T, Muller-Hocker J, Kadenbach B: The point mutation of mitochondrial DNA characteristic for MERRF disease is found also in healthy people of different ages. FEBS Lett 317: 27-30, 1993.

36. Munscher C, Muller-Hocker J, Kadenbach B: Human aging is associated with various point mutations in tRNA genes of mitochondrial DNA. Biol Chem Hoppe Seyler 374: 1099-1104, 1993.

37. Ames BN, Shigenaga MK, Hagen TM: Oxidants, antioxidants, and the degenerative diseases of aging. Proc Natl Acad Sci USA 90: 7915-7922, 1993.

38. Shigenaga MK, Hagen TM, Ames BN: Oxidative damage and mitochondrial decay in aging. Proc Natl Acad Sci USA 91: 10771-10778, 1994.

39. Yu BP, Suescun EA, Yang SY: Effect of age-related lipid peroxidation on membrane fluidity and phospholipase A2: modulation by dietary restriction. Mech Ageing Dev 65: 17-33, 1992.

40. Muller-Hocker J: Cytochrome c oxidase deficient fibers in the limb muscle and diaphragm of man without muscular disease: an age-related alteration. J Neurol Sci 100:14-21, 1990.

41. Flanigan KM, Lauria G, Griffin JW, Kund RW: Age-related biology and diseases of muscle and nerve. Neurol Clin 16: 659-669, 1998.

42. Sohal RS, Weindruch R: Oxidative stress, caloric restriction, and aging. Science 273: 59-63, 1996.

43. Mecocci P, Fanò G, Fulle S, MacGarvey U, Shinobu L, Polidori MC, Cherubini A, Vecchiet J, Senin U, Flint Beal M: Age-dependent increases in oxidative damage to DNA, lipids, and proteins in human skeletal muscle. Free Radical Biol & Med 26: 303-308, 1999.

44. Cormio A, Lezza AMS, Vecchiet J, Felzani G, Marangi L, Guglielmi FW, Francavilla A, Cantatore P, Gadaleta MN: MtDNA deletions in aging and in non-mitochondrial pathologies. Mol Cell Gerontol 908: 299-301, 2000.

45. Pansarasa O, Castagna L, Colombi B, Vecchiet J, Felzani G, Marzatico F: Age and sex differences in human skeletal muscle: role of reactive oxygen species. Free Rad Res 33: 287-293, 2000.

46. Vecchiet L, Giamberardino MA, de Bigontina P, Dragani L: Comparative sensory evaluation of parietal tissues in painful and nonpainful areas in fibromyalgia and myofascial pain syndrome, Progress in Pain Research and Management. Edited by GF Gebhart, DL Hammond, TS Jensen. IASP Press, Seattle, 1994, pp. 177-185.

47. Vecchiet L, Montanari G, Pizzigallo E, Iezzi S, de Bigontina P, Dragani L, Giamberardino MA: Sensory characterization of somatic parietal tissues in chronic fatigue syndrome. Neurosci Lett 208: 117-120, 1996.

48. Fulle S, Mecocci P, Fanò G, Vecchiet J, Vecchini A, Racciatti D, Cherubini A, Pizzigallo E, Vecchiet L, Senin U, Flint Beal M: Specific oxidative alterations in vastus lateralis muscle of patients with the diagnosis of chronic fatigue syndrome. Free Rad Biol & Med 29: 1252-1259, 2000.

49. National Health Nutrition Survey (NHANES) I Epidemiologic Follow-up Study (1982-1984). 1987 Plan and operation of the National Health and Nutrition Survey. I Epidemiological follow-up study, 1982-1984 Vital and health statistics, Series I, No. 22, DHS Pub. No. (PHS)87-1324.

The Neurobiology of Central Sensitization

Michael W. Salter

SUMMARY. Objectives: This review discusses plasticity of excitatory synaptic transmission in the spinal dorsal horn and the role of this plasticity in contributing to the pathogenesis of pain hypersensitivity.

Findings: In the dorsal horn pain transmission is mediated primarily through excitatory glutamatergic synapses. Glutamatergic synapses exhibit multiple forms of short-lasting and long-lasting forms of synaptic plasticity. The form of plasticity contributing to the persistent enhancement of pain transmission known as "central sensitization" is mechanis-

Michael W. Salter, MD, PhD, is CIHR Investigator, Programmes in Brain and Behavior and Cell Biology, Hospital for Sick Children. He is also Professor of Physiology and Director, University of Toronto, Centre for the Study of Pain, University of Toronto, Toronto, Ontario, Canada.

Address correspondence to: Michael W. Salter, MD, PhD, The Hospital for Sick Children, 555 University Avenue, Toronto, Ontario M5G 1X8, Canada [E-mail: mike.salter@ utoronto.ca].

The work of the author is supported by the Canadian Institutes of Health Research.

[Haworth co-indexing entry note]: "The Neurobiology of Central Sensitization." Salter, Michael W. Co-published simultaneously in *Journal of Musculoskeletal Pain* [The Haworth Medical Press, an imprint of The Haworth Press, Inc.] Vol. 10, No. 1/2, 2002, pp. 23-33; and: *The Clinical Neurobiology of Fibromyalgia and Myofascial Pain: Therapeutic Implications* [ed: Robert M. Bennett] The Haworth Medical Press, an imprint of The Haworth Press, Inc., 2002, pp. 23-33. Single or multiple copies of this article are available for a fee from The Haworth Document Delivery Service [1-800-HAWORTH, 9:00 a.m. - 5:00 p.m. [EST]. E-mail address: getinfo@haworthpressinc.com].

tically similar to long-term potentiation in other regions of the central nervous system. This synaptic potentiation is produced by calcium entry through the N-methyl-D-aspartate subtype of glutamate receptor which initiates intracellular signalling cascades that ultimately cause an increase in the number and function of the alpha-amino-3-hydroxy-5-methyl-4-isoxazoleproprionate/kainate subtypes of glutamate receptors.

Conclusions: Central sensitization is an expression of synaptic plasticity at glutamatergic synapses in pain transmission neurons in the dorsal horn. The resultant enhancement of synaptic responses increases the gain in pain pathways and contributes in a significant manner to the pain hypersensitivity. *[Article copies available for a fee from The Haworth Document Delivery Service: 1-800-HAWORTH. E-mail address: <getinfo@haworthpressinc.com> Website: <http://www.HaworthPress.com> © 2002 by The Haworth Press, Inc. All rights reserved.]*

KEYWORDS. Pain, glutamate receptors, tyrosine kinases, synaptic plasticity, spinal dorsal horn

One of the key insights in neuroscience over the past decade is that synaptic connections between neurons are in a near continual state of change and modification, and this modification is highly dependent upon the activating state of the pre- and postsynaptic neurons. During development, the biasing of these modifications by molecular signals is responsible for such diverse processes as axonal pathfinding and the formation, establishment, and consolidation of synaptic contacts. In the developed nervous system the continual interplay of modulatory processes subserves to produce synaptic modifications, or plasticity, that underlie physiological processes such as learning and memory. The same molecular signalling cascades that produce these normal forms of plasticity may, if aberrant, lead to pathological excitatory processes including epilepsy, neurodegeneration, and pain. The purpose of the present paper is to discuss the role of the commonalities in plasticity of excitatory synaptic transmission in the context of the function of the dorsal horn that may contribute to the pathogenesis of chronic pain.

GLUTAMATE MEDIATES FAST SYNAPTIC TRANSMISSION

Like the vast majority of excitatory synapses in the central nervous system [CNS], most presynaptic excitatory terminals in the dorsal horn release glutamate which activates ionotropic glutamate receptors that are strategically-localized in the postsynaptic neurons (1). The excitatory postsynaptic potentials [EPSPs] resulting from single presynaptic action potentials is caused primarily by activation of the alpha-amino-3-hydroxy-5-methyl-4-isoxazoleproprionate [AMPA] and kainate [KAI] subtypes of glutamate receptor. The N-methyl-D-aspartate [NMDA] subtype of glutamate receptor, which is also localized at excitatory synapses, contributes little to the responses to single presynaptic action potentials because these receptors are tonically suppressed by extracellular magnesium [Mg^{2+}] which blocks NMDA channels. This type of fast excitatory synaptic transmission occurs even at synapses of "slow" primary afferent which are predominantly nociceptors [Figure 1]. With low frequency activation of nociceptors produced by mild noxious stimuli, these EPSPs signal the onset, duration, intensity, and location of noxious stimuli to dorsal horn neurons.

"WINDUP" VERSUS "CENTRAL SENSITIZATION"

Discharge of primary afferent nociceptors at high frequencies, produced by more intense or sustained noxious stimuli, results in corelease of peptide neuromodulators such as substance P and calcitonin gene-related peptide from nociceptor central terminals which leads to slow synaptic potentials lasting tens of seconds (2) as illustrated in Figure 2. These slow EPSPs provide substantial opportunities for temporal summation of fast EPSPs (3) and the cumulative depolarization is boosted by the recruitment of NMDA receptor current upon removal of the Mg^{2+} blockade of the channels. The sustained depolarization also recruits voltage-gated calcium [Ca^{2+}] currents, triggering plateau potentials mediated by calcium-activated nonselective cation channels. The net effect of these multiple processes in dorsal horn pain transmission neurons is a progressive increase in the action potential discharge elicited by each stimulus, a phenomenon known as "windup" (4).

Nociceptive dorsal horns show an additional and mechanistically separable form of enhanced responsiveness to nociceptive inputs which is often referred to as "central sensitization" (5) which is a major component of inflammatory and neuropathic pain (6). Central sensitization, like windup, is initiated by peripheral nociceptor input but not by low-threshold peripheral inputs. In contrast to windup, sensitization of central pain pathway neurons outlasts, by up to many hours, the duration of the nociceptor inputs that initiates it. These inputs cause the en-

FIGURE 1. Activation of pain transmission neurons in the dorsal horn by glutamatergic fast excitatory postsynaptic potentials. Adapted from Woolf and Salter, 2000 [see text for definition of abbreviations].

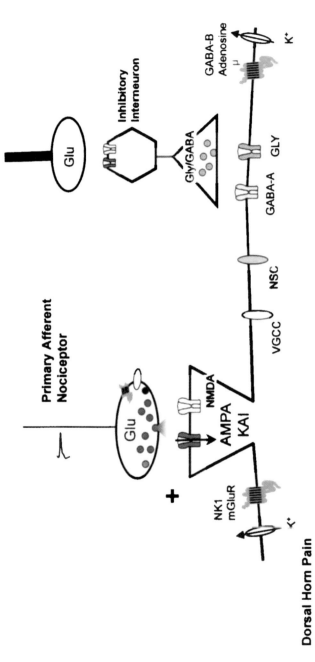

FIGURE 2. High frequency primary afferent discharges enhance glutamatergic responses through slow excitatory postsynaptic potentials, plateau potentials, and windup. Adapted from Woolf and Salter, 2000 [see text for definition of abbreviations].

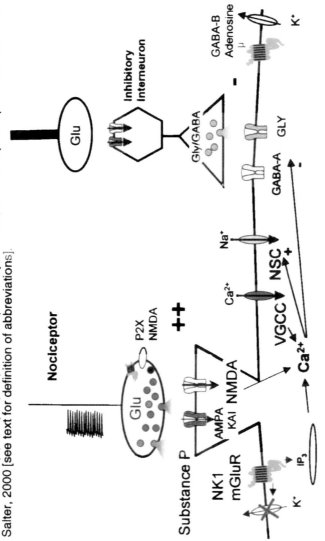

Reprinted with the permission from Woolf and Salter, 2000, *Science* 288, p. 1765. Copyright 2000 American Association for the Advancement of Science.

gagement of multiple intracellular signalling cascades, that were dormant during activation, leading to an orchestrated modification of neuronal behavior consisting of enhanced excitatory postsynaptic responses and depressed inhibition. The engagement of these signalling cascades functionally increases the gain of pain pathway neurons resulting in amplified responses to not only noxious but also to innocuous inputs. Most pain pathway neurons have a large excitatory subliminal fringe and the increased gain also results in unmasking of subthreshold inputs, causing the neurons to become sensitive to stimuli in surrounding regions of the periphery. Thus, not only are the responses of individual neurons amplified, but the number of pain pathway neurons is increased.

Central sensitization is initiated and sustained over the short-term primarily through posttranslational alterations in the function of the complement of gene-products already expressed by pain pathway neurons. However, the signalling cascades activated by nociceptor inputs also produce changes which maintain the increase in gain in the pain pathway on a long-term time scale through altering expression of a repertoire of genes which changes the phenotype of central transmission neurons and may even disrupt or kill inhibitory neurons (4).

ENHANCEMENT OF EXCITATORY SYNAPTIC TRANSMISSION

Conceptually, the simplest means to sensitize central pain transmission neurons is to increase the efficacy at the excitatory primary afferent inputs onto these neurons. In numerous studies primary afferent-evoked responses of pain pathway neurons have been shown to be enhanced by a wide variety of conditioning stimuli. But whether all of these represent enhanced efficacy at primary-afferent-to-second-order synapses is unclear because often the neurons studied received long-latency monosynaptic responses that overlap temporal with polysynaptic responses, or the responses were evoked by stimuli producing asynchronous discharge of primary afferents where the requisite timing information is lost. Nevertheless, with the most rigorous studies of monosynaptic responses, which have by necessity been done using superficial dorsal horn neurons, it is clear that brief duration, high frequency primary afferent stimulation may induce potentiation of AMPA-receptor mediated responses at synapses onto second order neurons (7). The potentiation is prevented by pharmacological blockade of NMDA receptors, and persists for as long as experimentally observable, up to many hours.

From these properties it is logical to propose that the lasting enhancement of excitatory synaptic responses at primary afferent-second order synapses in pain pathways shares a common signalling cascade with so-called NMDA receptor-dependent form of long-term potentiation [LTP] of excitatory synaptic transmission that is observed in many regions of the CNS. The mechanisms of NMDA receptor-dependent LTP have been examined in most detail for Schaffer collateral synapses onto CA1 neurons in the hippocampus, where a core signalling cascade for initiating LTP has been proposed (8,9). This requires Ca^{2+} influx through NMDA receptors during the tetanic stimulation which is accomplished by temporal summation of EPSPs, diminishing the Mg^{2+} blockade of the channel. Enhancement of NMDA channel function by the tyrosine kinase Src is also necessary and a coincident rise in postsynaptic sodium concentration may additionally contribute to boosting NMDA receptor activity (9). The resultant influx of Ca^{2+} sets off a cascade leading to activation of Ca^{2+}/calmodulin dependent kinase II [CAMKII] and phosphorylation of the AMPA receptor subunit protein [GluR1] which causes AMPA channels to move to a high conductance state. Phosphorylation of AMPA receptors may also cause increased cell surface expression of AMPA receptors and allows conversion of "silent synapses," those lacking AMPA receptors, into active ones.

The general form of this core signalling cascade–NMDA receptor activation leading to postsynaptic enhancement of AMPA receptor function or cell-surface expression–is likely applicable in spinal pain transmission neurons as illustrated in Figure 3. In particular there is evidence for silent synapses in dorsal horn neurons and for conversion of these to active synapses, a process requiring post-synaptic density-95, discs large, zonula occludens-1 domain interactions of AMPA receptors (10). As in many regions of the CNS silent synapses in the dorsal horn are most prominent at early developmental stages but there may be few if any silent synapses in the dorsal horn in the adult. Thus, in the adult dorsal horn LTP may be expressed primary by enhanced single-channel conductance of AMPA channels or enhanced cell-surface expression of AMPA receptors, although these mechanisms remain to be shown directly in the spinal dorsal horn.

The applicability of the entire signalling cascade described in CA1 is likely limited to a subpopulation of neurons in the dorsal horn. Administering exogenous CAMKII has been shown to enhance AMPA responses of dorsal horn neurons but expression of endogenous CAMKIIα is highly restricted within the dorsal horn. A protein kinase which is a

FIGURE 3. A model for the molecular mechanisms producing central sensitization through facilitating alpha-amino-3-hydroxy-5-ethyl-4-isoxazoleproprionate/kainate receptor function and/or cell-surface expression [see text for definition of abbreviations].

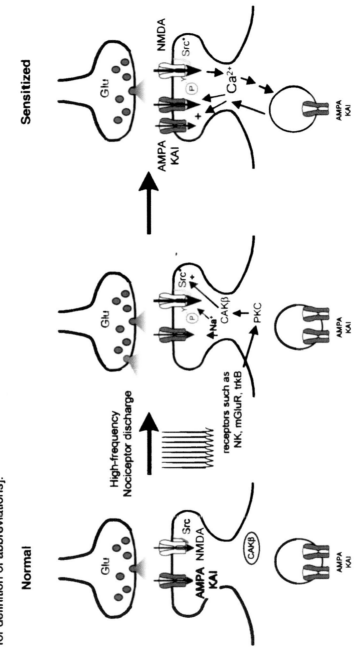

candidate to substitute for CAMKII is protein kinase C [PKC] which potentiates synaptic transmission in dorsal horn neurons and elsewhere. In CA1 PKC has been implicated in initiating LTP but recent evidence indicates that it is likely upstream of Src and its effects mediated via the protein tyrosine kinase [CAKβ/Pyk2] (11). In the dorsal horn PKC could play a dual role, phosphorylating AMPA receptors and stimulating CAKβ/Pyk2-Src signalling, or alternatively, phosphorylation of AMPA receptors may be produced by an as yet unidentified serine/threonine kinase.

Another kinase signalling cascade that appears required for induction of LTP in CA1 is the mitogen-activated protein kinase [MAPK, also known as ERK] pathway. The MAPK is activated upon phosphorylation by MEK and inhibitors of MEK block induction of LTP (8). Importantly, the early phase of LTP is prevented by MEK inhibition at times too early to be accounted for by changes in gene expression known to be induced by MAPK. In the superficial dorsal horn, MAPK phosphorylation increases following nociceptive stimulation and inhibiting MEK suppresses the second phase of the formalin test, indicative of suppression of central responsiveness (12). Thus, it has been hypothesized that the MAPK pathway is necessary for amplification in spinal pain pathways.

An additional mechanism for lasting enhancement of excitatory transmission is through activation of AMPA receptors lacking the edited form of the GluR2 subunit. Such GluR2-less AMPA receptors are permeable to Ca^{2+} which provides the potential to bypass a need for NMDA receptors to initiate synaptic plasticity dependent upon raising postsynaptic Ca^{2+}. Neurons expressing Ca^{2+}-permeable AMPA receptors are preferentially localized in the superficial dorsal horn. Lasting enhancement of synaptic transmission mediated by GluR2-less AMPA receptors by a postsynaptic mechanism has been demonstrated at dorsal horn synapses (13). Such enhancement may contribute to certain types of amplification of responsiveness of neurons in pain pathways.

In addition to the postsynaptic mechanisms described above presynaptic increase in the release of glutamate might also result in sustained increase in the gain of pain pathways. This could be produced by direct facilitation of transmitter release or by suppression of tonic presynaptic inhibition. Release of transmitter could be enhanced by stimulating receptors on primary afferent terminals, including P2X3 receptors and NMDA autoreceptors. However, the effects of such receptor stimulation may be relatively short-lived. In contrast, sustained enhancement of the release of glutamate may be produced by the neurotrophin brain-derived neurotropic factor [BDNF] which contribute to the known involvement of BDNF in inflammatory pain hypersensitivity (14).

PERSISTENT DEPRESSION OF INHIBITION

Potentially of equal importance as sustained enhancement of excitatory transmission is depression of spinal inhibitory mechanisms. Long-term depression [LTD] of transmission at primary afferent synapses onto inhibitory dorsal horn neurons is elicited by activation of Adelta primary afferents. The depression, which requires NMDA receptor activation and a subsequent rise in postsynaptic Ca^{2+}, is mechanistically similar to LTD in other regions, such as the hippocampus or cerebellum. The molecular basis for LTD in both hippocampus and cerebellum has emerged as due to clathrin-mediated endocytosis of synaptically localized AMPA receptors (15). Thus, it is likely that LTD at primary afferent synapses onto inhibitory dorsal horn neurons is due to internalization of cell-surface AMPA receptors.

An additional mechanism for suppressing glycine/gamma amino butyric acid [GABA] transmission in pain pathway neurons is down-regulation of postsynaptic receptors. There is little information specifically about control of these receptors in dorsal horn neurons but, by analogy with GABA receptor regulation in other CNS regions, sustained changes in receptor number or function are predicted.

CONCLUSIONS

Central sensitization is a form of synaptic plasticity that is mechanistically similar to persistent enhancement of excitatory synaptic transmission found in most regions of the CNS. The enhancement of excitatory responses in dorsal horn pain transmission neurons is one of the key active processes, which occur centrally and peripherally, leading to an increased gain of the pain transmission system and to pain hypersensitivity.

REFERENCES

1. Dingledine R, Borges K, Bowie D, Traynelis SF: The glutamate receptor ion channels. Pharmacol. Rev. 51:7-61, 1999.

2. De Koninck Y, Henry JL: Substance P-mediated slow excitatory postsynaptic potential elicited in dorsal horn neurons in vivo by noxious stimulation. Proc. Natl. Acad. Sci. U.S.A. 88:11344-11348, 1991.

3. Sivilotti LG, Thompson SW, Woolf CJ: Rate of rise of the cumulative depolarization evoked by repetitive stimulation of small-caliber afferents is a predictor of action potential windup in rat spinal neurons in vitro. J. Neurophysiol. 69:1621-1631, 1993.

4. Woolf CJ, Salter MW: Neuronal plasticity: increasing the gain in pain. Science 288:1765-1769, 2000.

5. Woolf CJ: Evidence for a central component of post-injury pain hypersensitivity. Nature 306:686-688, 1983.

6. Treede RD, Meyer RA, Raja SN, Campbell JN: Peripheral and central mechanisms of cutaneous hyperalgesia. Prog. Neurobiol. 38:397-421, 1992.

7. Randic M, Jiang MC, Cerne R: Long-term potentiation and long-term depression of primary afferent neurotransmission in the rat spinal cord. J. Neurosci. 13: 5228-5241, 1993.

8. Soderling TR, Derkach VA: Postsynaptic protein phosphorylation and LTP. Trends Neurosci. 23:75-80, 2000.

9. Ali DW, Salter MW: NMDA receptor regulation by Src kinase signalling in excitatory synaptic transmission and plasticity. Curr. Opin. Neurobiol. 11:336-342, 2001.

10. Zhuo M: Silent glutamatergic synapses and long-term facilitation in spinal dorsal horn neurons. Prog. Brain Res. 129:101-113, 2000.

11. Huang Y, Lu W, Ali DW, Pelkey KA, Pitcher GM, Lu YM, Aoto H, Roder JC, Sasaki T, Salter MW, MacDonald JF: CAKbeta/Pyk2 kinase is a signaling link for induction of long-term potentiation in CA1 hippocampus. Neuron 29:485-496, 2001.

12. Ji RR, Baba H, Brenner GJ, Woolf CJ: Nociceptive-specific activation of ERK in spinal neurons contributes to pain hypersensitivity. Nat. Neurosci. 2:1114-1119, 1999.

13. Gu JG, Albuquerque C, Lee CJ, MacDermott AB: Synaptic strengthening through activation of Ca^{2+}-permeable AMPA receptors. Nature 381:793-796, 1996.

14. Thompson SW, Bennett DL, Kerr BJ, Bradbury EJ, McMahon SB: Brain-derived neurotrophic factor is an endogenous modulator of nociceptive responses in the spinal cord. Proc. Natl. Acad. Sci. U.S.A. 96:7714-7718, 1999.

15. Carroll RC, Beattie EC, von Zastrow M, Malenka RC: Role of AMPA receptor endocytosis in synaptic plasticity. Nat. Rev. Neurosci. 2:315-324, 2001.

The Pharmacology of Central Sensitization

Rie Suzuki
Anthony H. Dickenson

SUMMARY. Objective: The purpose of this review is to show how central mechanisms of pain transmission relate to pharmacological systems that are responsible for the generation of central sensitization states.

Findings: Pain transmission is a complex process involving the interplay between excitatory and inhibitory systems acting at different levels of the central nervous system. A balance between excitatory and inhibitory receptor mediated events determines the level of excitability within spinal circuits capable of contributing to the transmission of noxious messages. All of these systems are subject to plasticity and other alterations in pharmacological functions that characterize pathological conditions.

Conclusions: A better understanding of the neuropharmacology of pain transmission within the spinal cord has the potential to improve the clinical management of pathologically severe and persistent pain. *[Article copies available for a fee from The Haworth Document Delivery Service: 1-800-HAWORTH. E-mail address: <getinfo@haworthpressinc.com> Website: <http://www.HaworthPress.com> © 2002 by The Haworth Press, Inc. All rights reserved.]*

KEYWORDS. Pain, inflammation, nerve injury, spinal cord, central sensitization

Rie Suzuki, BSc, PhD, and Anthony H. Dickenson, BSc, PhD, are affiliated with the Department of Pharmacology, University College London, Gower Street, London, UK, WC1E 6BT.

Address correspondence to: Rie Suzuki, PhD, Department of Pharmacology, University College London, Gower Street, London, UK, WC1E 6BT [E-mail: ucklrsu@ucl.ac.uk].

[Haworth co-indexing entry note]: "The Pharmacology of Central Sensitization." Suzuki, Rie, and Anthony H. Dickenson. Co-published simultaneously in *Journal of Musculoskeletal Pain* [The Haworth Medical Press, an imprint of The Haworth Press, Inc.] Vol. 10, No. 1/2, 2002, pp. 35-43; and: *The Clinical Neurobiology of Fibromyalgia and Myofascial Pain: Therapeutic Implications* [ed: Robert M. Bennett] The Haworth Medical Press, an imprint of The Haworth Press, Inc., 2002, pp. 35-43. Single or multiple copies of this article are available for a fee from The Haworth Document Delivery Service [1-800-HAWORTH, 9:00 a.m. 5.00 p.m. (EST). E-mail address: getinfo@haworthpressinc.com].

35

In recent years, considerable progress has been made with respect to our understanding of both acute and chronic pain mechanisms. This progress has largely been attributed to advancements in molecular biology and genomic techniques enabling us to explore potential targets for pain. The result has been a fundamentally improved understanding of the pathophysiology of pain mechanisms and a new hope for the development of novel analgesics. Despite this progress, however, the management of pain still remains inadequate in many cases and continues to be a significant problem.

The sequence of events which follow peripheral tissue/nerve injury, and consequently contribute to the development of inflammation or neuropathy, can be seen at various levels of the nervous system, both peripherally and more centrally. Following injury, plasticity is induced in the peripheral and central nervous system [anatomical, neurochemical, pharmacological, and electrophysiological changes], which may be related to the pathogenesis of these pain states [Figure 1]. This review will focus on the central mechanisms of pain transmission and in particular, we will discuss some of the pharmacological systems which are responsible for the generation of central sensitization states.

PHARMACOLOGY OF THE SPINAL CORD

Nociceptive sensory information arriving from primary afferent fibers enters via the dorsal horn [Figure 2]. The spinal cord is an important site at which various nociceptive signalling systems undergo convergence and modulation. Spinal neurons are controlled by peripheral inputs, interneurons, and descending controls, as first suggested in the gate theory of pain. Pain transmission is therefore a complex process involving the interplay between excitatory and inhibitory systems acting at different levels of the central nervous system. All these systems are subject to plasticity, and alterations in pharmacological systems may occur during pathological conditions.

EXCITATORY TRANSMISSION

Voltage Gated Calcium Channels

The vital link between activity in peripheral nerves and that in the spinal dorsal horn is transmitter release. Voltage gated calcium chan-

FIGURE 1. Neurophysiological events following peripheral tissue injury can lead to the development of pathological pain states. Peripheral neurological injury causes stimulation of the central nervous system which activates the process of central sensitization. Gene induction by acute pain leads transiently to decreased pain thresholds. With chronicity of the stimulus, that process becomes less reversible [plasticity] leading to persistently expanding receptive fields. Clinically, these changes can become physiologically manifested as hyperalgesia and allodynia.

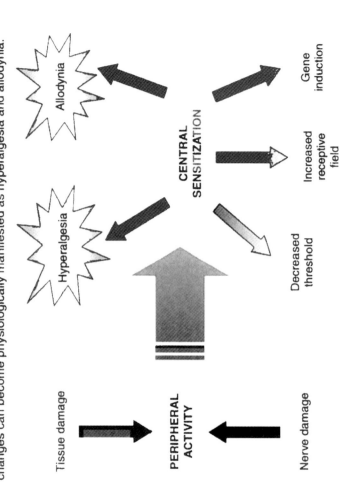

FIGURE 2. Regulation of nociception in the dorsal horn of the spinal cord. Nociceptive sensory information is delivered to the dorsal horn of the spinal cord by primary afferent C-fibers. Voltage-gated calcium channels [N- and P-type] are involved in controlling the release of neurochemicals [substance P, glutamate] into the synapse. These neurochemicals activate receptors, such as the alpha-amino-3-hydroxy-5-methyl-4-isoxazole-propionic acid receptor [AMPA-R], the neurokinin-1 receptor [NK1-R], or the N-methyl-D-aspartic acid receptor [NMDA-R]. The NMDA-R channel requires repeated stimulation [wind-up] by tachykinins, like substance P, to overcome blockade by physiological levels of magnesium at resting membrane potentials. Descending control of spinal nerve activation is mediated by serotonin [5HT], noradrenaline, and other neurochemicals. Gamma-aminobutyric acid [GABA] is another major inhibitory transmitter system. Nitric Oxide [NO] is a potent neuronal messenger which is produced on demand by the action of the enzyme nitric oxide synthase on L-arginine. There is increasing evidence to suggest that NO may be involved in the cascade of NMDA receptor-mediated central sensitization.

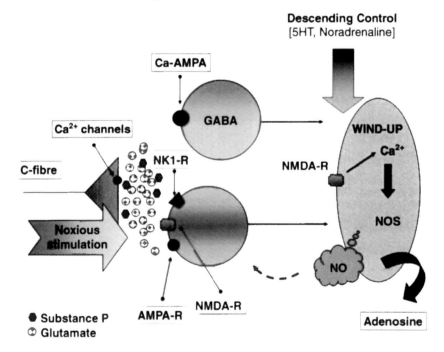

nels [VGCCs] are necessary to regulate calcium [Ca^{2+}] influx into nerve terminals. Several subtypes of channels have so far been identified, including the low voltage activated channels, such as the T-type, and the high voltage activated channels of the L-, N- and P/Q-type. In the spinal cord, the highest densities of N-type channels are found in the superficial dorsal horn, where they are found at synaptic sites, implicating a role of these channels in the release of neurotransmitters.

The influx of Ca^{2+} into neurons is important in persistent pain states where peripheral and/or central sensitization and plasticity are present. Thus changing the levels of Ca^{2+} or its mobilization has no effect on acute nociceptive tests in animal systems [e.g., tail-flick and hot plate assay]. However, in the presence of a more sustained stimulus in the same animals [assessed by the formalin test and the writhing tests], and in states of inflammation and neuropathy, Ca^{2+} channel blockers have been shown to exert effectiveness.

N- and P-type Ca^{2+} channel antagonists are effective against inflammatory pain models (1). In neuropathic states, intrathecally delivered N-type VGCC blockers, but not L- and P-type blockers, produce a blockade of tactile allodynia (2). This observation is further supported by electrophysiological evidence demonstrating that intrathecal N- and P-type VGCC blockers reduce the responses of spinal neurons to peripheral stimuli (3). Moreover, the effectiveness of the N-type blocker was enhanced in neuropathy suggesting a role for N-type Ca^{2+} channels in the plasticity that develops with this pain state.

Hence, the potent antinociceptive effects of Ca^{2+} channel antagonists, observed across various models of pain, would favor the use of these compounds for the treatment of pain states associated with central hyperexcitability. Since both N- and P-type Ca^{2+} channels are implicated in neurotransmission under both physiological and pathophysiological conditions, the therapeutic utility of these compounds would depend on the development of therapeutic agents that can selectively target pathophysiological activity, therefore avoiding undesirable side effects. Interestingly, the anticonvulsant, gabapentin, effective in neuropathic pain, appears to interact with Ca^{2+} channels and so may block transmitter release in a yet not fully understood manner.

N-Methyl-D-Aspartate Receptor System

The excitatory amino acids, glutamate and aspartate, have been implicated in the transmission of nociceptive information in acute and chronic pain states. Several receptors for glutamate have been identified, including the N-methyl-D-aspartate [NMDA], alpha-amino-3-hydroxy-5-methyl-4-isoxazole-propionic acid [AMPA], kainate, and metabotropic glutamate receptors.

The excitatory amino acids are found in most sensory fibers, including both large and small diameter fibers where, in the latter case, they are colocalized with neuropeptides such as substance P. Whilst AMPA receptors are activated in response to brief acute stimuli and are involved in the fast events of pain transmission, NMDA receptors are only activated following repetitive noxious inputs, under conditions where the incoming stimulus is maintained (4). The NMDA channel is blocked by physiological levels of magnesium at resting membrane potentials, thus the receptor can only operate after sufficient repeated depolarization. The removal of the magnesium block is likely to be mediated by tachykinins like substance P. The NMDA receptors have been implicated in the spinal events underlying 'windup,' whereby the responses of dorsal horn neurons are significantly increased after repetitive C-fiber stimulation despite the constant input (4). Thus, the activation of this class of receptors brings about a marked increase in neuronal excitability and is responsible for the amplification and prolongation of neuronal responses in the spinal cord (4,5).

The NMDA receptor is an ionotropic receptor coupled to a cation channel, and is formed from two subunit types; the NR1 and NR2 subunit [NR2A-D]. An example in which windup has been demonstrated clinically is the report by Staud and coworkers (6), who assessed the temporal summation of pain [i.e., windup], using repetitive thermal stimulation of the hand in patients with fibromyalgia syndrome. Patients with fibromyalgia syndrome were shown to have a higher baseline response to the initial first stimulus, and additionally, exhibited a higher degree of temporal summation, therefore suggesting an abnormal central processing in these subjects (6). Whilst the increased pain response to initial stimuli may indicate enhanced transmitter release via greater Ca^{2+} channel activity [see section on Ca^{2+} channels], the increase in temporal summation may reflect a greater NMDA receptor function.

To date, there is substantial evidence suggesting for the involvement of NMDA receptors in various pathological pain states, including inflammation, neuropathy, allodynia, and ischemia (4,5,7). Following nerve injury, there appears to be a greater contribution of the NMDA receptor system to neuronal activity, and this may play a role in the spinal hyperexcitability that underlies this condition (8).

One consequence of central sensitization is the expansion of receptive field size and this has been demonstrated after inflammation and peripheral nerve injury in dorsal horn neurons (9). Any increase in spinal excitability, will cause neurons to start to respond to inputs that are normally too weak to evoke activity–resulting in the expansion of receptive field size. Thereafter, a given stimulus will activate a greater number of spinal neurons. Similar observations have been seen clinically, where patients with osteoarthritis displayed an enlargement of the referred pain area following intramuscular infusion of hypertonic saline (10).

Nitric Oxide and Nitric Oxide Synthase

A comparatively new putative nociceptive transmitter is nitric oxide [NO]. Nitric oxide is a neuronal messenger which, unlike other messengers, is not stored in synaptic vesicles, but is produced on demand. Nitric oxide is synthesised from L-arginine by the enzyme nitric oxide synthase and is thought to act as an intercellular, and possibly an intracellular messenger. There is now evidence for the spinal role of NO in nociceptive processing during states of inflammation or neuropathy (11). This raises the possibility that NO may be involved in the cascade of events underlying NMDA receptor-mediated central sensitization.

INHIBITORY TRANSMISSION

In addition to these excitatory events, inhibitory systems also exist in the spinal cord where they are in dynamic equilibrium with other intrinsic systems to suppress nociceptive transmission and effectively produce analgesia.

Adenosine Receptor System

The purines, adenosine, and adenosine 5'-triphosphate have been implicated in the modulation of nociceptive transmission, both in the periphery and in the central nervous system (12).

Receptor sites for adenosine in the spinal cord have been identified in the substantia gelatinosa where they are localized primarily on intrinsic neurons. Two main subclasses of adenosine receptors [A_1 and A_2] have been described and it appears to be predominantly the A_1 receptor subtype which plays a major role in inhibiting the nociceptive input in the dorsal spinal cord (13). A_1 receptor agonists have been shown to inhibit windup, an NMDA receptor-mediated event (13). There is accumulating evidence for the antinociceptive effects of adenosine analogues (14). Furthermore, adenosine-mediated antinociception can be enhanced through the use of adenosine kinase and adenosine deaminase inhibitors, which prevent the degradation of adenosine.

Neuropathic and inflammatory pain states are associated with neuronal hyperexcitability; hence adenosine and adenosine kinase inhibitors may offer a beneficial approach in attenuating excessive neuronal activity through interactions with the NMDA receptor system

Gamma-Aminobutyric Acid System

Gamma-aminobutyric acid [GABA] forms the major inhibitory transmitter system within the spinal cord and appears to exert tonic inhibitory controls on excitatory transmission. Various receptors for GABA have been identified and these have been classified into two subtypes, the $GABA_A$ receptor and $GABA_B$ receptor.

There is increasing evidence for the role of GABA inhibitory system in the modulation of nociceptive transmission at the spinal level. Alterations in the disposition of GABA and glycine are therefore likely to lead to the generation or maintenance of persistent pain states (4,5). During inflammation, there is an increase in GABAergic inhibitory control, as demonstrated by an increase in GABA immunoreactivity, and this may possibly reflect a mechanism by which enhanced neuronal excitability is counteracted. In direct contrast, $GABA_B$ receptor binding and GABA immunoreactivity are seen to decrease in the dorsal horn following nerve injury. Changes in endogenous inhibitory controls may facilitate the generation of spontaneous activity in the spinal cord, and contribute to the induction of central hyperexcitability.

CONCLUSION

The existence of central sensitization may explain why pains of tissue damage are enhanced by peripheral sensitization to activate and maintain central mechanisms of windup. By contrast, neuropathic pains are often severe and chronic despite the fact that there must be relatively low levels of afferent input arriving in the spinal cord from the damaged nerve. Initial afferent barrages at high intensity after nerve damage induce windup which is then maintained by low ongoing activity.

Thus it would appear that a balance between excitatory and inhibitory receptor mediated events determines the level of excitability within spinal circuits contributing to the transmission of noxious messages. There is a good consensus between electrophysiological and behavioral approaches in animals and clinical studies in terms of building a picture of the pharmacology of transmission and modulation within the spinal cord. Plasticity within these systems has consequences for the understanding and better treatment of persistent pains.

REFERENCES

1. Diaz A, Dickenson AH: Blockade of spinal N- and P-type, but not L-type, calcium channels inhibits the excitability of rat dorsal horn neurones produced by subcutaneous formalin inflammation. Pain 69: 93-100, 1997.

2. Chaplan SR, Pogrel JW, Yaksh TL: Role of voltage-dependent calcium channel subtypes in experimental tactile allodynia. J Pharmacol Exp Ther 269: 1117-23, 1994.

3. Matthews E, Dickenson A: Effects of spinally delivered N- and P-type voltage-dependent calcium channel antagonists on dorsal horn neuronal responses in a rat model of neuropathy. Pain 92: 235-246, 2001.

4. Dickenson AH, Chapman V, Green GM: The pharmacology of excitatory and inhibitory amino acid-mediated events in the transmission and modulation of pain in the spinal cord. Gen Pharmacol 28: 633-8, 1997.

5. Millan MJ: The induction of pain: an integrative review. Prog Neurobiol 57: 1-164, 1999.

6. Staud R, Vierck C, Cannon R, Mauderli A, Price D: Abnormal sensitization and temporal summation of second pain (wind-up) in patients with fibromyalgia syndrome. Pain 91: 165-75, 2001.

7. McMahon S, Lewin G, Wall P: Central hyperexcitability triggered by noxious inputs. Curr Opin Neurobiol 3: 602-610, 1993.

8. Suzuki R, Matthews E, Dickenson A: Comparison of the effects of MK-801, ketamine and memantine on responses of spinal dorsal horn neurones in a rat model of mononeuropathy. Pain 91: 101-109, 2001.

9. Suzuki R, Kontinen V, Matthews E, Dickenson A: Enlargement of receptive field size to low intensity mechanical stimulation in the rat spinal nerve ligation model of neuropathy. Exp Neurol 163: 408-413, 2000.

10. Bajaj P, Bajaj P, Graven-Nielsen T, Arendt-Nielsen L: Osteoarthritis and its association with muscle hyperalgesia: an experimental controlled study. Pain 93: 107-114, 2001.

11. Malmberg A, Yaksh T: Spinal nitric oxide synthesis inhibition blocks NMDA-induced thermal hyperalgesia and produces antinociception in the formalin test in rats. Pain 54: 291-300, 1993.

12. Sawynok J: Adenosine receptor activation and nociception. Eur J Pharmacol 347: 1-11, 1998.

13. Reeve AJ, Dickenson AH: The roles of spinal adenosine receptors in the control of acute and more persistent nociceptive responses of dorsal horn neurones in the anaesthetized rat. Br J Pharmacol 116: 2221-2228, 1995.

14. Dickenson A, Suzuki R, Reeve A: Adenosine as a potential analgesic target in inflammatory and neuropathic pains. CNS Drugs 13: 77-85, 2000.

Is Fibromyalgia a Central Pain State?

Karl G. Henriksson

SUUMARY. Objective: To review the literature concerning pain mechanisms in fibromyalgia [FMS].

Findings and Conclusions: Thirteen investigations using different methods, comprising 250 patients with FMS, confirm a biological dysfunction of the nociceptive system, especially in the central nervous system in the majority of patients with FMS. The hyperexcitability in the nociceptive nervous system may have different causes in the individual patient. Localized long-standing muscle pain, chronic stress, genetic factors, and hormonal changes may all play a role. Pain generators in the muscle may not be specific for FMS but may be of importance for initiating and maintaining pain and allodynia/hyperalgesia. *[Article copies available for a fee from The Haworth Document Delivery Service: 1-800-HAWORTH. E-mail address: <getinfo@haworthpressinc.com> Website: <http://www. HaworthPress.com> © 2002 by The Haworth Press, Inc. All rights reserved.]*

KEYWORDS. Fibromyalgia, pain mechanisms, muscular pain, central sensitization

INTRODUCTION

According to the classification criteria proposed by the American College of Rheumatology [ACR] fibromyalgia [FMS] comprises one

Karl G. Henriksson, MD, PhD, is Associate Professor, Department of Rehabilitation Medicine, Pain Clinic and Neuromuscular Unit, Faculty of Health Sciences, Linköping University, Sweden.

Address correspondence to: Karl G. Henriksson, MD, PhD, Neuromuscular Unit, University Hospital, Linköping, S-581 85 Sweden [E-mail address: karl-g@telia.com].

[Haworth co-indexing entry note]: "Is Fibromyalgia a Central Pain State?" Henriksson, Karl G. Co-published simultaneously in *Journal of Musculoskeletal Pain* [The Haworth Medical Press, an imprint of The Haworth Press, Inc.] Vol. 10, No. 1/2, 2002. pp. 45-57; and: *The Clinical Neurobiology of Fibromyalgia and Myofascial Pain: Therapeutic Implications* [ed: Robert M. Bennett] The Haworth Medical Press, an imprint of The Haworth Press, Inc., 2002, pp. 45-57. Single or multiple copies of this article are available for a fee from The Haworth Document Delivery Service [1-800-HAWORTH, 9:00 a.m. - 5:00 p.m. [EST]. E-mail address. getinfo@haworthpressinc.com].

symptom–chronic multifocal pain–and one sign–generalized allodynia/ hyperalgesia (1). The patient who is diagnosed with FMS, however, is polysymptomatic. Besides pain there is fatigue, sleep disturbance, psychological distress, impaired muscle function, and symptoms that are usually regarded as stress-related. Fibromyalgia is an illness, a syndrome, that effects three systems that regulate our well being: the nociceptive system, the stress-regulating system, and the immune system. These systems interact with each other, making it difficult to determine which of them is primarily affected in an individual patient. Psychological factors, personality traits, and social circumstances play a role for the total clinical picture. Fibromyalgia is indeed a biopsychosocial syndrome. The biological part concerns mainly pain and allodynia/hyperalgesia as well as biological changes related to continuous physical and emotional stress. This article will deal only with pain and allodynia. Allodynia is pain elicited by normally nonpainful stimuli. Hyperalgesia is increased pain intensity and prolonged pain duration evoked by stimuli that normally are painful.

CHRONIC PAIN IN FIBROMYALGIA–A DISEASE?

A permanently disturbed function in an organ system that gives rise to symptoms of ill heath is a disease, which requires objective and standardized tests in order to be diagnosed. The pain in FMS is continuous in most patients. Short-lasting pain-free periods occur only in about a third of the patients. Pressure allodynia is generalized, pointing to a change in pain signal processing in the nervous system. A systematic search for pain mechanisms is rarely performed in spite of the fact that several studies have been published on pain mechanisms in FMS. Some of the methods used in these studies could be used not only in research but also in the clinic setting. The aim of this section of the article is briefly to present studies that show a pathologic function of the nociceptive system, especially in the central nervous system [CNS], in FMS. With respect to whether pain and allodynia/hyperalgesia in FMS are a disease or not, the results of the studies that will be presented below could be added together. Altogether, 250 patients with FMS [studies on substance P in the cerebrospinal fluid and studies using quantitative sensory testing not included] diagnosed according to the ACR criteria participated in the different studies.

Pharmacological Pain Analyses and Response
to Experimentally Induced Muscle Pain

We performed four studies to investigate pain mechanisms in FMS. The methods used were pharmacological pain analyses and test of the response to experimentally induced muscle pain.

In the first study, nine patients were given 10 mg morphine, 11 lidocaine [5 mg/kg] and 11 ketamine [0.3 mg/kg] intravenously (2). Ketamine [Ketalar® Park-Davis] is an N-methyl-D-aspartate [NMDA] receptor antagonist. The study was placebo controlled. A responder was defined as a person where pain intensity [visual analog scale] was reduced by 50 percent or more. None responded to morphine. The dose of morphine may have been too small. Four responded to lidocaine, whereas eight were responders in the ketamine test. Pressure pain threshold and tolerance thresholds measured by a dolorimeter increased significantly compared to placebo in the ketamine test.

In the second randomized, double-blind, cross-over study, all 18 patients received intravenous infusions of placebo, morphine, lidocaine, and ketamine (3). The doses were the same as in the first study, with the exception of morphine, which was 0.3 mg/kg. Here, 13 patients were responders to one or several drugs but not to the placebo. There were two placebo responders, whereas three were nonresponders. Pressure pain thresholds and tolerance thresholds increased significantly in responders.

The third study was done in cooperation with the Institute for Sensory-Motor Interaction, Aalborg University in Denmark (4). Muscle pain was experimentally induced by infusion of hypertonic saline [5.7 percent] in a muscle [anterior tibial muscle], where neither the FMS patients nor the healthy controls had any ongoing pain. The rate of infusion and the amount of saline infused were standardized and computer controlled. The 12 patients were all ketamine responders. Those with FMS differed from healthy controls with respect to the following:

- The patients had lower pressure pain threshold.
- The pain threshold to repeated electrical stimulation was lower than the threshold to a single stimulus, which means a facilitation of temporal summation [see next page].
- The pain evoked by hypertonic saline had longer duration compared to controls.
- The referred pain area was larger in the patients.

The fourth study was divided in two experiments. In the first experiment it was found that 17 of the 29 participants were ketamine responders (5). Fifteen of these took part in the second experiment. It was found that the area of referred pain, the temporal summation, the muscle hyperalgesia, and the muscle pain at rest were attenuated by ketamine but not by placebo.

We draw the following conclusions from the four investigations:

- The FMS population that meets the classification criteria proposed by ACR is not homogenous with respect to pain mechanisms.
- In the majority of FMS patients there are objective findings of hyperexcitability in the nociceptive system in the CNS. Central sensitization due to activation of NMDA receptors is part of this hyperexcitability.
- Pharmacological pain analyses and the method of inducing experimental muscle pain are standardized methods that can be used not only in research but also in the clinic.

Temporal Summation

Temporal summation means a progressive increase in action potential discharge from nociceptive nerve cells in the dorsal horn in response to repetitive stimulation by identical stimuli [windup]. Staud et al. recently published a study of 59 FMS patients and 65 normal controls, where the response to repetitive thermal stimulation was recorded (6). The stimuli were of equal intensity. The amount of temporal summation was greater in FMS patients than in controls. Staud et al. discuss both peripheral and central mechanisms as causes of the increased temporal summation.

Abnormal Responses to Electrocutaneous Stimulation

Arroyo and Cohen used electrocutaneous stimulation to determine perception thresholds and pain tolerance in the upper arm in 10 patients with FMS and 10 healthy controls (7). They found a reduction in pain tolerance and a spread and persistence of dysesthesia in patients with FMS. The authors conclude that the findings imply "perturbation of central nociceptive mechanisms."

Vecchiet et al. measured pain thresholds to electrical stimulation in the skin, subcutaneous tissue, and muscle in patients with FMS, patients with myofascial pain syndrome, and normal controls (8). The feature that distinguished FMS from myofascial pain was that, in FMS, hyperalgesia was found in the skin, subcutaneous tissue, and muscle, even outside painful sites.

Stimulus [Pressure]-Response [Pain] Function

Noxious stimuli activate high-threshold mechanosensitive neurons. Stimulus-response function is a power function (9). Activation by innoxious stimuli give a linear function.

Bendtsen et al. found that, in patients with FMS, the stimulus [pressure]-response [pain] function was linear in contrast to normal controls, who showed a power function (10). The authors interpret their findings as support for the notion that there are "abberant central pain mechanisms" in FMS.

Tests of Somatosensory Evoked Potentials

Two studies show increased amplitude of the cerebral somatosensory potentials evoked by laser heat stimuli to the dorsal surface of the hand in patients with FMS compared with controls. In the Gibson et al. investigation (11), the intensity of the stimulus was at the pain threshold and 1.5 times the pain threshold. In the study by Lorenz et al., the intensity was set to 20 W (12). Lorenz et al. conclude that the effect on one component [N170] of the laser-evoked potential can best be explained by "exogenous factors like peripheral and spinal sensitization or reduced cortical or subcortical inhibition of nociception."

Pain Modulation During Isometric Muscle Contraction and During Heterotopic Noxious Conditioning Stimulation

In a study by Kosek et al., 14 patients with FMS were compared with 14 healthy controls with respect to pressure pain threshold [PPT] measured with an algometer during isometric muscle contraction [25 percent of maximal voluntary contraction] (13). In controls, the PPT increased during contraction, whereas in patients, PPT decreased. The authors conclude that the decrease of PPT during isometric contraction could be due to "sensitization of mechanonociceptors caused by muscle ischemia and/or dysfunction in pain modulation during muscle contraction."

In another study by Kosek and Hansson, 10 patients with FMS and 10 controls were tested with a submaximal effort tourniquet test (14). Pain during ischemic work by muscles in the forearm was the heterotopic noxious conditioning stimulus. The PPT, measured in the thigh, was increased in controls but not in FMS patients. This finding was interpreted as a dysfunction of diffuse noxious inhibitory controls which involve supraspinal structures.

Reduced Regional Cerebral Blood Flow

In 1995, Mountz et al. reported that regional cerebral blood flow in the left and right hemithalami and left and right heads of the caudate nucleus were lower in patients with FMS than in healthy controls (15). Bradley et al. discuss these findings in an overview of the results of neuroimaging in patients with FMS (16). In this overview Bradley et al. contends that the reduced blood flow in the thalamus and the caudate nucleus is secondary to hypersensitivity in spinal and peripheral nociceptive neurons. In the thalamus and caudate nucleus, pain signals from the periphery are modulated. In acute pain, the blood flow in these structures is increased, whereas in chronic pain, such as cancer pain, neuropathic pain, and FMS, the blood flow is reduced.

Substance P in the Cerebrospinal Fluid

Increased levels of substance P in the cerebrospinal fluid are found in the majority of patients with FMS (17). The increase in substance P is an objective sign of subjective pain and may be due to activity in primary afferent nociceptive neurons, or activity in central neurons, or in both peripheral and central neurons.

Conclusions

The results of each of the investigations described above support the presence of a longstanding or permanent change in function of the nociceptive system in CNS in most patients with FMS. The change in function reflects neuroplasticity in nociceptive neurons. Taken together, the studies not only support, but also confirm, that there are changes in the function of the nociceptive system. These disturbances constitute a disease in the majority of patients with FMS. There is in FMS a state of permanent hyperexcitability in the nociceptive system. The pain and the increase in sensitivity to certain sensory stimuli have a biological explanation. With respect to these findings, pain and allodynia/hyperalgesia in FMS can not be regarded as signs of somatization.

FACTORS THAT CAUSE OR DETERMINE THE INTENSITY OF ALLODYNIA/HYPERALGESIA

First of all, more than one factor might contribute to allodynia/hyperalgesia in an individual patient, and some can be regarded as predisposing for the development of FMS. The causes may be different in different subgroups of FMS.

Development of Fibromyalgia from Localized or Regional Pain

In our patient material, which consists of patients referred to rheumatological clinics or pain clinics, the majority have developed FMS from localized or regional muscle pain conditions. In FMS patients with this history, the most likely cause of generalized allodynia/hyperalgesia is longstanding bombardment of the nociceptive system in the CNS by impulses in primary afferent C-fibers and, when allodynia is established, also by impulses in A-beta [touch, pressure] fibers. Findings, which show that longstanding allodynia/hyperalgesia and an increase in substance P in the cerebrospinal fluid can occur as a consequence of localized nociceptive pain conditions such as arthrosis, support the notion that longstanding hyperexcitability in the nociceptive system in the CNS can be secondary to tissue damage in the periphery (18). It is of further interest that longstanding changes in pain modulation in the CNS due to arthrosis disappeared after an operation that gave pain relief (19,20).

Genetic Factors

It is a common experience that FMS occurs in more than one member of a family (21), suggesting that genetic factors may predispose a person to FMS (22). Some personality traits may also be regarded as risk factors. For example, anxious sensitivity or somatic anxiety may influence the perception of pain (23,24).

Stress and Neuroendocrinological Aberrations

Neuroendocrinological aberrations compatible with chronic stress similar to those found in posttraumatic stress disorder have been found in a subgroup of FMS patients (25). Pain is both a physical and an emotional stressor, and chronic pain is always a chronic stress. Whether pain or stress comes first is a difficult question to answer. Temporary exacerbations of pain and allodynia can often be related to an increase in the level of stress. It is more doubtful whether permanent changes in the nociceptive system in CNS are primarily caused by changes in the stress-regulating systems.

The metabolism of serotonin [5HT] is abnormal in FMS. Changes in 5HT metabolism have been studied, in particular by Russell and his co-workers (26,27). Interestingly, studies by Ernberg et al. have shown that 5HT release in the masseter muscle upon trauma [muscle puncture] was higher in patients with FMS than in normal controls (28). Intramuscular microdialysis was used to sample 5HT. Whether the change in 5HT metabolism is a primary or secondary pathogenetic factor is presently not known.

Sex and Gender and Hormonal Changes

The female preponderance among FMS patients is still not explained. The difference in muscle strength may be of importance for the localized pain that often precedes FMS. Results from animal experiments suggest that estrogen is of importance for regulation of pain sensitivity. Estrogen receptors are found on neurons in the dorsal horn. Estrogen regulates the enkephalin transcription in these neurons (29).

The Role of Proinflammatory Agents and Cytokines

When discussing factors that could cause or contribute to generalized allodynia/hyperalgesia, it is important to consider new data on the role of proinflammatory agents and cytokines (30-32). These data tell us that the CNS can be told about pain in the periphery not only by signals in the nerves but also by blood-borne cytokines. Cytokines and prostanoids in the CNS induced by inflammation related to tissue injury in the periphery may contribute to pain hypersensitivity.

Are these findings relevant for hyperalgesia in human pain conditions like FMS? Presently we do not know. Certain observations might be of interest. Muscle damage in relation to exercise is accompanied by inflammation (33). Moreover, there are signs of neurogenic inflammation in skin biopsies from patients with FMS. The number of connective tissue mast cells was increased in patients with FMS compared to controls (34).

Peripheral Pain Generators

Muscular changes that could be related to pain are dismissed as unspecific and related to inactivity in most articles on FMS. This is an oversimplification. The pain in FMS may not be spontaneous, but evoked. Muscle pain is often increased in intensity during and after exercise.

Bengtsson et al. (35) reported that muscle pain and tender points completely disappeared in patients with FMS during epidural administration of lignocaine. This could support the notion that impulses in primary afferent neurons evoke the pain in FMS. Localized or regional muscle pain precedes the widespread pain in FMS in most patients. In Bengtsson et al. (36), 87 percent of FMS patients reported local pain before generalized pain. In another unpublished study on 191 FMS patients 80 percent reported the same. Lapossy et al., in a retrospective study, found that 25 percent of women with chronic low back pain developed FMS (37). In a prospective study Buskila et al. reported that 21.6 percent of persons who had been subjected to a trauma against the neck region developed FMS (38).

Muscle fibers are not provided with nociceptors. The nociceptors in the muscle are found along vessels, except capillaries (39). The stimuli that excite intramuscular nociceptors are the combination of hypoxia and energy-requiring muscle contraction or tension as well as any situation where energy production is insufficient with respect to energy demand. With this in mind, our findings described below are relevant. The tissue oxygen pressure was measured in the trapezius muscle in patients with FMS and in healthy controls with an oxygen electrode placed directly on the muscle surface (40). An average of 120 measurements per patient was collected and presented as a histogram. In the controls the histogram was bell-shaped, which signifies a normal microcirculation. In the patients the histogram was scattered or had the shape of a ski-slope. This indicates a disturbed regulation of the microcirculation. There are morphological changes in the capillary endothelium in the trapezius muscle in FMS (41). These changes cannot be explained by inactivity. The changes in intramuscular microcirculation could contribute to pain and sensitization of intramuscular nociceptors. Chemical analyses of energy-rich phosphates in the trapezius muscle showed decreased absolute levels of adenosine 5'-triphosphate [ATP] and phosphocreatine compared with controls (42). Some studies using magnetic resonance [MR] spectroscopy, where relative values were presented, did not confirm our findings (43). Park et al. (44) have more recently made new MR spectroscopy investigations on the quadriceps muscle. They found, that ATP and phosphocreatine levels at rest and at exercice [25 percent of MVC] were lower in patients with FMS compared with controls.

When allodynia/hyperalgesia is established in chronic muscle pain, be it regional or widespread, the intensity of stimuli that can excite C and A beta receptors can be low. It cannot be excluded that substances released during normal muscle contraction could give rise to pain. It should further be remembered that the factors that cause pain in the muscles may be different in different muscles and may change from one time to another. Elert et al. found that a subgroup of patients with FMS had an insufficient relaxation between contractions (45). It is possible that some patients with chronic muscle pain have a disturbed contraction-relaxation cycle. The reduced muscle strength and endurance found in patients with FMS is likely not of muscular origin. Inhibition of activation of motor units due to pain is a more plausible explanation.

In conclusion, the changes in muscle that could excite intramuscular nociceptors are not likely specific to FMS, but they could be of importance for maintaining pain and allodynia both in chronic localized muscle pain and in FMS. The muscle changes may be of particular importance in the group of patients with FMS where there is a gradual transition from localized to widespread pain.

CONCLUDING REMARKS

There is strong support for the notion that pain and allodynia/hyperalgesia in FMS have an organic cause. The hyperexcitability in the nociceptive nervous system is mainly due to changes in the CNS. Longstanding excitation of nociceptors and low threshold mechano-receptors in the muscle may initiate and maintain such hyperexcitability. The permanent changes constitute a disease. There are methods for objectively diagnosing this disease.

The psychological and social consequences of chronic pain in FMS are the main determinants for the degree of disability and handicap.

Many causes could initiate and maintain the disease: e.g., longstanding local or regional musculoskeletal pain, changes in stress-regulating systems, hormonal changes, changes in serotonin metabolisms, and genetic factors.

REFERENCES

1. Wolfe F, Smythe HA, Yunus MB, Bennett RM, Bombardier C, Goldenberg DL, Tugwell P, Campbell SM, Abeles M, Clark P, Fam AG, Farber SJ, Fiechtner JJ, Franklin CM, Gatter RA, Hamaty D, Lessard J, Lichtbroun AS, Masi AT, McCain GA, Reynolds WJ, Romano TJ, Russell IJ, Sheon RP: The American College of Rheuma-

tology 1990 criteria for the classification of fibromyalgia: Report of the Multicenter Criteria Committee. Arthritis Rheum 22: 160-172, 1990.

2. Sörensen J, Bengtsson A, Bäckman E, Henriksson KG, Bengtsson M: Pain analysis in patients with fibromyalgia. Effects of intravenous morphine, lidocaine and ketamine. Scand J Rheumatol 24: 360-365, 1995.

3. Sörensen J, Bengtsson A, Ahlner J, Henriksson KG, Ekselius L: Fibromyalgia–Are there different mechanisms in the processing of pain? J Rheumatology 24: 1615-1621, 1997.

4. Sörenson J, Graven-Nielsen T, Henriksson KG, Bengtsson M, Arendt-Nielsen L: Hyperexcitability in fibromyalgia. J Rheumatology 25: 152-155, 1998.

5. Graven-Nielsen T, Aspegren Kendall S, Henriksson KG, Bengtsson M, Sorensen J, Johnson A, Gerdle B, Arendt-Nielsen L: Ketamine reduces muscle pain, temporal summation, and referred pain in fibromyalgia patients. Pain 85: 483-491, 2000.

6. Staud R, Vierck CJ, Cannon RL, Mauderli AP, Price DD: Abnormal sensitization and temporal summation of second pain (wind-up) in patients with fibromyalgia syndrome. Pain 91: 165-175, 2001.

7. Arroyo JF, Cohen ML: Abnormal responses to electrocutaneous stimulation in fibromyalgia. J Rheumatol 20: 1925-1931, 1993.

8. Vecchiet L, Giamberardino MA, de Bigontina P, et al.: Comparative sensory evaluation of parietal tissues in painful and nonpainful areas in fibromyalgia and myofascial pain syndrome. Progress in Pain Research and Management. Eds.: GF Gebhart, DL Hammond and TS Jensen, IASP Press, Seattle, 1994, 2: pp 177-185.

9. Yu XM, Mense S: Response properties and descending control of rat dorsal horn neurons with deep receptive fields. Neuroscience 39: 823-831, 1990.

10. Bendtsen L, Norregaard J, Jensen R, Olesen J: Evidence of qualitatively altered nociception in patients with fibromyalgia. Arthritis Rheum 40(1): 98-102, 1997.

11. Gibson SJ, Littlejohn GO, Gorman MM, Helme RD, Granges G: Altered heat pain thresholds and cerebral event-related potentials following painful CO_2 laser stimulation in subjects with fibromyalgia syndrome. Pain 58: 185-193, 1994.

12. Lorentz J, Grasedck K, Bromm B: Middle and long latency somatosensory evoked potentials after painful laser stimulation in patients with fibromyalgia syndrome. Electroencephalography & Clin Neurophysiol 100: 165-168, 1996.

13. Kosek E, Ekholm J, Hansson P: Modulation of pressure pain thresholds during and following isometric contraction in patients with fibromyalgia and in healthy controls. Pain 64: 415-423, 1996.

14. Kosek E, Hansson P: Modulatory influence on somatosensory perception from vibration and heterotopic noxious conditioning stimulation [HNCS] in fibromyalgia patients and healthy subjects. Pain 70: 41-51, 1997.

15. Mountz JM, Bradley LA, Modell JG, Alexander RW, Triana-Alexander M, Aaron LA, Stewart KE, Alarcon GS, Mountz JD: Fibromyalgia in women. Abnormalities of regional cerebral blood flow in the thalamus and the caudate nucleus are associated with low pain threshold levels. Arthritis Rheum 38(7): 926-938, 1995.

16. Bradley LA, McKendree-Smith NL, Alberts KR, Alarcon GS, Mountz JM, Deutsch G: Use of neuroimaging to understand abnormal pain sensitivity in fibromyalgia. Current Rheumatology Reports 2: 141-148, 2000.

17. Russell IJ, Orr MD, Littman B Vipraio GA, Alboukrek D, Michalek JE, Lopez Y, MacKillip F: Elevated cerebrospinal fluid levels of substance P in patients with the fibromyalgia syndrome. Arthritis Rheum 37: 1593-1601, 1994.

18. Lindh C, Liu Z, Lyrenäs S, Ordeberg G, Nyberg F: Elevated cerebrospinal fluid substance P-like immunoreactivity in patients with painful osteoarthritis, but not in patients with rhizopatic pain from a herniated lumbar disc. Scand J Rheumatol, 1997.

19. Kosek E, Ordeberg G: Abnormalities of somatosensory perception in patients with painful osteoarthritis normalize following successful treatment. European J Pain 4: 229-238, 2000.

20. Kosek E, Ordeberg G: Lack of pressure pain modulation by heterotopic noxious conditioning stimulation in patients with painful osteoarthritis before, but not following, surgical pain relief. Pain 88: 69-78, 2000.

21. Buskila D, Neumann L, Hazanov I: Familiar aggregation in fibromyalgia syndrome. Semin Arthritis Rheum 26: 605, 1996.

22. Offenbaecher M, Bondy B. de Jonge S, Glatzeder K, Kruger M, Schoeps P, Ackenheil M: Possible association of fibromyalgia with a polymorphism in the serotonin transporter gene regulatory region. Arhritis Rheum 42: 2482-2488, 1999.

23. Ekselius L, Bengtsson A, von Knorring L: Personality traits as determined by means of the Karolinska Scales of Personality in patients with fibromyalgia. J Musculoske Pain 6(2): 35-49, 1998.

24. Keogh E, Mansoor L: Investigating the effects of anxiety sensitivity and coping on the perception of cold pressor pain in healthy women. European J Pain 5: 11-25, 2001.

25. Pillemer SR, Bradley LA, Crofford LJ, Moldofsky H, Chrousos GP: The neuroscience and endocrinology of fibromyalgia. Arthritis Rheum 40: 1928-1939, 1997.

26. Russell IJ, Vipraio GA: Serotonin [5HT] in serum and platelets [PLT] from fibromyalgia patients [FS] and normal controls [NC]. Arthritis Rheum 37 (suppl): S214, 1994.

27. Russell IJ: Neurochemical pathogenesis of fibromyalgia syndrome. J Musculoske Pain 7 (1/2): 183-191, 1999.

28. Ernberg M, Hedenberg-Magnusson B, Alstergren P, Kopp S: The level of serotonin in the superficial masseter muscle in relation to local pain and allodynia. Life Sci 65: 313-325, 1999.

29. Blomqvist A: Sex hormones and pain: A new role for brain aromatase? J Comparative neurology 423: 549-551, 2000.

30. Samad TA, Moore KA, Sapirstein A, Billet S, Allchorne A, Poole S, Bonventre JV, Woolf CJ: Interleukin-1β-mediated induction of Cox-2 in the CNS contributes to inflammatory pain hypersensitivity. Nature 410: 471-475, 2001.

31. Ek M, Engblom D, Saha S, Blomqvist A, Jakobsson PJ, Ericsson-Dahlstrand A: Pathway across the blood-brain barrier. Nature 410: 430-431, 2001.

32. Watkins LR, Maier SF, Goehler LE: Immune activation: the role of pro-inflammatory cytokines in inflammation, illness responses and pathological pain states. Pain 63: 289-302, 1995.

33. Roth SM, Martel GF, Rogers MA: Muscle biopsy and muscle fiber hypercontraction: a brief review. Eur J Appl Physiol 83: 239-245, 2000.

34. Eneström S, Bengtsson A, Frödin T: Dermal IgG deposits and increase of mast cells in patients with fibromyalgia–relevant findings or epiphenomena? Scand J Rheumatol 26: 308-313, 1997.

35. Bengtsson M, Bengtsson A, Jorfeldt L: Diagnostic epidural opioid blockade in primary fibromyalgia at rest and during exercise. Pain 39:171-180, 1989.

36. Bengtsson A, Henriksson KG, Jorfeldt L, Kagedal B, Lennmarken C, Lindstrom F: Primary fibromyalgia. A clinical and laboratory study of 55 patients. Scand J Rheumatol 15: 340-347, 1986.

37. Lápossy E, Maleitzke R, Hrycaj P, Mennet W, Muller W: The frequency of transition of chronic low back pain to fibromyalgia. Scand J Rheumatol 24: 29-53, 1995.

38. Buskila D, Neumann L, Vaisberg G, Alkalay D, Wolfe F: Increased rates of fibromyalgia following cervical injury. A controlled study of 161 cases of traumatic injury. Arthritis Rheum 29: 817-821, 1986.

39. Mense S: Nociception from skeletal muscle in relation to clinical muscle pain. Pain 54: 241-289, 1993.

40. Lund N, Bengtsson A, Thorborg P: Muscle tissue oxygen pressure in primary fibromyalgia. Scand J Rheumatol 15: 165-173, 1986.

41. Lindman R, Hagberg M, Bengtsson A, Soderlund K, Hultman E, Thornell LE: Capillary structure and mitochondrial volume density in the trapezius muscle of chronic trapezius myalgia, fibromyalgia and healthy subjects. J Musculoske Pain 3: 5-22, 1995.

42. Bengtsson A, Henriksson KG, Larsson J: Reduced high-energy phosphate levels in the painful muscles of patients with primary fibromyalgia. Arthritis Rheum 29: 817-821, 1986.

43. Simms RW, Ray SH, Hrovat M, Anderson JJ, Kimmels A, Zerbini CF, DeLuca C, Jolesz F: Lack of association between fibromyalgia syndrome and abnormalities in muscle energy metabolism. Arthritis Rheum 37: 794-800, 1994.

44. Park JH, Phothimat P, Oates CO, Hernanz-Schulman M, Olsen NJ: Use of P-31 magnetic resonance spectroscopy to detect metabolic abnormalities in muscles of patients with fibromyalgia. Arthritis Rheum 41(3): 406-413, 1998.

45. Elert J, Kendall SA, Larsson B, Mansson B, Gerdle B: Chronic pain and difficulty in relaxing postural muscles in patients with fibromyalgia and chronic whiplash associated disorders. J Rheumatol 28: 1361-1368, 2001.

Imaging Pain in the Brain:
The Role of the Cerebral Cortex
in Pain Perception and Modulation

M. Catherine Bushnell
Chantal Villemure
Irina Strigo
Gary H. Duncan

SUMMARY. Objectives: This review examines data from human neuro-imaging studies, in an effort to better understand the neural basis of the conscious appreciation of pain. Included is evidence from experimental studies of normal pain processing and pain modulation by psychological state. Also reviewed is evidence from studies of patients with chronic pain syndromes, such as neuropathic pain, central pain, and fibromyalgia, that may involve aberrant forebrain processing of nociceptive information.

M. Catherine Bushnell, PhD, is Harold Griffith Professor, Departments of Anesthesia and Physiology, McGill University, Montreal, Quebec, Canada.

Chantal Villemure, PhD, is Postdoctoral Fellow, Department of Anesthesia, McGill University, Montreal, Quebec, Canada.

Irina Strigo, BSc, is Graduate Student, Department of Physiology, McGill University, Montreal, Quebec, Canada.

Gary H. Duncan, DDS, PhD, is Professor Titulaire, McConnell Brain Imaging Centre, McGill University, Montreal, Quebec, Canada.

Address correspondence to: M. Catherine Bushnell, PhD, Anesthesia Research Unit, McGill University, 3655 Promenade Sir William Osler, Room 1220, Montreal, Quebec, Canada H3G 1Y6 [E-mail: catherine.bushnell@mcgill.ca].

[Haworth co-indexing entry note]: "Imaging Pain in the Brain: The Role of the Cerebral Cortex in Pain Perception and Modulation." Bushnell, M. Catherine et al. Co-published simultaneously in *Journal of Musculoskeletal Pain* [The Haworth Medical Press, an imprint of The Haworth Press, Inc.] Vol. 10, No. 1/2, 2002, pp. 59-72; and: *The Clinical Neurobiology of Fibromyalgia and Myofascial Pain: Therapeutic Implications* [ed: Robert M. Bennett] The Haworth Medical Press, an imprint of The Haworth Press, Inc., 2002, pp. 59-72. Single or multiple copies of this article are available for a fee from The Haworth Document Delivery Service [1-800-HAWORTH, 9:00 a.m. - 5:00 p.m. (EST). E-mail address: getinfo@haworthpressinc.com].

59

Findings: Both positron emission tomography and functional magnetic resonance imaging studies of experimental pain in normal subjects reveal a complex network of neural activity in the cerebral cortex that likely underlies the conscious appreciation of pain. The totality of sensory and emotional experience associated with pain varies among individuals and circumstances, and these dissimilarities are reflected in variations in patterns of neural activation observed among studies. However, striking commonalities are observed among studies, including the activation of sensory regions, such as primary and secondary somatosensory cortices and limbic areas such as anterior cingulate cortex and insular cortex. Studies of cognitive modulation of pain show that the degree of activation of these regions is dependent on cognitive factors, such as attentional state, that alter our perception of pain. Finally, imaging studies of patients with chronic pain states often reveal abnormalities of pain processing that result in the "cortical pain network" being activated by normally nonpainful stimuli, thus providing a neural basis for perceptual phenomena such as allodynia and hyperalgesia.

Conclusions: There is a common network of cortical and subcortical structures that subserves the pain experience. Whether this network is activated by tissue-damaging stimuli in a "normal" situation, or by non-noxious stimuli such as a light brush or cool breeze on the skin in pathological conditions, the final experience associated with its activation is pain. Finally, activity in this network can be modulated by cognitive state, as well as by pharmacological treatments, leading to an alteration of the pain experience. *[Article copies available for a fee from The Haworth Document Delivery Service: 1-800-HAWORTH. E-mail address: <getinfo@haworthpressinc.com> Website: <http://www.HaworthPress.com> © 2002 by The Haworth Press, Inc. All rights reserved.]*

KEYWORDS. Brain imaging, pain perception, neuropathic pain, fibromyalgia

Pain is a psychological term used to describe a subjective experience. Pain is sometimes experienced in the absence of the stimulation of nociceptors. One example of this is central pain, in which damage to the brain or the spinal cord can lead to excruciating pain, although nociceptors are not being activated. Another example that does not involve neural damage is the "thermal grill illusion." When people place their hands on an interlaced pattern of warm and cool metal they usually feel a burning pain sensation, although no potential tissue-damaging stimulus is presented (1,2).

NEUROPHYSIOLOGICAL MECHANISMS UNDERLYING THE CONSCIOUS APPRECIATION OF PAIN

Until recent years, there has been little consensus about the neural circuitry underlying the perception of pain. Although it is now generally believed that the cerebral cortex is most likely the site of the conscious perception of pain, this idea has not always been accepted. Early this century, Beecher and others observed that soldiers who had extensive injuries of the cerebral cortex continued to perceive pain, leading them to conclude that the cortex played only a minimal role in pain perception (3). Nevertheless, despite these observations, we now have anatomical and physiological evidence that information about pain reaches a number of cortical areas. Recent studies of the human brain, using positron emission tomography [PET] to measure the relative cerebral blood flow [rCBF] and functional magnetic resonance imaging [fMRI] to measure changes in blood oxygenation, now reveal that a number of cortical regions are activated during pain. Human brain imaging studies show that even during a brief tolerable pain, such as that produced by touching the skin with a hot metal plaque, a number of cortical and subcortical brain regions are activated (4-8), including the primary and secondary somatosensory cortices [S1 and S2], the anterior cingulate cortex [ACC], and the insular cortex [IC]. Figure 1 shows fMRI scans revealing activation of these four cortical areas by a noxious heat stimulus presented to an individual's leg.

Researchers have demonstrated cerebral blood flow changes related to a number of different painful stimuli, including painful cooling of the skin (8,10), the application of irritating chemicals such as capsaicin (11,12), electrical stimulation of muscles (13), and distension of visceral tissue, including the rectum and esophagus (14-16). Although some differences are found among studies, S1, S2, ACC and IC are activated by most painful stimuli. The consistent activation of these brain regions during painful stimulation shows that they are important for producing the experience of pain.

Although other cortical regions, including parts of prefrontal cortex and premotor areas such as the supplemental motor cortex, are activated in some pain studies (6,10,17), these responses are less reliable, suggesting that their activation may not be directly related to the essential pain experience. Neurophysiological and anatomical studies further support a direct role of S1, S2, ACC, and IC in pain perception. Data from anesthetized animals reveal neurons in each of these regions that respond best when noxious stimuli, such as pinching or heating the skin,

FIGURE 1. Functional and anatomical magnetic resonance imaging of a single subject exposed to a 46°C noxious heat stimulus on the left leg. Ten nine-sec noxious heat stimuli and 10 nine-sec neutral warm stimuli [36°C] were presented sequentially with nine-sec interstimulus intervals. The circled color-coded areas represent regions with significantly greater activation during the noxious heat than during the warm stimuli [Spearman's rank order correlation]. In this subject and others, there was significant pain-related activation in [1A] primary somatosensory cortex [S1], [1B] secondary somatosensory cortex [S2], anterior insular cortex [IC], and cingulate cortex [ACC]. Panels 1A and 1C show coronal slices [right side of brain depicted on right], and panel 1B shows a sagittal slice. Adapted from Bushnell et al. (9).

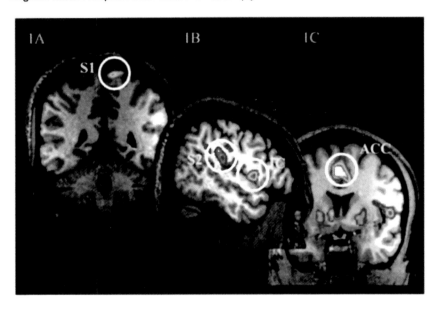

are presented (18-21). Similar nociceptive neurons have been recorded in the ACC of awake human subjects undergoing neurosurgical procedures (22).

The fact that several parts of the brain are activated when a person feels pain reflects the complex nature of the experience. Pain perception has been classified into sensory-discriminative, affective-motivational, and autonomic components (23). The sensory-discriminative component of pain includes the sensation a person feels, such as burning, pricking, or aching, as well as the localization of that sensation to a specific part of the body. In addition, there are emotional [affective] and behavioral [motivational] reactions to pain, both of which can vary during different circumstances. Autonomic responses, such as increased heart rate, blood pressure, and sweating, can occur when a person experiences pain. The IC may be important for affective responses to pain by integrating the sensory information with memories of previous pain. The ACC is probably involved in affective, behavioral and/or autonomic reactions to pain, and S1 and S2 cortices may be most important for pain sensations. However, these brain regions are anatomically connected, and discrete damage to any one region does not produce a precise, permanent deficit in pain perception. Chronic pain may be temporarily alleviated by lesions to discrete cortical regions, but usually the pain returns after several months. These observations suggest that pain is processed by complex brain networks. Further, the resilience of chronic pain may involve a plasticity in pain pathways, whereby functions usually performed by one region are taken over by another. Such redundancy and resiliency are of obvious evolutionary value, since nociception is essential for survival.

NEURAL BASIS OF ABERRANT PAIN PROCESSING

Brain imaging studies now allow us to ask questions about pain that is experienced without actually stimulating pain receptors in the skin or other tissues of the body. Is central pain real or imaginary? Does the pain of fibromyalgia have a neurophysiological basis? Is the "illusion" of pain produced by the thermal grill "real"? Human brain imaging studies show that there is a real neurophysiological basis for these aberrant types of pain. For example, PET studies reveal that when people experience the thermal grill pain illusion, produced by stimulating the skin with an alternating grid of warm and cool bars, regions of the cerebral cortex normally activated by noxious stimulation are activated during the "illusion" of pain (2).

Several investigators have used PET in patients with peripheral neuropathic pain or central pain to determine changes in pain processing that could account for such symptoms as ongoing pain, hyperalgesia, and allodynia. Possibly because of the difficulties of applying PET to small heterogeneous populations of patients, or possibly because of differential pathologies, no consistent effects have emerged. In examining patients with peripheral neuropathic pain, one group found a unilateral decrease in thalamic activity (24), and another group found increases in blood flow to a number of pain-related cortical regions, including ACC and IC (25). In studying patients with central pain, one imaging study associated the pain with hyperexcitability in the thalamus (26) and another with hyperexcitability in the cerebral cortex (27).

Some data suggest that allodynia, whether related to neuropathic pain or capsaicin application, is processed differently in the cerebral cortex than is nociceptive pain. Whereas the ACC is almost always activated in PET or fMRI studies of nociceptive pain, Peyron et al. (28, 29) failed to find ACC activation during allodynia in central pain patients. Similarly, Baron et al. (12) also did not observe ACC activation when examining dynamic tactile allodynia during a capsaicin model in normal subjects and suggested that Aβ-mediated pain has a unique cortical presentation. Nevertheless, other data do not support this interpretation, but rather suggest that pain arising from aberrant or normal processes ultimately activates the same cortical structures. For example, Iadarola et al. (11) reported ACC activation during dynamic tactile allodynia after capsaicin injection in normal subjects, and Craig et al. (2) found ACC activation during the thermal grill pain illusion, an experimental model for central pain [see above]. Further, results from a patient studied in our laboratory indicate that tactile allodynia associated with central pain does in some cases activate normal cortical pain-processing regions, including ACC, prefrontal cortex [PFC] and S2 (30) [Figure 2].

Fibromyalgia is a chronic pain syndrome characterized by widespread spontaneous pain, lowered pain thresholds, and muscle stiffness, in addition to other symptoms (31). At least two studies have examined neural changes related to fibromyalgia. Using single photon emission tomography, Kwiatek et al. (32) found a reduction in thalamic rCBF, consistent with brain imaging findings of other chronic pain conditions. They also observed a reduced pontine tegmental activation, which has not been observed in other conditions and the significance of which is not known. Lekander et al. (33) correlated PET blood flow measures with immune function in five fibromyalgia patients and found that natural killer cell activity correlated negatively with neural activity in S2, motor cotices, thalamus, and posterior cingulate cortex, suggesting a possible role of immune dysfunction in the pain of fibromyalgia.

ROLE OF CEREBRAL CORTEX IN COGNITIVE MODULATION OF PAIN PERCEPTION

Several lines of evidence show a role of the cerebral cortex in pain modulation. For example, direct stimulation of the motor cortex has

FIGURE 2. Functional magnetic resonance imaging during painful tactile stimulation in a hemispherectomized patient. Nine-sec periods of brushing the skin [2 Hz] were alternated with nine-sec rest periods. The circled color-coded areas represent regions with significantly greater activation during brushing than during rest. Whereas brushing the right hand [contralateral to the intact hemisphere] produced normal tactile sensation and activated the primary somatosensory cortex and the secondary somatosensory cortex [not shown], brushing the left hand produced burning pain and additional activation of limbic pain-related areas, including the anterior cingulate cortex [red circles] and medial prefrontal cortex [blue circle]. Adapted from Olausson et al. (30).

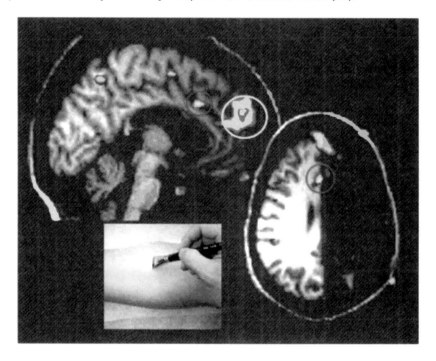

been shown to reduce chronic intractable pain (34-36). In addition, evidence suggests that some of the pain-relieving effects of opiates may involve cortical receptor sites (37,38). Finally, both clinical and experimental studies show that psychological factors can alter pain perception. This review will examine evidence from imaging studies showing the involvement of cerebral cortex in cognitive modulation of pain.

Both clinical and experimental evidence shows that an individual's psychological state alters pain perception. Many studies have shown that cognitive manipulations, such as hypnosis, behavioral modification, relaxation training, biofeedback, operant conditioning, and cognitive-behavioural therapy, can change a person's experience of pain. One simple variable that is common to many of these psychological procedures is the attentional state. Experimental studies show that people report lower pain when they are distracted from the pain (39-42).

Other cognitive manipulations that do not necessarily involve distraction can also alter pain. Hypnosis has been used as a cognitive intervention to produce analgesia in a variety of settings, including dental treatments, such as third molar extraction (43). Experimental studies of hypnotic analgesia show that not only does hypnosis reduce pain, but that different hypnotic suggestions can be used to reduce independently the perceived intensity of a painful stimulus [sensory dimension] and its perceived unpleasantness [affective dimension] (44,45).

What is the physiological basis of cognitive modulation of pain? Human brain imaging studies reveal that there is a clear neurophysiological basis for psychological modulation of pain. When attention is directed away from a painful heat stimulus presented on a person's arm, his evaluation of the intensity of the pain is decreased, and the activity of SI cortex elicited by the painful stimulus is dramatically reduced (46). Other studies have found attention-related modulation of pain in other pain processing areas, such as thalamus, ACC, and IC (47-49). These findings are consistent with other evidence that the afferent nociceptive signals are reduced by a cognitively activated descending control system in the brain. When subjects report less pain while distracted, they have not just learned to ignore the pain signal; the pain signal reaching the cortex has been diminished by the subject's attentional state, just as it can be diminished by pharmacological analgesic treatments.

Other imaging data show that hypnotic suggestions alter pain-evoked cortical activity and that this alteration depends on the nature of the hypnotic suggestions (44,45). Hypnotic suggestions can be given that reduce how much a painful stimulus bothers the person [i.e., the unpleasantness], while the person still feels the burning sensations. Figure 3 shows that when subjects are given such suggestions, activity in the ACC is reduced, but activity in SI is not. However, when the subjects are given suggestions to reduce the intensity of the burning pain sensation, SI activity is dramatically reduced, just as it is when subjects are distracted.

There is also evidence confirming that cognitive factors other than attention or hypnotic suggestion, such as mood, emotional state, attitudes, and expectations, can alter pain perception. Clinical studies show

FIGURE 3. Modulation of pain by hypnotic suggestions. Changes in pain-related activity associated with hypnotic suggestions of high [left images] and low [right] pain intensity [A] and pain unpleasantness [B]. Suggestions for increased or decreased pain intensity preferentially altered pain-evoked activity in the primary somatosensory cortex [A], whereas suggestions for increased or decreased pain unpleasantness preferentially altered pain-evoked activity in the anterior cingulate cortex [B]. Data from positron emission tomography were recorded when the subject's hand was submerged in thermally neutral water [35°C] or in painfully hot [47°C] water during hypnotic suggestions of high or low pain intensity or unpleasantness. Adapted from Hofbauer et al. (45) [part A] and Rainville et al. (44) [part B].

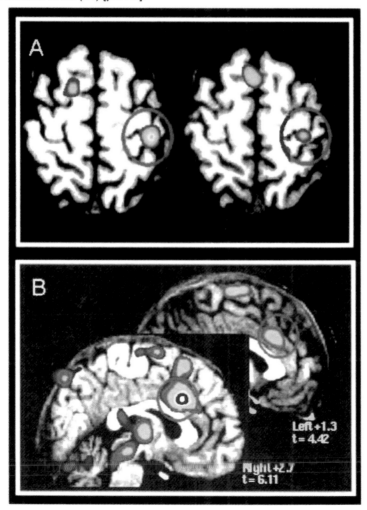

that emotional states and attitudes of patients have an effect on post-surgical analgesic requirements (50) and pain associated with chronic diseases (51-54). In the experimental context, manipulations that alter mood or emotional state, such as pleasant music or humorous films, reduce pain perception (55-58). Nevertheless, such studies do not clearly dissociate changes in mood from changes in attention, anxiety, or relaxation. Further, the neural circuitry underlying such pain modulation is not known. The findings from the hypnosis studies described above suggest that ACC might be an important region for hedonic modulation of pain. Further, a recent study revealed a region in the PFC that is activated by stimuli with either positive or negative hedonic value, independent of stimulus modality (59). This region is also sometimes activated by pain (10,25,30,60), so that it may possibly be important for hedonic alterations in pain states.

In conclusion, there appears to be a common network of cortical and subcortical structures, the activation of which may underlie the pain experience. Whether this network is activated by acute noxious stimuli in an experimental setting, or by stimuli such as gentle stroking or a cool breeze on the skin in clinical conditions of aberrant pain processing, the final experience associated with its activation is pain. Moreover, activity in this network can be modulated by changes in cognitive state, as well as by pharmacological treatments, resulting in an alteration of the pain experience.

REFERENCES

1. Craig AD, Bushnell MC: The thermal grill illusion: Unmasking the burn of cold pain. Science 265:252-255, 1994.

2. Craig AD, Reiman EM, Evans AC, Bushnell MC: Functional imaging of an illusion of pain. Nature 384:258-260, 1996.

3. Beecher HK: Pain in men wounded in battle. Ann Surg 123:96-105, 1946.

4. Talbot JD, Marrett S, Evans AC, Meyer E, Bushnell MC, Duncan GH: Multiple representations of pain in human cerebral cortex. Science 251:1355-1358, 1991.

5. Jones AKP, Brown WD, Friston KJ, Qi LY, Frackowiak RSJ: Cortical and subcortical localization of response to pain in man using positron emission tomography. Proc R Soc Lond [Biol] 244:39-44, 1991.

6. Coghill RC, Talbot JD, Evans AC, Meyer E, Gjedde A, Bushnell MC, Duncan GH: Distributed processing of pain and vibration by the human brain. J Neurosci 14:4095-4108, 1994.

7. Derbyshire SW, Jones AK, Devani P, Friston KJ, Feinmann C, Harris M, Pearce S, Watson JD, Frackowiak RS: Cerebral responses to pain in patients with atypical fa-

cial pain measured by positron emission tomography. J Neurol Neurosurg Psychiatry 57:1166-1172, 1994.

8. Casey KL, Minoshima S, Morrow TJ, Koeppe RA: Comparison of human cerebral activation patterns during cutaneous warmth, heat pain, and deep cold pain. J Neurophysiol 76:571-581, 1996.

9. Bushnell MC, Duncan GH, Ha B, Chen J-I, Olausson H: Non-invasive brain imaging during experimental and clinical pain. Proceedings of the 9th World Congress in Pain Research and Management, Vol. 16, Edited by M Devor, MC Rowbotham, Z Wiesenfeld-Hallin. IASP Press, 2000, pp. 485-495.

10. Craig AD, Chen K, Bandy D, Reiman EM: Thermosensory activation of insular cortex. Nat Neurosci 3:184-190, 2000.

11. Iadarola MJ, Berman KF, Zeffiro TA, Byas-Smith MG, Gracely RH, Max MB, Bennett GJ: Neural activation during acute capsaicin-evoked pain and allodynia assessed with PET. Brain 121 (Pt 5):931-947, 1998.

12. Baron R, Baron Y, Disbrow E, Roberts TP: Brain processing of capsaicin-induced secondary hyperalgesia: a functional MRI study. Neurology 53:548-557, 1999.

13. Svensson P, Minoshima S, Beydoun A, Morrow TJ, Casey KL: Cerebral processing of acute skin and muscle pain in humans. J Neurophysiol 78:450-460, 1997.

14. Silverman DH, Munakata JA, Ennes H, Mandelkern MA, Hoh CK, Mayer EA: Regional cerebral activity in normal and pathological perception of visceral pain. Gastroenterology 112:64-72, 1997.

15. Aziz Q, Andersson JL, Valind S, Sundin A, Hamdy S, Jones AK, Foster ER, Langstrom B, Thompson DG: Identification of human brain loci processing esophageal sensation using positron emission tomography. Gastroenterology 113:50-59, 1997.

16. Binkofski F, Schnitzler A, Enck P, Frieling T, Posse S, Seitz RJ, Freund HJ: Somatic and limbic cortex activation in esophageal distention: a functional magnetic resonance imaging study. Ann Neurol 44:811-815, 1998.

17. Derbyshire SW: Exploring the pain "neuromatrix." Curr Rev Pain 4:467-477, 2000.

18. Sikes RW, Vogt BA: Nociceptive neurons in area 24 of rabbit cingulate cortex. J Neurophysiol 68:1720-1732, 1992.

19. Dong WK, Salonen LD, Kawakami Y, Shiwaku T, Kaukoranta EM, Martin RF: Nociceptive responses of trigeminal neurons in SII-7b cortex of awake monkeys. Brain Res 484:314-324, 1989.

20. Kenshalo DR, Jr., Isensee O: Responses of primate SI cortical neurons to noxious stimuli. J Neurophysiol 50:1479-1496, 1983.

21. Burkey AR, Carstens E, Wenniger JJ, Tang JW, Jasmin L: An opioidergic cortical antinociception triggering site in the agranular insular cortex of the rat that contributes to morphine antinociception. Journal of Neuroscience 16:6612-6623, 1996.

22. Hutchison WD, Davis KD, Lozano AM, Tasker RR, Dostrovsky JO: Pain-related neurons in the human cingulate cortex. Nat Neurosci 2:403-405, 1999.

23. Melzack R, Casey KL: Sensory, motivational and central control determinants of pain: a new conceptual model. The Skin Senses. Edited by DR Kenshalo. Springfield, IL, 1968, pp. 423-443.

24. Iadarola MJ, Max MB, Berman KF, Byas-Smith MG, Coghill RC, Gracely RH, Bennett GJ: Unilateral decrease in thalamic activity observed with positron emission tomography in patients with chronic neuropathic pain. Pain 63:55-64, 1995.

25. Hsieh JC, Belfrage M, Stone-Elander S, Hansson P, Ingvar M: Central representation of chronic ongoing neuropathic pain studied positron emission tomography. Pain 63:225-236, 1995.

26. Cesaro P, Mann MW, Moretti JL, Defer G, Roualdès B, Nguyen JP, Degos JD: Central pain and thalamic hyperactivity: a single photon emission computerized tomographic study. Pain 47:329-336, 1991.

27. Canavero S, Pagni CA, Castellano G, Bonicalzi V, Bello' M, Duca S, Podio V: The role of cortex in central pain syndromes: preliminary results of a long-term technetium-99 hexamethylpropyleneamineoxime single photon emission computed tomography study. Neurosurgery 32:185-191, 1993.

28. Peyron R, Garcia-Larrea L, Gregoire MC, Convers P, Lavenne F, Veyre L, Froment JC, Mauguiere F, Michel D, Laurent B: Allodynia after lateral-medullary (Wallenberg) infarct. A PET study. Brain 121 (Pt 2):345-356, 1998.

29. Peyron R, Garcia-Larrea L, Gregoire MC, Convers P, Richard A, Lavenne F, Barral FG, Mauguiere F, Michel D, Laurent B: Parietal and cingulate processes in central pain. A combined positron emission tomography (PET) and functional magnetic resonance imaging (fMRI) study of an unusual case. Pain 84:77-87, 2000.

30. Olausson H, Marchand S, Bittar RG, Bernier J, Ptito A, Bushnell MC: Central pain in a hemispherectomized patient. Eur J Pain 5:209-218, 2001.

31. Wolfe F, Ross K, Anderson J, Russell IJ, Hebert L: The prevalence and characteristics of fibromyalgia in the general population. Arthritis Rheum 38:19-28, 1995.

32. Kwiatek R, Barnden L, Tedman R, Jarrett R, Chew J, Rowe C, Pile K: Regional cerebral blood flow in fibromyalgia: single-photon-emission computed tomography evidence of reduction in the pontine tegmentum and thalami. Arthritis Rheum 43: 2823-2833, 2000.

33. Lekander M, Fredrikson M, Wik G: Neuroimmune relations in patients with fibromyalgia: a positron emission tomography study. Neurosci Lett 282:193-196, 2000.

34. Katayama Y, Tsubokawa T, Yamamoto T: Chronic motor cortex stimulation for central deafferentation pain: experience with bulbar pain secondary to Wallenberg syndrome. Stereotact Funct Neurosurg 62:295-299, 1994.

35. Peyron R, Garcia-Larrea L, Deiber MP, Cinotti L, Convers P, Sindou M, Mauguière F, Laurent B: Electrical stimulation of precentral cortical area in the treatment of central pain: electrophysiological and PET study. Pain 62:275-286, 1995.

36. Katayama Y, Fukaya C, Yamamoto T: Poststroke pain control by chronic motor cortex stimulation: neurological characteristics predicting a favorable response. J Neurosurg 89:585-591, 1998.

37. Casey KL, Svensson P, Morrow TJ, Raz J, Jone C, Minoshima S: Selective opiate modulation of nociceptive processing in the human brain. J Neurophysiol 84: 525-533, 2000.

38. Zubieta JK, Smith YR, Bueller JA, Xu Y, Kilbourn MR, Jewett DM, Meyer CR, Koeppe RA, Stohler CS: Regional mu opioid receptor regulation of sensory and affective dimensions of pain. Science 293:311-315, 2001.

39. Miron D, Duncan GH, Bushnell MC: Effects of attention on the intensity and unpleasantness of thermal pain. Pain 39:345-352, 1989.

40. Leventhal H, Brown D, Shacham S, Engquist G: Effects of preparatory information about sensations, threat of pain, and attention on cold pressor distress. J Pers Soc Psychol 37:688-714, 1979.

41. Levine JD, Gordon NC, Smith R, Fields HL: Post-operative pain: effect of extent of injury and attention. Brain Res 234:500-504, 1982.

42. McCaul KD, Haugtvedt C: Attention, distraction, and cold-pressor pain. J Pers Soc Psychol 43:154-162, 1982.

43. Enqvist B, Fischer K: Preoperative hypnotic techniques reduce consumption of analgesics after surgical removal of third mandibular molars: a brief communication. Int J Exp Hypn 45:102-108, 1997.

44. Rainville P, Duncan GH, Price DD, Carrier B, Bushnell MC: Pain affect encoded in human anterior cingulate but not somatosensory cortex. Science 277:968-971, 1997.

45. Hofbauer RK, Rainville P, Duncan GH, Bushnell MC: Cortical representation of the sensory dimension of pain. J Neurophysiol 86:402-411, 2001.

46. Bushnell MC, Duncan GH, Hofbauer RK, Ha B, Chen J, Carrier B: Pain perception: is there a role for primary somatosensory cortex? Proc Natl Acad Sci USA 96:7705-7709, 1999.

47. Longe SE, Wise R, Bantick S, Lloyd D, Johansen-Berg H, McGlone F, Tracey I: Counter-stimulatory effects on pain perception and processing are significantly altered by attention: an fMRI study. NeuroReport 12:2021-2025, 2001.

48. Petrovic P, Petersson KM, Ghatan PH, Stone-Elander S, Ingvar M: Pain-related cerebral activation is altered by a distracting cognitive task. Pain 85:19-30, 2000.

49. Peyron R, Garcia-Larrea L, Gregoire MC, Costes N, Convers P, Lavenne F, Mauquire F, Michel D, Laurent B: Haemodynamic brain responses to acute pain in humans: sensory and attentional networks. Brain 122:1765-1780, 1999.

50. Yang JC, Clark WC, Tsui SL, Ng KF, Clark SB: Preoperative Multidimensional Affect and Pain Survey (MAPS) scores predict postcolectomy analgesia requirement. Clin J Pain 16:314-320, 2000.

51. Schanberg LE, Sandstrom MJ, Starr K, Gil KM, Lefebvre JC, Keefe FJ, Affleck G, Tennen H: The relationship of daily mood and stressful events to symptoms in juvenile rheumatic disease. Arthritis Care Res 13:33-41, 2000.

52. Kvaal SA, Patodia S: Relations among positive affect, negative affect, and somatic symptoms in a medically ill patient sample. Psychol Rep 87:227-233, 2000.

53. Haythornthwaite JA, Benrud-Larson LM: Psychological aspects of neuropathic pain. Clin J Pain 16:S101-S105, 2000.

54. Fernandez E, Milburn TW: Sensory and affective predictors of overall pain and emotions associated with affective pain. Clin J Pain 10:3-9, 1994.

55. Weisenberg M, Raz T, Hener T: The influence of film-induced mood on pain perception. Pain 76:365-375, 1998.

56. Good M: Effects of relaxation and music on postoperative pain: a review. J Adv Nurs 24:905-914, 1996.

57. Zillmann D, De Wied M, King-Jablonski C, Jenzowsky S: Drama-induced affect and pain sensitivity. Psychosom Med 58:333-341, 1996.

58. Magill-Levreault L: Music therapy in pain and symptom management. J Palliat Care 9:42-48, 1993.

59. Royet JP, Zald D, Versace R, Costes N, Lavenne F, Koenig O, Gervais R: Emotional responses to pleasant and unpleasant olfactory, visual, and auditory stimuli: a positron emission tomography study. J Neurosci 20:7752-7759, 2000.

60. Coghill RC, Sang CN, Maisog JM, Iadarola MJ: Pain intensity processing within the human brain: a bilateral, distributed mechanism. J Neurophysiol 82:1934-1943, 1999.

Brain Mechanisms of Persistent Pain States

Donald D. Price
G. Nicholas Verne

SUMMARY. Objectives: The objective of this review is to explain the relationships between neural mechanisms of persistent pain and neural representations of these conditions in brains of animal models and in brains of human pain patients.

Findings: Animal models of persistent pain, such as that which results from constrictive injury to the sciatic nerve or from intradermal injections of formalin, are accompanied by spatially widespread yet somatotopically organized increases in spinal cord dorsal horn neural activity and by similar widespread somatotopically organized increases in several pain-related areas of the brain. Consistent with these animal studies, human brain imaging studies that examine neural representations of visceral and cutaneous hyperalgesia have found that both forms of hyperalgesia are represented in many of the same multiple brain regions that are activated during acute normal pain, yet have a more extensive representation.

Conclusions: Hyperalgesic states are represented by increased activity in the same pathways and centers that are involved in acute normal pain. Additional areas activated during clinically relevant pain include

Donald D. Price, PhD, is affiliated with the Departments of Oral and Maxillofacial Surgery, and Neuroscience, McKnight Brain Institute, University of Florida, FL 32610 USA.

G. Nicholas Verne, MD, is affiliated with the Division of Gastroenterology, Hepatology, and Nutrition, Department of Medicine, University of Florida, FL 32610 USA.

Address correspondence to: Dr. Donald D. Price, Department of Oral and Maxillofacial Surgery, University of Florida College of Dentistry, Box 100416, Gainesville, FL 32610 [E-mail: dprice@dental.ufl.edu].

[Haworth co-indexing entry note]: "Brain Mechanisms of Persistent Pain States." Price, Donald D., and G. Nicholas Verne. Co-published simultaneously in *Journal of Musculoskeletal Pain* [The Haworth Medical Press, an imprint of The Haworth Press, Inc.] Vol. 10, No. 1/2, 2002, pp. 73-83; and: *The Clinical Neurobiology of Fibromyalgia and Myofascial Pain: Therapeutic Implications* [ed: Robert M. Bennett] The Haworth Medical Press, an imprint of The Haworth Press, Inc., 2002, pp. 73-83. Single or multiple copies of this article are available for a fee from The Haworth Document Delivery Service [1-800-HAWORTH, 9:00 a.m. 5:00 p.m. [EST]. E mail address: getinfo@haworthpressinc.com].

prefrontal cortical regions, possibly in association with psychological factors that are prevalent in clinical pain [e.g., anxiety, fear, depression, frustration]. *[Article copies available for a fee from The Haworth Document Delivery Service: 1-800-HAWORTH. E-mail address: <getinfo@haworthpressinc. com> Website: <http://www.HaworthPress.com> © 2002 by The Haworth Press, Inc. All rights reserved.]*

KEYWORDS. Persistent pain, cutaneous and visceral hyperalgesia, brain imaging

INTRODUCTION

Until recently, our understanding of brain mechanisms of persistent pain conditions has been almost nonexistent. With the advent of neuroimaging studies [i.e., positron emission tomography [PET], functional magnetic resonance imaging [fMRI]] of both human pain disorders and animal models of persistent pain, the cortical representations of persistent pain conditions have begun to be understood and related to their possible neural mechanisms. The purpose of this review is to explain how brain-imaging studies advance our knowledge about brain mechanisms of persistent pain conditions. First, a very brief and general review is presented of what has been learned in the last twenty years about physiological mechanisms of persistent pain states. We then focus on how this knowledge can be extended by neural imaging studies of persistent pain states.

GENERAL MECHANISMS OF PERSISTENT PAIN

Although multiple types of persistent pain conditions exist, new knowledge of these types of pain has been largely derived from studies of neuropathic pain and other forms of pathophysiological pain. Critical advances in understanding neural mechanisms underlying neuropathic pain have taken place as a result of recently developed animal models of neuropathic pain. Perhaps the most notable one is that which models complex regional pain syndrome [CRPS], the rat chronic constrictive injury [CCI] model of Bennett and Xie (1). In this model, four ligatures are placed around the sciatic nerve in a manner that partially constricts the nerve. This partial constriction results in impulse conduction block in large myelinated axons and causes tonic impulse discharge in thin myelinated and unmyelinated axons that innervate peripheral nociceptors (2). Rats who have this chronic constrictive injury display mechanical allodynia and hyperalgesia, hot and cold allodynia and hyperalgesia, and spontaneous pain-related behavior [e.g., guarding of the hindpaw associated with the constricted sciatic nerve], all of which are observed in human CRPS patients. Similar to some patients with neuropathic pain, mechanical allodynia also occurs in skin territories outside those innervated by the injured sciatic nerve in this same model (3). For example, this CCI rat model shows thermal hyperalgesia on the foot related to the injured nerve and mechanical hyperalgesia on both hindpaws (3,4). Pain models such as CCI are of enormous importance because they allow the investigation of physiological mechanisms underlying persistent pain states in general and neuropathic pain in particular.

Studies of animal models of neuropathic pain and patients with neuropathic pain show that ongoing pain and hyperalgesia/allodynia are codetermined by two major factors: 1. tonic impulse input from nociceptive afferents in damaged or otherwise dysfunctional nerves and 2. central sensitization mechanisms mediated by N-methyl-D-aspartate [NMDA]/substance P receptor mechanisms, including sensitization of postsynaptic membrane glutamate receptors and excitotoxic loss of inhibitory mechanisms (5,6). The interrelationships between these two general factors are evident in several ways. For example, bupivicaine applied to the rat's injured sciatic nerve in the rat CCI model eliminates the widespread hyperalgesia that is normally present as does spinal application of small doses of MK-801, a NMDA glutaminergic receptor antagonist (7). However, combining the local anesthetic block with antagonism of spinal NMDA receptors produced a reversal of hyperalgesia and pain-behaviors that long outlasted the duration of either the peripheral [local anesthesia] or central [MK-801] manipulation given alone. Thus, zones of allodynia and hyperalgesia that extend well beyond the cutaneous territory innervated by the injured nerve, indicative of altered central processing, are dynamically maintained by ongoing nociceptor input. Complementary evidence for this mechanism comes from experiments in patients who have one or more foci of unusually high sensitivity and areas of allodynic and hyperalgesic skin that are spatially remote from these small foci (8). Local anesthesia of these small foci was found to eliminate the patient's ongoing pain and eliminate the allodynia and hyperalgesia in areas of skin spatially remote from the local injections of anesthetics.

Physiological, neurochemical, and pharmacological studies that have utilized animal models of neuropathic pain have provided new insight into the pathophysiology of neuropathic pain (3,5,9). Pain associated with nerve injury and with inflammation results, at least in part, from long-term increases in sensitivity of spinal cord nerve cells that transmit nociceptive messages. These increases in responsiveness of these nerve cells are likely to at least partially account for the hyperalgesia and allodynia observed in some persistent pain states. Increased sensitivity is initiated peripherally by tonic impulse activity in primary nociceptive afferent neurons, particularly those that have unmyelinated axons and respond to intense thermal, mechanical, and chemical stimulation of body tissues (2,9). Such tonic impulse input to dorsal horn nociceptive neurons is associated with sustained release of excitatory amino acid neurotransmitters, specifically glutamate and aspartate, as well as neuropeptides such as substance P (10,11). The sustained release of these neuropeptides and neurotransmitters leads to persistent increases in sensitivity of postsynaptic membranes of nociceptive neurons through activation of specific types of postsynaptic membrane receptors to glutamate/aspartate and the intracellular neurochemical events triggered by activation of these receptors (12).

Cellular and molecular studies of persistent pain present a valuable yet limited explanation of the functional significance of central sensitization mechanisms that lead to hyperalgesia. A more complete explanation requires consideration of how these central sensitizing mechanisms lead to patterns of increased neural activity that is distributed throughout the central nervous system. The remainder of this review focuses on the neural representations of pain and their functional significance with emphasis on brain areas involved in persistent pain. Neural imaging studies provide much of this information.

NEURAL IMAGING OF PERSISTENT PAIN CONDITIONS

Recent neuroimaging studies of pain have confirmed increases in neural activity within multiple pain-related pathways and brain regions. These studies provide a three dimensional view of the central nervous system regions activated during pain. Two types of neural imaging experiments conducted so far include mapping of pain-related neural activity in animals with a persistent pain condition and human neuroimaging studies of pain. The results from both types of studies are complementary and will be discussed in turn.

Mapping Spinal Cord Neural Activity in Persistent Pain

The use of the radioactive 2-deoxyglucose [2-DG] tracer in the CCI model has provided maps of increased neural activity that occur in the spinal cord and brain of the rat CCI model (13,14). Such maps are instructive in illustrating the specific regions of the central nervous system that have increased neural activity as a result of this persistent pain condition. These regions include those previously implicated in pain processing in general, as well as those not predicted by previous knowledge of pain mechanisms. The central sensitizing mechanisms discussed earlier result not only in increased responses of dorsal horn neurons to nociceptive and non-nociceptive inputs, but also to expansion of their receptive fields so that they extend across multiple dermatomes (15). The expanded receptive fields and enhanced responsiveness of dorsal horn nociceptive neurons result in a *greater number* of neurons responding to a nociceptive or non-nociceptive stimulus than they would otherwise. The increased activation of more dorsal horn neurons along the rostral-caudal axis of the spinal cord may be associated with enhanced pain and spatial radiation of the painful sensation.

To test the prediction of increased activation along the rostral-caudal axis of the spinal cord, the 2-DG mapping technique was used to map spinal cord neural activity in CCI rats (13). This analysis revealed extensive rostro-caudal elevations in neural activity of the dorsal horn extending from L1 to L5 as well as both ipsilateral and contralateral elevations in dorsal horn neuron activity. This was so despite the fact that only the right sciatic nerve was constricted. As expected, peak activity was in the dorsal horn of L4 ipsilateral to the injured sciatic nerve. These results suggest that sensitization mechanisms recruit neurons across several spinal segments and neurons that are in the dorsal horn contralateral to the sciatic nerve injury. Such recruitment is accompanied by thermal and mechanical hyperalgesia/allodynia in zones that are remote from the original source of injury. Similar widespread zones of hyperalgesia occur in human CRPS patients (5,8,9) and patients with other types of painful diseases such as fibromyalgia (16) and even irritable bowel syndrome [IBS] (17).

Neural Mapping Studies of Brain Activity in Chronic Constrictive Injury Rats

Given the extensive rostro-caudal and bilateral representation of elevated neural activity in the spinal cord of CCI rats, a similar extensive representation of elevated activity would be expected in several brain areas of CCI rats. An extensive representation of increased neural activity in brains of CCI rats could have important functional implications for persistent pain conditions in humans. Regional increases in brain neural activity were examined in CCI rats by using the 2-DG method (14). The pattern of activation based on statistical analysis of group data revealed that significant increases in neural activity were found in all brain areas known to receive input from ascending pain-related pathways. Thus, increases in neural activity were found in central targets of the following known ascending pathways for pain (9,18,19): 1. *spinopontoamygdaloid pathway*–pontine parabrachial nucleus and amygdala; 2. *spinohypothalamic pathway*–ventral posteriomedial and arcuate hypothalamic nuclei; 3. *spinomesencephalic and spinoreticular pathways*–deep layers of the superior colliculus, central grey matter, pontine reticular formation, medullary gigantocellular nucleus, and paragigantocellular nucleus; 4. *spinothalamocortical pathways*–ventral posterior lateral nucleus, posterior thalamic nucleus, hindlimb region of S-I and S-II somatosensory areas, anterior cingulate cortex, retrosplenial granular cortex.

Several findings were predicted from the spinal cord studies of CCI rats. Consistent with patterns of spinal cord dorsal horn activation, thalamic ventral posteriolateral/posterior nuclear complex nuclei and S-I/S-II somatosensory areas contralateral to the injured nerve revealed larger increases in neural activity than corresponding ipsilateral brain regions, yet significant bilateral increases occurred within these regions. Although the peak area of increased S-1 somatosensory parietal cortical activity was in the contralateral hindlimb area, diffuse increases were seen throughout the somatosensory cortex and this pattern occurred bilaterally. Again, this widely distributed pattern with a peak in the somatotopically appropriate area is a predicted consequence of spinal cord patterns of increased activity. Similar increases were not present in cortical areas unrelated to somatosensory processing, such as the visual or auditory areas.

Cortical areas heavily interconnected with subcortical limbic structures also were activated and are likely to reflect affective, motivational, attentional, and motoric aspects of persistent pain. These included the amygdala, anterior cingulate cortex [within frontal lobes], and the retrosplenial granular cortex. Sciatic nerve injury-induced increases in neural activity within extensive brain regions previously implicated in sensory and affective-motivational dimensions of pain are likely to reflect neural representations of spontaneous pain as well as activation of brain areas involved in the modulation of pain.

These patterns of increased brain neural activity following CCI are similar in many respects to those induced by intradermal formalin injection that produces a temporary persistent pain condition in rats. Thus, Porro et al. (20) observed similar patterns of brain metabolic activity in response to subcutaneous formalin injection and Morrow et al. (21) have shown very similar patterns of regional cerebral blood flow in CCI rats as well as in rats given intradermal formalin injections. Increases in cortical areas involved in somatosensory processing and increases in cortical areas heavily interconnected with subcortical limbic structures are common findings across all of these studies. The correspondence between results using regional cerebral blood flow mapping and 2-DG in animals is important because it helps to validate and interpret the results of human studies using neuroimaging to measure regional cerebral blood flow.

Human Neural Imaging Studies of Persistent Pain Conditions

The specific cortical areas that mediate acute and chronic pain in humans have been poorly understood until recently. Functional neuroimaging in humans employing PET and fMRI have begun to provide some insight into cortical participation in the processing of pain (18,22). Functional brain imaging techniques can measure regional changes in cerebral blood flow, which reflect local changes in neuronal activity. Functional MRI provides a noninvasive method for measuring brain responses to sensory, motor, affective, and cognitive responses in humans. When employed in human subjects, it has the potential advantage of being able to relate brain activation and function to subjective dimensions of pain.

Similar to neural imaging studies of persistent pain states in rats, several neural imaging studies have shown increases in neural activity in areas of the brain that are functionally similar to those found in animal studies described above (22). Although there are modest differences in imaging techniques and forms of experimental pain across studies, brain areas most commonly activated include the lateral and/or medial thalamus, S-1 and S-II somatosensory cortex, anterior/posterior insular cortex, anterior cingulate area 24b, perigenual cingulate, posterior cingulate, supplementary motor area, periaqueductal grey, prefrontal cortical areas, and cerebellum (22). Early neural imaging studies using mild to moderate pain intensities found activation in only one to four of these areas, whereas later studies that used more intense or long-term painful stimuli found activation in most if not all areas just mentioned. A pivotal study showed part of the basis for these variable and controversial findings (23). It provided clear evidence that the number of brain regions activated and their overall areas of activation increase as a function of the intensity of pain. This unique PET study used four graded temperatures of 35 degrees, 46 degrees, 48 degrees, and 50 degrees centigrade to determine nociceptive stimulus-neural response relationships for several brain areas that may be involved in pain processing. Precise stimulus-response relationships were obtained for several functionally diverse brain areas, including those involved in motor control, affect, pain sensation, and attention. These stimulus-response functions occurred bilaterally in the anterior cingulate cortex, thalamus, insula, cerebellum, putamen, and somatosensory cortex. Exclusive contralateral pain intensity encoding occurred in the primary somatosensory cortex and supplemental motor area. These results suggest that the precise coding of the intensity of nociceptive stimulation is common to all functions associated with pain, including sensory, affective, attentional, and motoric components. However, quantitative differences in neural activation are reflected by increases in the magnitude of the neural signal, the additional recruitment of more brain structures, and the spatial distribution of that signal.

The vast majority of human neuroimaging studies of pain have evaluated regional cerebral activation in response to stimuli eliciting brief pain in healthy subjects. Early imaging studies of clinical pain states have found unpredictable patterns of brain activity, ones that include decreases in areas that normally increase during pain, or increases in very few areas (22). However, more recent studies show patterns of brain activity are more consistent with those of animal models of persistent pain. For example, we and others have begun to examine patterns of brain activation in patients with persistent pain from IBS in response to experimental visceral and cutaneous heat stimuli (24-26). We found that IBS patients, in comparison to age/sex matched control subjects, exhibited enhanced activation in virtually all known pain-related areas listed above in human pain neural imaging studies. These include those at early levels of pain processing such as lateral thalamus and S-1 cortex (26). This enhanced activation was found both in response to pain from rectal distension and to pain from nociceptive heat stimulation of the foot. The latter result is consistent with cutaneous heat hyperalgesia in IBS patients (17). However, in comparison to heat stimulation, rectal distension evoked much greater activity in prefrontal cortical areas, a result that may reflect greater anxiety in response to a more clinically relevant pain.

These patterns of a distributed network of increased pain-related activity in IBS patients suggest two very simple principles about neural representations of persistent clinical pain conditions. First, the brain areas activated are, in general, the same ones activated by experimental pain and therefore do not require activation of ascending pathways or central centers that are different from that utilized in normal pain processing. This similarity is expected because neurons of origin of ascending spinal pathways for pain respond to *both* brief nociceptive stimuli and to experimental manipulations that produce persistent pain, such as nerve injury or intradermal formalin injection (5,6,15,21). Second, the difference between neural representations of persistent clinical pain and acute experimental pain may reflect psychological factors such as pain-related anxiety, fear, depression, and other emotions in the case of the former. Future neuroimaging studies may relate different dimensions of pain, such as perceived sensory intensity, unpleasantness, and pain-related emotions, to neural activities in specific brain regions. Such studies should allow us to advance our knowledge of altered central pain processing mechanisms in chronic disorders such as IBS and fibromyalgia.

On a final note, it is important to recognize that neural imaging is not destined to be confined to global measures of neural activity, as described for studies reviewed here, but may eventually include measures of activation, release, and effects of specific neurotransmitters and neuromodulators [e.g., glutamate, opioids]. If such is the case, then we may well witness a merging of cellular and molecular approaches discussed at the beginning with approaches that provide three dimensional views of increased neural activity throughout multiple regions of the central nervous system. This merging of approaches may have profound consequences for the neuroscience and psychology of pain and for the care of pain patients.

REFERENCES

1. Bennett GJ, Xie YK: A peripheral mononeuropathy in rat that produces disorders of pain sensation like those seen in man. Pain 33: 87-107, 1988.

2. Kajander KC, Bennett GJ: The onset of a painful peripheral neuropathy in rat: a partial and differential deafferentation and spontaneous discharge in A-beta and A-delta primary afferent neurons. J Neurophysiol 68: 734-744, 1992.

3. Bennett GJ: Animal models of neuropathic pain. In: Proceedings of the 7th World Congress on Pain, Progress in Pain Research and Management, Vol. 2. Edited by GF Gebhart, DL Hammond and TS Jensen. IASP Press: Seattle, 1994, pp. 495-510.

4. Bennett G J, Kajander KC, Sahara Y, Iadarola MJ, Sugimoto T: Neurochemical and anatomical changes in the dorsal horn of rats with an experimental painful peripheral neuropathy. In: Proceedings of Sensory Information in the Superficial Dorsal Horn of the Spinal Cord. Edited by F Cervero, GJ Bennett and PM Headley. Plenum Press: New York, 1989, pp. 463-471.

5. Price DD, Mao J, Mayer DJ: Central neural mechanisms of normal and abnormal pain states. In: Pharmacological Approaches to the Treatment of Pain: New Concepts and Critical Issues, Progress in Pain Research and Management, Vol. 1. Edited by HL Fields and JC Liebeskind. IASP Press: Seattle, 1994, pp. 61-84.

6. Dubner R: Neuronal plasticity and pain following peripheral tissue inflammation or nerve injury. In: Proceedings of Vth World Congress on Pain. Pain Research and Clinical Management. Vol 5. Edited by M Bond, E Charlton, and CJ Woolf. Amsterdam: Elsevier, 1991, pp. 263-276.

7. Mao J, Price DD, Mayer DJ, Lu J, Hayes RL: Intrathecal MK 801 and local nerve anesthesia synergistically reduce nociceptive behaviors in rats with experimental peripheral mononeuropathy. Brain Res 576: 254-262, 1992.

8. Gracely RH, Lynch SA, Bennett G J: Painful neuropathy: altered central processing maintained dynamically by peripheral input. Pain 51: 175-194, 1992.

9. Price DD: Psychological Mechanisms of Pain and Analgesia. IASP Press, Seattle, 1999.

10. Thompson SWN, Woolf CJ: Primary afferent-evoked prolonged potentials in the spinal cord and their central summation: role of the NMDA receptor. In: Proceedings of the VIth World Congress on Pain. Edited by MR Bond, J Carlton, and CJ Woolf. Amsterdam: Elsevier, 1990, pp. 150-163.

11. Urban L, Randic M: Slow excitatory transmission in rat dorsal horn: possible mediation by peptides. Brain Res. 1984;290:336-341.

12. Mayer ML, Miller RJ: Excitatory amino acid receptors, second messengers and regulation of intracellular Ca^{2+} in mammalian neurons. Trends Pharmacol Sci 11: 254-260, 1990.

13. Mao J, Price DD, Coghill RC, Mayer DJ, Hayes RL: Spatial patterns of spinal cord [^{14}C]-2-deoxyglucose metabolic activity in a rat model of painful peripheral mononeuropathy. Pain 50: 89-100, 1992.

14. Mao J, Mayer DJ, Price DD: Patterns of increased brain activity indicative of pain in a rat model of peripheral mononeuropathy. J Neurosci 13(6): 2689-2702, 1993.

15. Palecek J, Paleckova V, Dougherty PM: Responses of spinothalamic tract cells to mechanical and thermal stimulation of skin in rats with experimental peripheral neuropathy. J Neurophysiology 67: 1562-1573, 1992.

16. Staud R, Vierck CJ, Cannon RL, Mauderli AP, Price DD: Abnormal sensitization and temporal summation of second pain (wind-up) in patients with fibromyalgia syndrome. Pain 91(1-2): 165-175, 2001.

17. Verne GN, Robinson ME, Price DD: Hypersensitivity to visceral and cutaneous pain in the irritable bowel syndrome. Pain 93: 7-14, 2001.

18. Price DD: Psychological and neural mechanisms of the affective dimension of pain. Science 288: 1769-1772, 2000.

19. Willis WD: The Pain System. Karger: New York, 1985.

20. Porro CA, Cavazzuti M, Baraldi P, Giuliani D, Panerai AE, Corazza R: CNS pattern of metabolic activity during tonic pain: evidence for modulation by beta-endorphin. European Journal of Neurosci 11: 874-888, 1999.

21. Morrow TJ, Paulson, PE, Danneman PJ, Casey KL: Regional changes in forebrain activation during the early and late phase of formalin nociception: analysis using cerebral blood flow in the rat. Pain 75(2-3): 355-365, 1998.

22. Casey, KL and Bushnell, MC: Pain Imaging. Progress in Pain Research and Management. Volume 18. IASP Press: Seattle, 2000, 248 pages.

23. Coghill RC, Mayer DJ, Price DD: Spinal cord coding of pain: the role of spatial recruitment and discharge frequency in nociception. Pain 53: 295-309, 1993.

24. Mertz H, Morgan V, Tanner G, Pickens D, Price R, Shyr Y, Kessler R: Regional cerebral activation in irritable bowel syndrome and control subjects with painful and nonpainful rectal distension. Gastroenterology 118: 842-848, 2000.

25. Silverman DHS, Munakata JA, Ennes H, Mandelkern MA, Hoh CK, Mayer EA: Regional cerebral activity in normal and pathological perception of visceral pain. Gastroenterology 112: 64-72, 1997.

26. Verne GN, Himes NC, Robinson ME, Briggs RW, Gopinath KS, Weng L, Price DD: Central representation of cutaneous and visceral pain in the irritable bowel syndrome. Gastroenterology 120: A3844, 2001.

Suffering and Dysfunction
in Fibromyalgia Syndrome

Dennis C. Turk

SUMMARY. Objectives: To describe the plight of the person with fibromyalgia syndrome [FMS], the psychosocial and behavioral factors that contribute to the extent of suffering experienced, and the heterogeneity of patient subgroups that characterize adaptation and response to treatment.

Findings: People diagnosed with FMS are confronted with a range of factors the influence there perception, adaptation, and response to treatment. Three subgroups of FMS patients have been identified using cluster analytic procedures. One subgroup is characterized by high levels of pain, perceived interference of symptoms with life, affective distress and social support, and low levels of perceived control and activity–"Dysfunctional." The unique characteristics of a second subgroup, relative to other FMS patients, relates to their perceptions of little support from significant others and a high degree of negative responses to their reports of symptoms–"Interpersonally Distressed." Compared to the other two groups, the third group reported lower levels of pain, emotional distress,

Dennis C. Turk, PhD, John & Emma Bonica Professor of Anesthesiology & Pain Research, University of Washington, Seattle, Washington.

Preparation of this manuscript was supported in part by grants from the National Institute of Arthritis and Musculoskeletal and Skin Diseases [AR/AI44724, AR47298] and the National Institute of Child Health and Human Development/National Center for Medical Rehabilitation Research [HD33989].

Address correspondence to: Dr. Dennis C. Turk, Department of Anesthesiology, Box 356540, University of Washington, Seattle, WA 98195 [E-mail: turkdc@u.washington.edu].

[Haworth co-indexing entry note]: "Suffering and Dysfunction in Fibromyalgia Syndrome." Turk, Dennis C. Co-published simultaneously in *Journal of Musculoskeletal Pain* [The Haworth Medical Press, an imprint of The Haworth Press, Inc.] Vol. 10, No. 1/2, 2002, pp. 85-96; and: *The Clinical Neurobiology of Fibromyalgia and Myofascial Pain: Therapeutic Implications* [ed: Robert M. Bennett] The Haworth Medical Press, an imprint of The Haworth Press, Inc., 2002, pp. 85-96. Single or multiple copies of this article are available for a fee from The Haworth Document Delivery Service [1-800-HAWORTH, 9:00 a.m. - 5:00 p.m. [EST]. E mail address: getinfo@haworthpressinc.com].

85

and higher levels of perceived control over symptoms, and were more active–"Adaptive Copers." The percentage of patients classified within each of the three groups were roughly equivalent. The three subgroups respond differentially to a standard interdisciplinary rehabilitation program.

Conclusions: Successful treatment of patients diagnosed with FMS will require attention to important individual differences in patients' perceptions, modes of responding, and responses by significant others in addition to physical factors associated with FMS. *[Article copies available for a fee from The Haworth Document Delivery Service: 1-800-HAWORTH. E-mail address: <getinfo@haworthpressinc.com> Website: <http://www. HaworthPress.com> © 2002 by The Haworth Press, Inc. All rights reserved.]*

KEYWORDS. Disability, expectations, pain behaviors, patient heterogeneity, treatment matching

THE PLIGHT OF THE PERSON WITH CHRONIC PAIN

Despite advances in the understanding of anatomy and physiological processes and innovative and technically sophisticated pharmacological, medical, and surgical treatments; pain continues to be a perplexing puzzle for health care providers and a source of significant distress for individual pain sufferers. No treatments are currently available that consistently and permanently relieve pain for all.

People with chronic pain often feel rejected by the very elements of society who exist to serve them. They lose faith and become frustrated with the healthcare system. At the same time that returning to work becomes less of a possibility and medical bills for unsuccessful treatments accumulate, chronic pain sufferers may begin to feel they are being blamed by their physicians, employers, and even family members when their condition does not respond to treatment. The legitimacy of reported symptoms may be challenged and third-party payers may even suggest that the person is fabricating symptoms in order to receive financial gain. Thus, the emotional distress that is commonly observed in chronic pain patients may be attributed to a variety of factors, including fear, maladaptive support systems, inadequate coping resources, overuse of potent medications, inability to work, financial difficulties, and prolonged litigation. Moreover, the experience of "medical limbo"–the presence of a painful condition that eludes diagnosis and that carry the implication of either psychiatric causation or malingering–is itself a source of stress.

People with persistent pain become enmeshed in the medical community as they migrate from doctor to doctor, laboratory test to laboratory test, and imaging procedure to imaging procedure in a continuing search to have their symptoms diagnosed and treated. For many patients the pain becomes the central focus of their lives. As patients withdraw from society, they lose their jobs, alienate family and friends, and become isolated. The quest for relief often remains elusive. Thus, it should hardly be surprising that patients experience feelings of demoralization, helplessness, frustration, anger, and depression–*suffering*.

In contrast to acute pain, chronic pain confronts people not only with the stress created by pain but also with a cascade of ongoing stressors that compromise all aspects of their lives. Living with persistent pain conditions requires considerable resilience and tends to deplete people's emotional reserves, and taxes not only the individual sufferer but also the capacity of family, friends, coworkers, and employers to provide support.

Pain is a subjective perception. There is no objective method currently available to determine how much pain someone is experiencing. The only way to determine how much of a subjective symptom, such as pain, that a patient is experiencing is to ask them for a verbal report or to observe their behavior [e.g., facial expressions, ambulation, posture]. To cite Ellen Scarry (1): "To have great pain is to have certainty, to hear that another person has pain is to have doubt."

In this paper, I will focus on one chronic pain syndrome, fibromyalgia syndrome [FMS]. What has been learned about chronic pain, in general, over the past three decades is relevant for FMS sufferers. I will emphasize the role of subjective interpretation and environmental responses to the experience and response to chronic pain and treatments offered. Further, I will suggest that there is a need to recognize that not all patients with the same medical diagnosis will respond in the same way to the identical treatments. To treat patients with FMS requires that treatment be individualized to meet both the psychosocial and behavioral, as well as physical characteristics of patients.

SYMPTOMS AND DISABILITY

Functional Disability

Exercise intolerance, reports of weakness, and functional disabilities are significant problems in FMS (2). Previous research has demonstrated that one of the cardinal criteria for the classification of FMS, painful tender points, are more prevalent in physically deconditioned people (3). Moreover, exercise programs often reduce pain sensitivity (4,5) suggesting that reduced physical conditioning may be an important contributing factor in FMS. Some studies of FMS patients suggest that they exhibit significantly lower levels of muscle strength and endurance than do other chronic myofascial pain patients (6), and healthy people (7,8).

Research on physical conditioning and activity performance of FMS patients, however, has provided inconsistent results. Daily physical exertions, based upon patients' recall, have been reported to be significantly lower in FMS patients compared to healthy people (9). Moreover, despite comparable levels of cardiovascular reactivity, FMS patients tend to terminate exercise at lower workloads than healthy people due to perceived exhaustion (10) do. Several studies report below average levels of aerobic conditioning in the majority of FMS patient (11,12) other studies, however, report that FMS patients' aerobic capacity does not differ significantly from age-matched healthy people although FMS patients consistently rate the exercise as more fatiguing (10,13).

Studies investigating muscle physiology, blood flow, and bioenergetics have also not been consistent in identifying specific abnormalities in FMS (14,15). Surface electromyographic activity during isokinetic tasks reveals no specific abnormality in the fatigue mechanisms in the local muscles of FMS patients (16). Thus, these studies are not capable of explaining the decreased level of muscle conditioning observed in people with FMS. Fibromyalgia syndrome patients may be as aerobically fit as others but *report* reduced activity levels, *perceive* the exercise as more demanding, and show reduced *voluntary* endurance and strength.

Effects of Expectancy in Physical Functioning

Physical performance on exercise tasks relies on subjects' voluntary effort. Research shows that reports of physical exertion can be influenced by motivation based on expectations about physical capability (17), suggesting that cognitive and affective factors need to be taken into account when evaluating physical functioning in people with chronic pain. Expectations typically develop as a result of prior experiences. Thus, a dynamic process may be initiated by a deficit in the central processing of physical sensations, resulting in 1. underestimation of physical functioning, 2. lowered expectations for performing physical activity, 3. inhibition of activity, and 4. eventually leading to physical deconditioning. The increased deconditioning may lead to even greater fatigue and reduced activity–a vicious circle.

Expectations about one's physical ability play an important role in coping and adaptation since degree of disability is influenced by peoples' assessments of the adequacy of their resources to match situational demands–self-efficacy beliefs (18). Studies (19) have shown that FMS patients' self-efficacy beliefs about performance of activities are related to impaired performance on physical tasks. The importance of FMS patients' self-efficacy beliefs have been supported in several studies demonstrating that pretreatment self-efficacy beliefs predict posttreatment activity. Moreover, improvements in self-efficacy have been shown to be associated with FMS patients' performance of physical activities following completion of a rehabilitation program (19,20).

Perceptions of Cause of Symptoms

Symptom perception in chronic pain may be affected by beliefs of having been "injured." These beliefs may be associated with the traumatic onset of an illness, and the thought that activity will lead to additional harm and symptom exacerbation. The acknowledgement that symptoms followed a specific pathological cause appears to greatly increase fear (21,22). Hypervigilance may predispose patients to attend selectively to all somatic perturbations that might otherwise be ignored and to avoid activities that they believe will contribute to further problems [i.e., fear avoidance]. Moreover, exposure to noxious agents [events, pathogens] may alter how one interprets physical sensations. Patients may identify any physical sensation as abnormal, harmful, and noxious, thereby increasing anxiety. These changes may, consequently, lower pain threshold and tolerance, increase activity avoidance, and exacerbate general deconditioning and fatigue commonly observed in FMS sufferers.

Experiencing a traumatic injury may also alter how people evaluate sensory information. For example, Lee and colleagues (21) observed that post-motor vehicle accident victims reported lower pain tolerance compared with healthy subjects. It is not known whether decreased pain tolerance among posttrauma patients is due to subtle, if not gross, changes in anatomy, which could result in hypersensitivity to nociception and consequently reports of pain. This could also be due to changes in psychological processes involving selective attention and fear appraisals. Elevated body awareness and anticipation of pain may result in a pain-sensitive perceptual system, in which one may focus more on physical sensations and interpret relatively benign sensory input as pain.

A substantial number of patients with diverse chronic pain syndromes attribute the onset of their pain to some type of precipitating event. My colleague and I (22) examined a heterogeneous sample of chronic pain patients and determined that 75 percent attributed the onset of their symptoms to a physical trauma, most commonly a motor vehicle accident or work-related injury. We found no significant differences in the physical findings between the groups who reported a traumatic onset compared with those who reported an insidious onset. In order to eliminate the possible confound of compensation status, we performed analyses of the relationships between the two types of onset and chronic pain for the subset of patients who were not receiving or actively seeking compensation. The results indicated that the patients who attributed their pain to a specific trauma reported significantly higher levels of emotional distress, life interference, and higher levels of pain severity than did the patients who indicated that their pain had a gradual onset. We found no differences in physical pathology between these groups that would likely explain the results.

My colleague and I (23) replicated the results on perceptions of the causes of symptoms with a sample of patients with FMS. Once again, we found no significant difference in physical pathology between those with a sudden traumatic versus gradual onset of symptoms. Again, controlling for compensation status and physical pathology, we found that the patients with traumatic onset of symptoms reported greater pain severity, greater life interference, physical disability, and affective distress.

PAIN BEHAVIORS

A specific set of behaviors has been labeled as *pain behaviors* (24). Pain behaviors consist of overt expressions of pain, distress, and suffering. The fact that these behaviors are observable means that they have the potential to elicit a response from others. A number of studies have supported the important role of the contingencies of reinforcement on the maintenance of pain behaviors independent of physical impairments (25).

Health care providers may inadvertently reinforce patient behavior by their responses. That is, patients learn that their behavior elicits a response from the health care provider, and if the response results in relief of pain, the patients may come to report pain in order to obtain the medication or to avoid physical therapy exercises. Consider what happens when pain medication is prescribed on *prn* [as needed] basis. The patient must indicate that the pain has increased in order to take the medication. If the medication provides relief, then the attention to and self-rating of pain may be maintained by the anticipated outcome of pain relief. Assume that a patient is being encouraged to exercise to build up his or her physical conditioning. If the patient does engage in the exercise and as a result feels increased pain, he or she may avoid exercise in the future. Increased avoidance of exercise has a reinforcing effect–the patient may avoid increased pain–but there is a consequence, namely, increased physical deconditioning. If a family member observes from the patient's behavior that the patient is having a "bad day" the family member may express concern and provide attention. As a consequence, a patient learns that displaying a particular set of pain behaviors results in attention, sympathy, and support.

SYMPTOM ATTRIBUTION AND TREATMENT

Patient interpretation of symptoms and presentation to health care providers may influence the behavior of the health care providers. In one of the studies cited earlier, my colleague and I (23) found that patients who attribute symptoms to a physical trauma were significantly more likely to receive physical treatments for symptoms including nerve blocks, physical therapy, and transcutaneous electrical nerve stimulation. The traumatic-onset patients were five times more likely to be prescribed opioid medication even though they did not reveal greater physical pathology. Thus, patients who report sudden, traumatic onset to their symptoms, independent of objective indications of physical pathology, are treated differently by physicians. In a second study, we (22) observed that physicians were more likely to prescribe opioid medication based on patients reports of disturbed mood, reports of greater impact on their lives, and behavioral presentation but, once again, not physical pathology or even reported pain severity. The role of physician's behaviors in the maintenance of symptoms and disability of pain sufferers has been frequently noted (e.g., 26,27).

The attribution of pain and related symptoms to a physical trauma seems to add an additional emotional burden and to exacerbate the problems of FMS patients (28). In addition, patients whose painful symptoms follow an accident have been shown to be more refractory to treatment than patients with nontraumatic onset (29,30).

PATIENT HETEROGENEITY

Despite the extensive research efforts, however, no treatment has proven to be universally effective for FMS. We do not understand why treatments may be effective for some but not others with the same diagnosis, nor can we reliably predict what works best for whom. One of the problems in the current literature may be related to the lack of appreciation of the heterogeneity of the population and appreciation of subtypes of suffers on any number of factors [e.g., precipitating events, emotional distress, coping and adjustment] (31). Several investigators (32,33) recommend a dual-diagnostic system for chronic pain disorders, allowing for both a physical and psychosocial diagnoses.

In order to clarify the heterogeneity of FMS, my colleagues and I (34) examined whether FMS patients could be classified into subgroups based upon their psychological adaptation to pain using the Multidimensional Pain Inventory [MPI] (35). We identified three subgoups of patients: Dysfunctional [DYS: high levels of pain, functional limitation, and affective distress], Interpersonally Distressed [ID: similar to DYS but further characterized by low levels of support from their significant other], and Adaptive Coper [AC: low levels of pain, distress, and disability]. In contrast to other chronic pain syndromes where we found disproportionate percentages of patients in the dysfunctional subgroup [42 percent and 62 percent for headache and chronic back pain, respectively], patients with FMS were roughly distributed equally within each of the three profiles. The percentage of FMS patients in the ID subgroup was substantially higher than observed in other pain syndromes [e.g., 33 percent vs. 18 percent and 25 percent for FMS, back pain, and headache, respectively].

Validity of the Multidimensional Pain Inventory Classification

In order to ascertain the discriminant validity of Multidimensional Pain Inventory [MPI] subgroups, my colleagues and I (36) compared them on physical functioning, pain, depressive moods, perceived functional limitation, and quality of interpersonal relationships. As expected, the three groups did not differ in the observed physical functioning such as lumbar flexion and cervical range of motion. However, the analyses revealed that: 1. the DYS patients reported significantly higher levels of pain than AC patients, 2. the DYS and ID groups reported significantly higher levels of depressed mood and perceived disability, and 3. the ID patients rated their interpersonal relationships with significant others to be significantly lower in quality compared to the DYS and AC patients. Posthoc analysis of the co-occurring symptoms demonstrates that the three groups did not differ in the prevalence of other symptoms. The results reinforce the suggestion that psychosocial dimensions of FMS may be independent of biomedical-physical dimension.

TREATMENT EFFICACY OF AN INTERDISCIPLINARY REHABILITATION PROGRAM

Given the multiple symptoms of FMS, many have advocated the importance of employing a multicomponent rehabilitation approach. In a preliminary study, my colleagues and I (34) examined the efficacy of an interdisciplinary treatment program for FMS patients, including six-month follow-up. The treatment program consisted of six, half-day sessions, spaced over four weeks. Each session included medical [education, medication, management], physical [aerobic and stretching exercise], occupational [pacing, body mechanics], and psychological [pain and stress management] components. The comparisons between the pretreatment and posttreatment scores revealed significant improvement in the targeted areas of pain severity, sense of control, depression, and fatigue, but remained at the pretreatment levels for nontargeted variables such as support from significant others. Results at follow-up revealed that the majority of treatment gains were sustained for six months following completion of treatment, although there was a statistically significant relapse in reported fatigue.

In order to delineate factors that would predict improvement in FMS pain, we (36) conducted a discriminant analysis with six pretreatment variables that were considered to be particularly relevant in pain reports: pretreatment levels of pain, depression, activity, perceived disability, solicitous responses from others, and whether FMS onset was attributed to a known cause or not [idiopathic]. All variables except the pretreatment level of pain yielded meaningful associations. Thus, patients who reported an idiopathic onset, who were relatively active and coping well, and who have solicitous partners tended to report significant improvement in pain. With these six variables, 77 percent of the patients could be accurately classified as responders or nonresponders.

DIFFERENTIAL TREATMENT RESPONSES AS A FUNCTION OF THE MULTIDIMENSIONAL PAIN INVENTORY PROFILES

Based upon the significant differences in adaptation to the chronic pain condition across psychosocial subgroups of FMS patients, we (37) hypothesized that the MPI subgroups would respond differently to a standard rehabilitation protocol. Patients who completed the FMS program were classified into one of the three MPI subgroups described earlier. Overall, the patients in the DYS group improved in most areas, whereas the ID patients, who reported comparable levels of pain and disability to the DYS group, failed to respond to the treatment. There was little change in the AC patients, possibly due to a ceiling effect. The results further support the need for different treatments targeting characteristics of subgroups and suggest that psychosocial characteristics of FMS patients are important predictors of treatment responses and may be used to customize treatment.

CONCLUDING COMMENTS

People with FMS need to have realistic goals. Health care providers should address the patients' concerns, provide reassurance, and clarify what can reasonably be expected. It is demoralizing to tell a patient that he or she has a *chronic* illness, because chronic has the connotation of forever. The patient and provider must have congruent goals and the provider must be cautious to avoid attitudes and behaviors that may *delegitimize* patients' experience. Health care providers should consider the unique characteristics of patients and attempt to match treatments both to patients' physical and psychosocial needs. Greater attention needs to be given to patients' interpretations and beliefs and to the role of significant others, including health care providers, in contributing to the maintenance of distress and disability.

REFERENCES

1. Scarry E: The Body in Pain. Oxford University Press, New York, 1985.

2. Bengtsson A, Henriksson KG, Jorfeldt L: Primary fibromyalgia. A clinical and laboratory study of 55 patients. Scand J Rheumatol 15: 340-347, 1986.

3. Granges G, Littlejohn GO: A comparative study of clinical signs in fibromyalgia/fibrositis syndrome, healthy and exercising subjects. J Rheumatol 20: 344-351, 1993.

4. Martin L, Nutting A, MacIntosh BR, Edworthy SM, Butterwick D, Cook J: An exercise program in the treatment of fibromyalgia. J Rheumatol 2: 1050-1053, 1996.

5. Wigers SH, Stiles TC, Vogel PA: Effects of aerobic exercise versus stress management treatment in fibromyalgia. A 4.5 year prospective study. Scand J Rheumatol 25: 77-86, 1996.

6. Jacobsen S, Danneskiold-Samsoe B: Dynamic muscular endurance in primary fibromyalgia compared with chronic myofascial pain syndrome. Arch Phys Med Rehabil 73: 170-173, 1992.

7. Lindh MH, Johansson LG, Hedberg M, Grimby GL: Studies on maximal voluntary muscle contraction in patients with fibromyalgia. Arch Phys Medi Rehabil 5: 1217-1222, 1994.

8. Norregaard J, Bulow PM, Danneskiold-Samsoe B: Muscle strength, voluntary activation, twitch properties, and endurance in patients with fibromyalgia. J Neurol. Neurosurg, Psychiat 57: 1106-1111, 1994.

9. Norregaard J, Bulow PM, Mehlsen J, Danneskiold-Samsose B: Biochemical changes in relation to a maximal exercise test in patients with fibromyalgia. Clin Physiol 14: 159-167, 1994.

10. van Denderen JC, Boersma JW, Zeinstra P, Hollander AP, van-Neerbos BR: Physiological effects of exhaustive physical exercise in primary fibromyalgia syndrome [PFS]: Is PFS a disorder of neuroendocrine reactivity? Scand J Rheumatol 21: 35-37, 1992.

11. Bennett RM, Clark SR, Campbell SM, Burckhardt CS: Low levels of somatomedin C in patients with the fibromyalgia syndrome. A possible link between sleep and muscle pain. Arthritis Rheumat 35: 1113-1116, 1993.

12. Mannerkorpi K, Burckhardt CS, Bjelle A: Physical performance characteristics of women with fibromyalgia. Arthritis Care Res 7: 123-129, 1994.

13. Mengshoel AM, Forre O, Komnaes HB: Muscle strength and aerobic capacity in primary fibromyalgia. Clin Exp Rheumatol, 8: 475-479, 1990.

14. Joos E, De Meirleir K, Vandenborne K: ^{31}P magnetic resonance muscle spectroscopy in fibromyalgia. J Rheumatol 20: 1985-1986, 1993.

15. Simms RW, Roy SH, Hrovat M: Lack of association between fibromyalgia syndrome and abnormalities in muscle energy metabolism. Arthritis Rheumat 37: 794-800, 1994.

16. Elert JE, Rantapaa-Dahlqvist SB, Henriksson-Larsen K, Gerdle B: Muscle performance, electromyography and fibre type composition in fibromyalgia and work-related myalgia. Scand J Rheumatol 21: 28-34, 1992.

17. Blalock S, DeVellis B, DeVellis R: Psychological well-being among people with recently diagnosed rheumatoid arthritis. Do self-perceptions of abilities make a difference? Arthritis Rheumat 35: 1267-1272, 1992.

18. Bandura A: Self-efficacy: Toward a unifying theory of behavioral change. Psychol Rev 84: 191-215, 1977.

19. Buckelew SP, Murray SE, Hewett JE, Johnson J, Huyser B: Self-efficacy, pain, and physical activity among fibromyalgia subjects. Arthritis Care Res 8: 43-50, 1995.

20. Buckelew SP, Huyser B, Hewett JE, Parker JC, Johnson JC, Conway R, Kay DR: Self-efficacy predicting outcome among fibromyalgia subjects. Arthritis Care Res 9: 97-1104, 1996.

21. Lee J, Giles K, Drummond PD: Psychological disturbance and exaggerated response to pain in patients with whiplash injury. J Psychosom Res 37: 105-110, 1993.

22. Turk DC, Okifuji A: What factors affect physicians' decisions to prescribe opioids for chronic noncancer pain patients? Clin J Pain 13: 330-336, 1997.

23. Turk DC, Okifuji A: Perception of traumatic onset, compensation status, and physical findings: impact on pain severity, emotional distress, and disability in chronic pain patients. J Behav Medi 19: 435-453, 1996.

24. Fordyce WE: Behavioral Methods for Chronic Pain and Illness. CV Mosby, St. Louis, MO, 1976.

25. Romano JM, Turner JA, Jensen MP, Friedman LS, Bulcroft RA, Hops H, Wright SF: Chronic pain patient–spouse behavioral interaction predict disability. Pain 63: 353-360, 1995.

26. Hadler NM: Fibromyalgia, chronic fatigue, and other iatrogenic diagnostic algorithms. Do some labels escalate illness in vulnerable patients? Postgrad Med 102: 161-172, 1997.

27. Reilly PA: How should we manage fibromyalgia? Ann Rheumat Dis 58: 325-326, 1999.

28. Greenfield S, Fitzcharles MA, Esdaile JM: Reactive fibromyalgia syndrome. Arthritis Rheumat 35: 678-681, 1992.

29. DeGood DE, Kiernan B: Perception of fault in patients with chronic pain. Pain 64: 153-159, 1996.

30. Tsushima W, Stoddard V: Ethnic group similarities in the biofeedback treatment of pain. Med Psychotherapy 3: 69-75, 1990.

31. Turk DC, Flor H: Primary fibromyalgia is greater than tender points: Toward a multiaxial taxonomy. J Rheumatol 16: 80-86, 1989.

32. Scharff L, Turk DC, Marcus DA: Psychosocial and behavioral characteristics in chronic headache patients: Support for a continuum and dual-diagnostic approach. Cephalalgia 15: 216-223, 1995.

33. Turk D: Customizing treatment for chronic pain patients: Who, what, and why. Clin J Pain 6: 255-270, 1990.

34. Turk DC, Okifuji A, Sinclair JD, Starz TW: Interdisciplinary treatment for fibromyalgia syndrome: Clinical and statistical significance. Arthritis Care Res 11: 186-195, 1998.

35. Kerns RD, Turk DC, Rudy TE: The West Haven-Yale Multidimensional Pain Inventory [WHYMPI]. Pain 23: 345-356, 1985.

36. Turk DC, Okifuji A, Sinclair JD, Starz TW: Pain, disability, and physical functioning in subgroups of patients with fibromyalgia. J Rheumatol 23: 1255-1262, 1996.

37. Turk DC, Okifuji A, Sinclair JD, Starz TW. Differential responses by psychosocial subgroups of fibromyalgia syndrome patients to an interdisciplinary treatment. Arthritis Care Res 11: 397-404, 1998.

REGIONAL PAIN SYNDROMES

Deep Tissue Hyperalgesia

Lars Arendt-Nielsen
Thomas Graven-Nielsen

SUMMARY. Objectives: The aim of this paper is to give a brief introduction to the mechanisms and manifestations related to muscle hyperalgesia. It has become increasingly evident that muscle hyperalgesia plays an important role in chronic musculoskeletal pain. Better understanding of the involved basic mechanisms and better methods to assess muscle pain in the clinic might provide new possibilities for designing rational therapies and for targeting the pharmacological intervention optimally.

Results: Increased muscle sensitivity can be manifested as either

Lars Arendt-Nielsen, DrmedSci, PhD, and Thomas Graven-Nielsen, PhD, are affiliated with the Laboratory for Experimental Pain Research, Center for Sensory-Motor Interaction, Aalborg University, Fredrik Bajers Vej 7, D3, DK-9220 Aalborg, Denmark.

Address correspondence to: Prof. dr. Lars Arendt-Nielsen, Aalborg University, Center for Sensory-Motor Interaction, Laboratory for Experimental Pain Research, Fredrik Bajers Vej 7, D3, DK-9220 Aalborg, Denmark [E-mail: LAN@smi.auc.dk].

The Danish National Research Foundation and the Danish Research Council are acknowledged for supporting the time spent by the authors to write this paper.

[Haworth co-indexing entry note]: "Deep Tissue Hyperalgesia." Arendt-Nielsen, Lars, and Thomas Graven-Nielsen. Co-published simultaneously in *Journal of Musculoskeletal Pain* [The Haworth Medical Press, an imprint of The Haworth Press, Inc.] Vol. 10, No. 1/2, 2002, pp. 97-119; and: *The Clinical Neurobiology of Fibromyalgia and Myofascial Pain: Therapeutic Implications* [ed: Robert M. Bennett] The Haworth Medical Press, an imprint of The Haworth Press, Inc., 2002, pp. 97-119. Single or multiple copies of this article are available for a fee from The Haworth Document Delivery Service [1-800-HAWORTH, 9:00 a.m. - 5.00 p.m. [EST]. E-mail address: getinfo@haworthpressinc.com].

1. pain evoked by a normally nonnociceptive stimulus [allodynia], 2. increased pain intensity evoked by nociceptive stimuli [hyperalgesia], or 3. increased referred pain areas with associated somatosensory changes. For basic experimental studies quantitative sensory testing provides the possibility to evaluate these manifestations in a standardized way in patients suffering from musculoskeletal pain or in healthy volunteers.

Conclusions: Increased muscle sensitivity is present in musculoskeletal pain conditions and may play a role for chronification of pain, and interventions should take this aspect into consideration. *[Article copies available for a fee from The Haworth Document Delivery Service: 1-800-HAWORTH. E-mail address: <getinfo@haworthpressinc.com> Website: <http://www. HaworthPress.com> © 2002 by The Haworth Press, Inc. All rights reserved.]*

KEYWORDS. Muscle hyperalgesia, referred pain, experimental muscle pain, musculoskeletal disorders

INTRODUCTION

Acute and chronic pain originating from deep somatic structures represent a major part of pain complaints in patients. Deep pain is a diagnostic and therapeutic problem, and further insights into the peripheral and central neurophysiological mechanisms are necessary to improve diagnosis and therapy. The focus of this paper is to discuss the possible mechanisms underlying deep tissue hyperalgesia and how these mechanisms can be assessed under experimental conditions or in patients suffering from chronic musculoskeletal pain. The terminology "hyperalgesia" will be used for pain evoked by normally nonnociceptive or nociceptive stimuli [i.e., including allodynia].

It is beyond the scope of this paper to describe in detail the complicated pathophysiological mechanisms involved in acute and in particular chronic muscle pain, and to a large extent, most mechanisms are unfortunately unknown. However, more recent research has disclosed some new aspects of muscle hyperalgesia, and some of these findings will be highlighted in the following.

Paradoxically, most experimental pain research has been on cutaneous pain although cutaneous pain is far less important than deep tissue pain. In contrast to sharp, localized characteristics of cutaneous pain, muscle pain is described as aching and cramping with diffuse localization. Kellgren (1) was one of the pioneers to study experimentally the diffuse characteristics of muscle pain and the actual locations of referred pain to selective activation of specific muscle groups. Firm neurophysiologically based explanations for referred pain do not exist, but it has been shown that wide dynamic range neurons as well as nociceptive specific neurons in the spinal cord and in the brain stem receive convergent afferent input from the mucosa, skin, muscles, joints, and viscera. This may cause misinterpretation of the afferent information coming from muscle afferents and reaching higher levels in the central nervous system, and hence be one reason for the diffuse and referred characteristics. The sensation of acute muscle pain is the result of activation of group III [Aδ-fiber] and group IV [C-fiber] polymodal muscle nociceptors. The nociceptors can be sensitized by release of neuropeptides from the nerve endings. This may eventually lead to central hyperexcitability of dorsal horn neurons manifested as prolonged neuronal discharges, increased responses to defined noxious stimuli, response to non-noxious stimuli, and expansion of the receptive field (2). Wall and Woolf (3) have shown that muscle nociceptive afferents seem particularly effective to induce such neurofunctional changes in the spinal cord. Therefore, it is most likely that muscular hyperalgesia plays an important role for muscle pain disorders. Extensive animal experiments have supported this notion by showing that hyperexcitability of dorsal horn neurons may be a possible cause for muscular hyperalgesia and referred pain (2).

In humans little information is available on the peripheral neuronal correlate of muscle nociceptor sensitization and only few microneurographic studies have been published (4,5). The reason is difficulties in recording and directly activation of the muscle nociceptors. Other more indirect but still quantitative techniques are therefore needed, and quantitative sensory testing may help to assess muscle pain and hence muscle hyperalgesia. As there have been made substantial achievements in this field in recent years, a short update will be given in the following.

ASSESSMENT OF MUSCLE PAIN
AND HYPERALGESIA IN HUMANS

The ultimate goal of advanced human experimental pain research is to obtain a better understanding of mechanisms involved in pain transduction, transmission, and perception under normal and pathophysiological conditions.

Experimental muscle pain research involves two separate topics: 1. Standardized activation of the muscle nociceptive system and 2. Measurements of the evoked responses. Experimental approaches can be applied in the laboratory for basic studies [e.g., central hyperexcitability or preclinical screening of drug efficacy] but also in the clinic to characterize patients with sensory dysfunctions and/or, e.g., musculoskeletal pain.

As pain is a multidimensional perception, it is obvious that the reaction to a single standardized stimulus of a given modality can only represent a very limited fraction of the entire pain experience. It is therefore a necessity to combine different stimulation and assessment approaches to gain advanced differentiated information about the nociceptive system under normal and pathophysiological conditions. For muscle pain research we need to assess both muscle sensitivity and possible modality specific somatosensory changes in the referred areas. A major advantage of experimental muscle pain models is that isolated aspects of muscle pain mechanisms can be investigated in a standardized setting without confounding factors.

Various methods can be used to induce and assess muscle pain. Usually, the methods are classified into two groups: 1. endogenous [without external stimuli] and 2. exogenous [external stimuli] methods (6).

Endogenous Models

The endogenous methods are characterized by high response rate and are suitable to study general muscle pain states. However, they have the disadvantage of involving several or all muscle groups within the region investigated, and often pain from other somatic tissues cannot be excluded.

Ischemic muscle pain is a classical experimental pain model and has been used for many years as an unspecified pain stimulus. The method is found to be reliable (7) and has been used for human analgesic assay (8). This is a very efficient model to induce pain in muscles but skin, periosteum, and other tissues will contribute to the overall pain perception. The model is applicable in experimental studies requiring a general tonic pain stimulus.

Various forms of heavy and unaccustomed exercise can evoke exercise-induced pain in specific muscles. Together with overloading and insufficient resting periods, concentric dynamic and isometric contractions will elicit muscle pain, which may share the same physiopathogenetic mechanisms as ischemic pain (9).

In contrast, eccentric contractions induce a delayed onset of muscle pain or soreness (10-13). The mechanisms underlying this kind of postexercise muscle pain seem to be entirely different from those of ischemic muscle pain. The mechanism underlying delayed onset muscle soreness is probably related to ultrastructural damage resulting in the release of algogenic substances (14,15). This may produce an inflammatory reaction, as anti-inflammatory drugs [NSAID] appear to have an effect on this type of jaw muscle soreness (16,17). Howell et al. (18) were, however, unable to demonstrate an NSAID effects on delayed soreness in limb muscles.

Exogenous Models

Mechanical stimulation is another method for excitation of muscle nociceptors. Pressure algometry is the most generally applied technique for quantification of tenderness, which in clinical practice is assessed by palpation. Using this technique, it can be difficult to distinguish between peripheral and central sensitization, unless the sensitization is restricted to a single muscle/joint. Therefore, control determinations from nonaffected, extra-segmental areas are important. The pain threshold and tolerance threshold can be measured easily but also the stimulus-response functions can give important information on muscle hyperalgesia. Normally hand-held algometers are used (19) where the rate of pressure increase and absolute values can be monitored. It has been difficult to compare thresholds from various clinical pressure pain studies as different instrumentations, different probe diameters/shapes, and different force increase rates have been used. The diameter is of utmost importance as there is not necessarily a simple relation between diameter and threshold because spatial summation plays an important role for pain. The shape and contour of the probe are important as sharp edges may excite more cutaneous receptors due to high shear forces compared with blunt probes (20). Recent attempts to standardize the technique and normal values for various muscles have been published (19), and hopefully quantitative techniques will be more applicable and standardized for clinical applications in the future.

Intraneural stimulation of muscle afferents (21) is a laboratory model, which elicits selectively muscle pain accompanied by referred pain, which actually increases in size for increasing pain intensity. Intramuscular electrical stimulation (22-24) can evoke deep pain, but the sensation is confounded by concurrent activated muscle twitches. The method is adequate for studies where muscle pain and related referred areas should to be turned on and off momentarily. This provides the possibility to follow a given intervention over time [e.g., what happens before and after a referred area is anesthetized (25,26)]. Electrical stimulation has, however, the disadvantage that it is not nociceptive specific. Vecchiet et al. (27) found that determination of pain thresholds to electrical stimulation from different parietal tissues [muscle, subcutis, skin] rendered different degrees of hyperalgesia and as such could distinguished sensitization of the three parietal tissues.

Chemical stimulation by, e.g., intramuscular infusion of hypertonic saline causes local and referred pain (1,28-32). Unfortunately the saline does not selectively activate nociceptors (33), and the pain lasts for minutes once the saline is infused. Recent animal studies have shown that the method does not cause any muscle toxicity (34) and therefore the method is adequate for human experimentation. A major advantage of the hypertonic saline model is that a detailed description of sensory and motor effects can be obtained as the pain lasts for minutes. Furthermore, the model is reliable for studying referred pain from musculoskeletal structures due to the longer lasting pain.

In most of the earlier studies manual bolus infusions of hypertonic saline have been used. However, standardization of the infusion of small volumes is easier to accomplish by computer-controlled infusion pumps (35,36). A systematic evaluation of the infusion parameters [infusion concentration, volume, rate, and tissue] has been studied on pain intensity, quality, and local and referred pain patterns (36).

Intramuscular injections of algesic substances such as capsaicin (5,37-39), bradykinin [BK], serotonin [5HT] (40-43), potassium chloride (30), glutamate (44), levo-ascorbic acid (45), and acid phosphate buffer (46) have also been used experimentally to induce muscle pain in humans. In general, these methods elicit mild to moderate intense levels of pain.

MUSCLE HYPERALGESIA

Many clinical studies report increased sensitivity to painful stimuli of deep tissues within (47-54) and outside (48,49,52,53,55) muscle pain areas in patients compared to controls. Peripheral mechanisms [sensitization of receptors] may explain deep tissue hyperalgesia whereas modulation of somatosensory sensitivity at referred sites without obvious tissue pathologies is mediated by central mechanisms. This is obvious, as anesthetizing the referred area does not abolish totally the referred muscle pain (25,26).

Referred pain has been known and described for more than a century and has been used extensively as a diagnostic tool in the clinic. Head initially used the term referred tenderness and pain in 1893 (56). It has since then been used to describe pain perceived at a site adjacent to or at a distance from the site of origin. The taxonomy committee of the International Association for the Study of Pain has not made a definition of the term. However, several authors have defined it in different ways. In this paper, the definition "pain felt at a site remote from the site of origin/stimulation" will be used.

Several neuroanatomical and neurophysiological theories regarding the appearance of referred pain have been suggested, and basically they state that nociceptive dorsal horn or brain stem neurons receive convergent inputs from various tissues, thus higher centers cannot identify correctly the actual input source. Most recently the models have included newer theories where sensitization of dorsal horn and brainstem neurons plays a central role. Similar sensitization might be involved in deep tissue hyperalgesia at a site distant from the pain locus. The association between referred pain and degree of sensitization seems evident as correlation between degree of pain/nociception and referred pain areas are found in many studies. In the following experimental and clinical examples of as well peripheral as central deep tissue sensitization will be given.

Peripheral Sensitization

Experimental Findings

Sensitization of muscle nociceptors might explain deep tissue hyperalgesia as this phenomenon decreases the mechanical excitation threshold and increases responses to noxious stimuli. Experimentally this has been seen as decreased pressure pain thresholds after intramuscular injections of capsaicin (37). Intra-arterial injections of 5HT, BK, and prostaglandin E2 have been found effective in sensitizing nociceptors in animals (2). In humans, the deep tissue hyperalgesia is reflected in a decrease in the pressure pain threshold after combined intramuscular injections of 5HT and BK (42) [Figure 1]. Recently, Ernberg et al. (57) found that co-injection of 5HT and the 5HT3 receptor antagonist granisetron into the masseter muscle reduced the spontaneous pain evoked

FIGURE 1. Preripheral sensitization in humans leads to an increase in maximal pain intensity [visual analog scale, VAS, peak, top panel] when intramuscular injections of serotonin [5HT] are given before bradykinin [BK] compared to the sequence of isotonic saline before BK. Mean [± standard error, N = 10] VAS peak after the first and second infusion is shown. *: P < 0.05 compared to BK after isotonic saline. The area infiltrated with 5HT and BK shows [lower panel] decreased pressure pain thresholds [i.e., muscle hyperalgesia]. The pressure pain thresholds [PPT] are normalized to the PPT prior to infusion of 5HT and BK [mean ± standard error, N = 10, *: P < 0.05 compared to preinfusion]. Modified from (42).

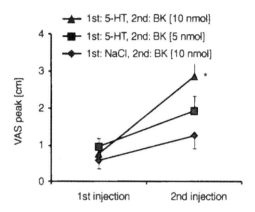

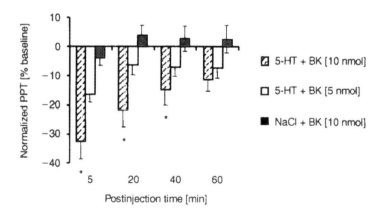

by injection of 5HT and prevented allodynia/hyperalgesia to mechanical pressure stimuli. Thus, peripheral serotonergic receptors could be involved in the regulation of musculoskeletal pain disorders.

The ionotropic and metabotropic glutamate receptors are other receptor types, which are found on peripheral unmyelinated sensory afferents in the skin (58,59). Intramuscular injections of glutamate produce muscle hyperalgesia to pressure stimuli in humans (44) and sensitize rat muscle afferents (60). Injection of selective metabotropic glutamate receptor agonists into the mouse hind paw causes a dose-dependent decrease in thermal thresholds lasting up to 150 min after administration (59). This thermal hyperalgesia can be attenuated by administration of selective metabotropic glutamate receptor antagonists, whereas other noncompetitive glutamate receptor antagonists and N-methyl-D-aspartate [NMDA] receptor antagonists have less or no effect (61,62). Du et al. (63) demonstrated a significant excitation of Aδ-fiber and C-fiber nociceptors, but not Aβ units in the glabrous skin of rats, by application of glutamate. Furthermore, they found evidence of sensitization to thermal stimuli, but not to punctuate mechanical stimuli. Further, there is some evidence from behavioral studies that glutamate and substance P work synergistically to sensitize primary afferents (64). Therefore, it is conceivable that glutamate-induced mechanical sensitization of muscle afferents may, in part, result from the actions of released neuropeptides such as substance P.

Svensson et al. (50) performed an experimental study in which increased tenderness assessed by pressure algometry was observed after the jaw muscle had been exposed to experimental muscle pain [hypertonic saline]. Moreover, pain thresholds to intramuscular electrical stimulation are significantly lower in muscles 24 hours after they have been exposed to hypertonic saline (22). Such findings on pressure and intramuscular electrical pain thresholds are, however, also seen after infusion of isotonic saline in the leg muscles (65). The findings on muscular sensitivity in saline-induced muscle pain areas are not clear, as hyperalgesia (22,30,50,66), hypoalgesia (67), or unaffected (68) sensitivity has been detected. Muscular hyperalgesia has mainly been detected on the masticatory muscles or brachioradialis muscle, whereas hypoalgesia or unchanged sensitivity is found in studies on the larger tibialis anterior muscle. This could suggest that the development of muscular hyperalgesia is dependent on the size of the muscle and, hence, possibly the level of afferent barrage. This is supported by the fact that pressure pain thresholds are higher for a large muscle such as tibialis anterior compared to a smaller muscle such as brachioradialis (50). From many clinical studies one would expect to observe muscle hyperalgesia in the presence of experimental muscle pain (69,70). For the superficial tissue overlying the saline-induced muscle pain area, increased sensitivity to electrical stimulation (22) and to pinprick stimulation (71) is found. In contrast, decreased responses to pinprick stimuli (36) and unchanged pain thresholds to pinch stimulation (65) have been reported. These findings might be related to central mechanisms discussed in the following section.

Another model on deep tissue hyperalgesia is the soreness developed after eccentric muscle work [delayed onset of muscle soreness] with peak soreness after 24-48 hours (9,11,12,14,72). Another feature of delayed onset of muscle soreness is the fact that there is no pain at rest, but pain is evoked by muscle function and during palpation [i.e., allodynia/hyperalgesia]. An example of delayed onset muscle soreness from a model of deep tissue pain in wrist extensors with characteristics similar to lateral epicondylalgia (13) is shown in Figure 2.

The phenomenon of neurogenic inflammation [axon reflex] caused by a noxious stimulus is well-known and studied as the flare reaction in human skin, but is most likely also important for muscles [Figure 3]. Neurogenic inflammation in a muscle may cause release of peptides that can increase the blood flow locally. Edema and/or plasma extravasation may be the result and as such the phenomenon may play a role in development of localized muscle hyperalgesia.

Clinical Findings

Pressure pain sensitivity is the most common technique to assess painful musculoskeletal conditions such as, e.g., tender points, fibromyalgia, work related myalgia, myofacial pain, strain injuries, myositis, chronic fatigue syndrome, arthritis/orthroses, and other muscle/tendon/joint inflammatory conditions (19). The technique is adequate to quantify and follow the development of given diseases but has also proven to be instrumental for documentation of treatment outcome such as local/systemic administration of NSAIDs. An example could be recording of the joint pain threshold before and weeks after topical application of an NSAID to patients suffering from unilateral finger joint inflammation and pain [arthritis] (73). Stimulus response functions can provide more information than just a threshold as sensitization to as well low as high intensities can be assessed, and a shift in parallel towards left together with an increased slope has been found in patients

FIGURE 2. An example of postexercise muscle soreness as a model of deep tissue hyperalgesia. Mean [± standard error, N = 12] pressure pain thresholds assessed on the extensor carpi radialis brevis muscle before and after eccentric work with the wrist. Significantly decreased thresholds compared to the unexercised arm [*: P < 0.05]. Based on data from (13).

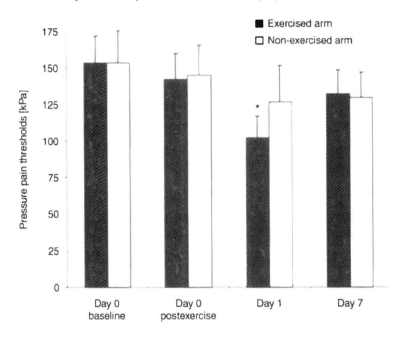

with myofacial pain (50). After anesthetizing the muscle, the curve was shifted towards the right with a reduced slope (50).

Referred Pain and Central Sensitization

Experimental Findings

Referred pain is probably a combination of central processing and peripheral input as it is possible to induce referred pain to limbs with complete sensory loss due to spinal injury (74) or an anesthetic block (26,66). However, the involvement of peripheral input from the referred pain area is not clear as anesthetizing this area shows inhibitory or no effects on the referred pain intensity (25,74-77). Central sensitization may be involved in the generation of referred pain. Animal studies show a development of new and/or expansion of existing receptive fields by

FIGURE 3. An illustration of neurogenic inflammation in a muscle. When a muscle nociceptor is stimulated, the action potentials travel towards the spinal cord, but runs also antidromically in the peripheral network and cause release of vasoactive substances from other nociceptors in the vicinity of the injury.

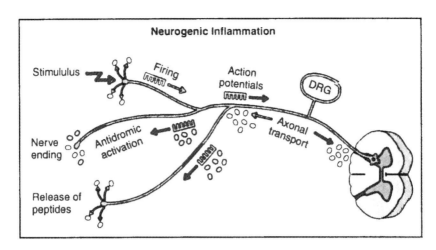

noxious muscle stimuli (78-80) [Figure 4]. Recordings from a dorsal horn neuron with a receptive field located in the biceps femoris muscle show new receptive fields in the tibialis anterior muscle and at the foot after intramuscular injection of bradykinin into the tibialis anterior muscle (79). In the context of referred pain, the unmasking of new receptive fields due to central sensitization could mediate referred pain (81). This has been suggested to be the phenomenon of secondary hyperalgesia in deep tissue. A number of studies have found that the area of the referred pain correlated with the intensity of the muscle pain (21,24,28,32,76,82) which parallels the observations for cutaneous secondary hyperalgesia where the hyperalgesic area is related to the capsaicin-induced pain intensity (83). This type of plasticity of the central nervous system may also alter somatosensory sensitivity and account for deep tissue hyperalgesia. The somatosensory sensitivity in the referred pain area may give additional information about the mechanisms involved in generation of referred pain [e.g., referred pain together with increased sensitivity in the referred pain area suggest that central sensitization is involved in the referred pain mechanisms] (67). In general, it is accepted that muscle pain can result in hyperalgesia in the referred somatic structures, and the somatosensory sensitivity in the

FIGURE 4. An example of expanded convergent receptive to touch and pinch after injection of mustard oil into the rat masseter muscle. The receptive fields are related to wide dynamic range neurons in the caudalis laminae V and VI. [Redrawn after data from (80)].

Expansion of cutaneous receptive fields

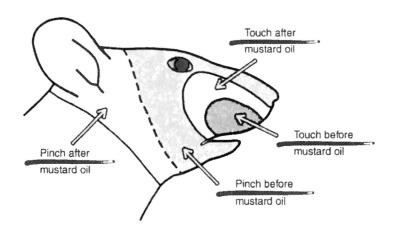

Touch after mustard oil

Touch before mustard oil

Pinch after mustard oil

Pinch before mustard oil

WDR neurons in caudalis laminae [V, VI]
Mustard oil in masseter muscle

referred pain area may give additional information about the mechanisms involved in generation of referred pain.

In referred areas of experimentally induced muscle pain, Kellgren (1) and Feinstein et al. (66) found tenderness to pressure, but Steinbrocker et al. (84) did not. Similarly, different findings on skin sensitivity in the referred pain area have been reported depending on the stimulus modality tested (66,67,85,86,87). Increased visual analog scale response to electrical cutaneous stimulation and decreased sensitivity to radiant heat stimulation have been reported in referred pain areas (85). This modality specific somatosensory change found in the referred muscle area is similar to findings in secondary hyperalgesic areas of the skin.

The mechanisms behind sensitivity changes in referred muscle pain areas may be of peripheral or central origin. Infiltration of the muscle tissue with anesthetics 30 minutes after injection of hypertonic saline [i.e., no ongoing pain] completely reverses cutaneous and muscular hyperalgesia (22). This effect of a peripheral block on the muscle hyperalgesia may suggest peripheral sensitization. Alternatively, the mechanisms responsible for deep and especially cutaneous hyperalgesia after muscle pain may be caused by a central mechanism where peripheral input is needed, which is also a necessary condition for referred pain (1,85). Recently, we found hyperalgesia to pressure distal to the referred pain area produced by experimental pain induced in the tibialis anterior muscle (88) [Figure 5]. The referred hyperalgesic area was innervated by the deep peroneous nerve, which also innervates the tibialis anterior muscle. This suggests involvement of summation be-

FIGURE 5. An illustration of somatosensory changes [N = 14, pressure stimulation] segmentally and extrasegmentally after induction of muscle pain in a lower limb muscle. In most areas hypoalgesia are found, most likely caused by muscle pain induced pain inhibitory mechanisms. In areas with common nerve supply, hyperalgesia are seen due to central summation. In the local muscle pain area, summation and inhibition seem to cancel each other with constant sensitivity as net result [data from (88)].

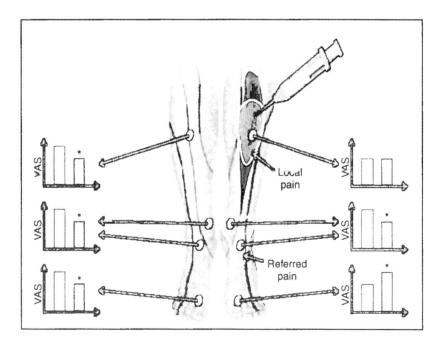

tween muscle afferents and the somatosensory afferents from the hyperalgesic area eventually facilitated by central sensitization.

Central sensitization of dorsal horn or brainstem neurons initiated by nociceptive activity from muscles may explain the expansion of pain with referral to other areas and probably also hyperalgesia in these areas. However, facilitated neurons cannot account for the decreased sensation to certain sensory stimuli in the referred area. Descending inhibitory control of the dorsal horn neurons may explain the decreased response to additional noxious stimuli in the referred pain area. Recently, we found that saline-induced muscle pain resulted in deep tissue hypoalgesia in extrasegmental areas [including the area of referred pain] distant from the pain focus (68,71). In addition, segmental inhibition at the spinal cord or brainstem level may contribute to the decreased sensitivity. In animals intramuscular capsaicin injections have shown to produce inhibition of C-fiber activity from the contralateral leg. This inhibition was blocked by cooling the spinal cord (89) and by spinal cord application of naloxone and phentolamine (90). Descending inhibitory mechanisms might, therefore, mask any eventual increase in somatosensory sensitivity caused by experimental pain.

Clinical Findings

Substantial clinical knowledge exists concerning the patterns of referred muscle pain from various skeletal muscles and after activation of trigger/tender points (91-93), and this aspect will not be covered further. Relatively few clinical studies have, however, aimed to study central sensitization in combination with chronic musculoskeletal pain.

The contribution of neuropathic pain in musculoskeletal disorders has been largely neglected until recently, when Mense et al. (93) dedicated one chapter in their book on "Muscle Pain" to this topic. Patients with, e.g., peripheral nerve lesions may experience as well cutaneous, subcutaneous as muscle hyperalgesia, or allodynia. The role of central sensitization and neuroplasticity is evident for neuropathic pain, but in all studies so far only the cutaneous components have been assessed. In a preliminary experiment we have investigated how patients [N = 6] with postapoplexy chronic pain responded to intramuscular injection of hypertonic saline in affected areas versus nonaffected areas [Figure 6]. The preliminary data showed that they rated the pain stronger and with a longer duration from the affected area compared to the non-affected area. This may imply that clinical examinations of patients suffering from neuropathic pain should include more detailed investigation of

FIGURE 6. The mean [N = 6] pain intensity ratings from postapoplexy patients suffering from unilateral neurogenic pain. Hypertonic saline [0.5 ml] was given intramuscularly on the affected side and contralateral unaffected side, and the pain intensity rating was scored continuously. Higher pain rating and longer pain duration were seen when injected into the affected painful area [unpublished results].

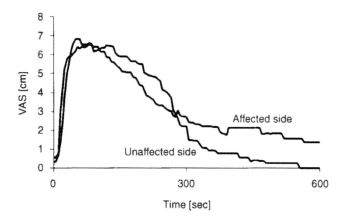

deep tissue hyperalgesia and possibly in future take it into consideration for planning the most rational therapies.

A number of recent studies have provided the first evidence of central sensitization in chronic musculoskeletal pain. In the first study Sörensen et al. (94) found that fibromyalgic patients experienced stronger pain and larger referred areas after intramuscular injection of hypertonic saline. The most interesting aspect was the fact that these manifestations were present in lower limb muscles where the patients normally do not experience ongoing pain. One could argue that the subjective pain ratings could be a result of, e.g., hypervigilance, but the patients had no clues of the normal referred pain area to injection of hypertonic saline in the tibialis anterior muscle. Moreover, the expanded referred pain areas in fibromyalgia patients have recently been reduced by ketamine [an NMDA-antagonist] targeting central sensitization (95). Normally pain from the tibialis anterior is projected distally to the ankle and never proximally. In the patients substantial proximal spread of the referred areas was found. This corresponds to basic neurophysiological experiments in rats, where dorsal horn neuron recordings from various spinal segments were investigated before and after muscle inflammation (79). In these experiments the inflammation caused a proximal spread of hyperexcitability, which explains the clinical findings.

Later these manifestations of central sensitization to experimental painful muscle stimulation have been shown in patients suffering from chronic whiplash pain (96) and from chronic osteoarthritic pain (97).

Another manifestation of central sensitization may be the number of palpable trigger points and recently, we found a significantly higher number of these points in lower limb muscles in patients suffering from knee osteoarthritis compared to controls (98). The presence of central sensitization may facilitate low intensity input [could be muscle allodynia] and, hence, result in the experience of pain when a possible latent trigger point is activated. This may also be one of the reasons why a localized painful condition can spread and become generalized.

CONCLUSIONS

An important part of the pain manifestations related to chronic musculoskeletal disorders may be due to peripheral and central sensitization. Better knowledge and evaluation possibilities of the mechanisms involved in chronic musculoskeletal pain may provide better clues to revise and optimize treatment regimes. Some manifestations of sensitization, such as expanded referred muscle pain areas in chronic musculoskeletal pain patients, have been explained from animal experiments by extra-segmental spread of sensitization.

REFERENCES

1. Kellgren JH: Observations on referred pain arising from muscle. Clin Sci 3: 175-190, 1938.

2. Mense S: Nociception from skeletal muscle in relation to clinical muscle pain. Pain 54: 241-289, 1993.

3. Wall PD, Woolf CJ: Muscle but not cutaneous C-afferent input produces prolonged increase in the excitability of the flexion reflex in the rat. J Physiol 356: 443-458, 1984.

4. Simone DA, Marchettini P, Caputi G, Ochoa JL: Identification of muscle afferents subserving sensation of deep pain in humans. J Neurophysiol 72: 883-889, 1994.

5. Marchettini P, Simone DA, Caputi G, Ochoa JL: Pain from excitation of identified muscle nociceptors in humans. Brain Res 740: 109-116, 1996.

6. Arendt-Nielsen L: Induction and assessment of experimental pain from human skin, muscle and viscera. Proceedings of the 8th World Congress on Pain. Edited by TS Jensen, JA Turner, Z Wiesenfeld-Hallin. Seattle: IASP Press, 1997, pp. 393-425.

7. Smith GM, Lowenstein E, Hubbard JH, Beecher HK: Experimental pain produced by the submaximum effort tourniquet technique: Further evidence of validity. J Pharmacol Exp Therapeut 63: 468-474, 1968.

8. Smith GM, Egbert LD, Markowitz RA, Mosteller F, Beecher HK: An experimental pain method sensitive to morphine in man. The submaximal effort tourniquet technique. J Pharmocol Exp Therapeut 154: 324-332, 1966.

9. Vecchiet L, Giamberardino MA, Marini I: Immediate muscular pain from physical activity. Pain and Mobility. Edited by M Tiengo, J Eccles, AC Cuello, D Ottoson. Raven Press, New York, 1987, pp. 193-218.

10. Abraham WM: Factors in delayed muscle soreness. Med Sci Sports 9: 11-20, 1977.

11. Asmussen E: Observations on experimental muscular soreness. Acta Rheumatol Scand 2: 109-116, 1956.

12. Bajaj P, Graven-Nielsen T, Arendt-Nielsen L: Post-exercise muscle soreness after eccentric exercise: Psychophysical effects and implications on mean arterial pressure. Scand J Med Sci Sport, 11(5):266-273, 2001.

13. Slater H, Arendt-Nielsen L, Wright A, Graven-Nielsen T: Deep tissue pain in wrist extensors–A model of lateral epicondylalgia. J Musculoske Pain 9(Suppl 5): 95, 2001.

14. Newham DJ: The consequences of eccentric contractions and their relation to delayed onset muscle pain. Eur J Appl Physiol 57: 353-359, 1988.

15. Newham DJ, Edwards RHT, Mills KR, Wall PD, Melzack R: Skeletal muscle pain. Textbook of Pain. Third Edition. Churchill Livingstone, Edinburgh, 23: 423-440, 1994.

16. Svensson P, Arendt-Nielsen L: Effect of topical NSAID on post-exercise jaw muscle soreness: A placebo controlled experimental study. Journal of Musculoskeletal Pain 3(4): 41-58, 1994.

17. Svensson P, Houe L, Arendt-Nielsen L: Effect of systemic versus topical nonsteroidal anti-inflammatory drugs on postexercise jaw-muscle soreness: A placebo-controlled study. J Orofacial Pain 11(4): 353-362, 1997.

18. Howell JN, Conatser RR, Chleboun GS, Karapondo DL, Chila AG: The effect of nonsteroidal anti-inflammatory drugs on recovery from exercise-induced muscle injury. 2. Ibuprofen. J Musculoskel Pain 6: 69-84, 1998.

19. Fischer AA (ed.). Muscle pain syndromes and fibromyalgia. Pressure algometry for quantification of diagnosis and treatment outcome. The Haworth Medical Press, New York, USA, 1998, 1-158.

20. Greenspan JD, McGillis SL: Thresholds for the perception of pressure, sharpness, and mechanically evoked cutaneous pain: effects of laterality and repeated testing. Somatosens Mot Res 11(4): 311-317, 1994.

21. Torebjörk HE, Ochoa JL, Schady W: Referred pain from intraneural stimulation of muscle fascicles in the median nerve. Pain 18: 145-156, 1984.

22. Vecchiet L, Galletti R, Giamberardino MA, Dragani L, Marini F: Modifications of cutaneous, subcutaneous and muscular sensory and pain thresholds after the induction of an experimental algogenic focus in the skeletal muscle. Clin J Pain 4: 55-59, 1988.

23. Kawakita K, Miura T, Iwase Y: Deep pain measurement at tender points by pulse algometry with insulated needle electrodes. Pain 44: 235-239, 1991.

24. Laursen RJ, Graven-Nielsen T, Jensen TS, Arendt-Nielsen L: Quantification of local and referred pain in humans induced by intramuscular electrical stimulation. European Journal of Pain 1: 105-113, 1997.

25. Laursen RJ, Graven-Nielsen T, Jensen TS, Arendt-Nielsen L: Referred pain is dependent on sensory input from the periphery: A psycophysical study. European Journal of Pain 1: 261-269, 1997.

26. Laursen R, Graven-Nielsen T, Jensen TS, Arendt-Nielsen L: The effect of compression and regional anaesthetic block on referred pain intensity in humans. Pain 80(1-2): 257-263, 1999.

27. Vecchiet L, Giamberardino MA: Referred pain. Clinical significance, pathophysiology, and treatment. Phys Med Rehabil Clinics, North Am 8: 87-100, 1997.

28. Inman VT, Saunders JBCM: Referred pain from skeletal structures. J Nerv Ment Dis 99: 660-667, 1944.

29. Wolff BB, Potter JL, Vermeer WL, McEwen C: Quantitative measures of deep somatic pain: Preliminary study with hypertonic saline. Clin Sci 20: 345-350, 1961.

30. Jensen K, Norup M: Experimental pain in human temporal muscle induced by hypertonic saline, potassium and acidity. Cephalalgia 12: 101-106, 1992.

31. Vecchiet L, Dragani L, De Bigontina P, Obletter G, Giamberardino MA: Experimental referred pain and hyperalgesia from muscles in humans. In New trends in referred pain and hyperalgesia. Edited by L Vecchiet, D Albe-Fessard, U Lindblom, MA Giamberardino. Elsevier Science Publishers B.V., Amsterdam, 1993, pp. 239-249.

32. Graven-Nielsen T, Arendt-Nielsen L, Svensson P, Jensen TS: Quantification of local and referred muscle pain in humans after sequential i.m. injections of hypertonic saline. Pain 69: 111-117, 1997.

33. Iggo A: Non-myelinated afferent fibres from mammalian skeletal muscle. J Physiol (Lond) 155: 52-53, 1961.

34. Svendsen O, Edwards CN, Rasmussen AD: Hypertonic saline: Study on muscle tissue toxicity in erythrocytes, rat myocyte culture and in rabbits after intramuscular injection. Proceedings, 2nd World Institute of Pain Congress, Istanbul, June, 2001.

35. Stohler CS, Lund JP: Psychophysical and orofacial motor response to muscle pain–validation and utility of an experimental model. In Brain and oral functions. Edited by T Morimoto, T Matsuya, K Takada. Elsevier Science B.V., Amsterdam, 1995, pp. 227-237.

36. Graven-Nielsen T, Arendt-Nielsen L, Svensson P, Jensen TS: Experimental muscle pain: A quantitative study of local and referred pain in humans following injection of hypertonic saline. J Musculoske Pain 5(1): 49-69, 1997.

37. Witting N, Svensson P, Gottrup H, Arendt-Nielsen L, Jensen TS: Intramuscular and intradermal injection of capsaicin: A comparison of local and referred pain. Pain 84: 407-412, 2000.

38. Sohn MK, Graven-Nielsen T, Arendt-Nielsen L, Svensson P: Inhibition of motor unit firing during experimental muscle pain in humans. Muscle Nerve 23: 1219-1226, 2000.

39. Arima T, Svensson P, Arendt-Nielsen L: Capsaicin-induced muscle hyperalgesia in the exercised and non-exercised human masseter muscle. J Orofac Pain 14: 213-223, 2000.

40. Jensen K, Tuxen C, Pedersen-Bjergaard U, Jansen I, Olesen J: Pain and tenderness in human temporal muscle induced by bradykinin and 5-hydroxytryptamine. Peptides 11: 1127-1132, 1990.

41. Ernberg M, Lundeberg T, Kopp S: Pain and allodynia/hyperalgesia induced by intramuscular injection of serotonin in patients with fibromyalgia and healthy individuals. Pain 85: 31-39, 2000.

42. Babenko V, Graven-Nielsen T, Svensson P, Drewes AM, Jensen TS, Arendt-Nielsen L: Experimental human muscle pain and muscular hyperalgesia induced by combinations of serotonin and bradykinin. Pain 82: 1-8, 1999.

43. Babenko V, Graven-Nielsen T, Svensson P, Drewes AM, Jensen TS, Arendt-Nielsen L: Experimental human muscle pain induced by intramuscular injections of bradykinin, serotonin, and substance P. Eur J Pain 3: 93-102, 1999.

44. Cairns BE, Hu JW, Arendt-Nielsen L, Sessle B, Svensson P: Human pain perception and rat afferent discharge evoked by injection of glutamate into the masseter muscle: Evidence of sex-related differences. J Neurophysiol 86: 782-791, 2001.

45. Rossi A, Decchi B: Changes in Ib heteronymous inhibition to soleus motoneurones during cutaneous and muscle nociceptive stimulation in humans. Brain Res 774: 55-61, 1997.

46. Issberner U, Reeh PW, Steen KH: Pain due to tissue acidosis: A mechanism for inflammatory and ischemic myalgia? Neurosci Lett 208: 191-194, 1996.

47. Vecchiet L, Giamberardino MA, Saggini R: Myofascial pain syndromes: Clinical and pathophysiological aspects. Clin J Pain 7: 16-22, 1991.

48. Lautenbacher S, Rollman GB, McCain GA: Multi-method assessment of experimental and clinical pain in patients with fibromyalgia. Pain 59: 45-53, 1994.

49. Vecchiet L, Giamberardino MA, de Bigontina P, Dragani L: Comparative sensory evaluation of parietal tissues in painful and nonpainful areas in fibromyalgia and myofascial pain syndrome. Proceedings of the 7th World Congress on Pain. Edited by GF Gebhart, DL Hammond, TS Jensen. IASP Press, Seattle, 1994, pp. 177-185.

50. Svensson P, Arendt-Nielsen L, Nielsen H, Larsen JK: Effect of chronic and experimental jaw muscle pain on pain-pressure thresholds and stimulus-response curves. J Orofac Pain 9: 347-356, 1995.

51. Bendtsen L, Jensen R, Olesen J: Qualitatively altered nociception in chronic myofascial pain. Pain 65: 259-264, 1996.

52. Kosek E, Ekholm J, Hansson P: Modulation of pressure pain thresholds during and following isometric contraction in patients with fibromyalgia and in healthy controls. Pain 64: 415 423, 1996.

53. Nørregaard J, Bendtsen L, Lykkegaard J, Jensen R: Pressure and heat pain thresholds and tolerances in patients with fibromyalgia. J Musculoske Pain 5(2): 43-53, 1997.

54. Sörensen J, Bengtsson A, Ahlner J, Henriksson KG, Ekselius L, Bengtsson M: Fibromyalgia—are there different mechanisms in the processing of pain? A double blind crossover comparison of analgesic drugs. J Rheumatol 24: 1615-1621, 1997.

55. Gibson SJ, Littlejohn GO, Gorman MM, Helme RD, Granges G: Altered heat pain thresholds and cerebral event-related potentials following painful CO_2 laser stimulation in subjects with fibromyalgia syndrome. Pain 58: 185-193, 1994.

56. Head H: On disturbances of sensation with especial reference to the pain of visceral disease. Brain 16: 1-136, 1893.

57. Emberg M, Lundeberg T, Kopp S: Effect of propranolol and granisetron on experimentally induced pain and allodynia/hyperalgesia by intramuscular injection of serotonin into the human masseter muscle. Pain 84: 339-346, 2000.

58. Carlton SM, Hargett GL and Coggeshall RE: Localization and activation of glutamate receptors in unmyelinated axons of rat glabrous skin. Neuroscience Lett 197: 25-28, 1995.

59. Bhave G, Karim F, Carlton SM, Gereau RW: Peripheral group I metabotropic glutamate receptors modulate nociception in mice. Nature Neurosci 4: 417-423, 2001.

60. Cairns BE, Gambarota G, Svensson P, Arendt-Nielsen L, Berde CB: Glutamate-induced sensitization of rat masseter muscle afferents. Neuromodulation, 2002.

61. Walker K, Reeve A, Bowes M, Winter J, Wotherspoon G, Davis A, Schmid P, Gasparini F, Kuhn R, Urban L: mGlu5 receptors and nociceptive function II. mGlu5 receptors functionally expressed on peripheral sensory neurones mediate inflammatory hyperalgesia. Neuropharmacology 40: 10-19, 2001.

62. Walker K, Bowes M, Panesar M, Davis A, Gentry C, Kesingland A, Gasparini F, Spooren W, Stoehr N, Pagano A, Flor PJ, Vranesic I, Lingenhoehl K, Johnson EC, Varney M, Urban L, Kuhn R: Metabotropic glutamate receptor subtype 5 (mGlu5) and nociceptive function. I. Selective blockade of mGlu5 receptors in models of acute, persistent and chronic pain. Neuropharmacology 40: 1-9, 2001.

63. Du J, Koltzenburg M, Carlton SM: Glutamate-induced excitation and sensitization of nociceptors in rat glabrous skin. Pain 89: 187-198, 2001.

64. Carlton SM, Shou S, Coggeshall RE: Evidence for the interaction of glutamate and NK1 receptors in the perihery. Brain Res 790: 160-169, 1998.

65. Graven-Nielsen T, Fenger-Grøn LS, Svensson P, Steengaard-Pedersen K, Arendt-Nielsen L, Jensen TS: Quantification of deep and superficial sensibility in saline-induced muscle pain–A psychophysical study. Somatosens Mot Res 5: 46-53, 1998.

66. Feinstein B, Langton JNK, Jameson RM, Schiller F: Experiments on pain referred from deep tissues. J Bone Joint Surg 36: 981-997, 1954.

67. Arendt-Nielsen L, Graven-Nielsen T, Svensson P, Jensen TS: Temporal summation in muscles and referred pain areas: an experimental human study. Muscle Nerve 20: 1311-1313, 1997.

68. Graven-Nielsen T, Babenko V, Svensson P, Arendt-Nielsen L: Experimentally induced muscle pain induces hypoalgesia in heterotopic deep tissues, but not in homotopic deep tissues. Brain Res 787: 203-210, 1998.

69. Reid KI, Gracely RH, Dubner RA: The influence of time, facial side, and location on pain-pressure thresholds in chronic myogenous temporomandibular disorder. J Orofacial Pain 8: 258-265, 1994.

70. Ohrbach R, Gale EN: Pressure pain thresholds, clinical assessment, and differential diagnosis: reliability and validity in patients with myogenic pain. Pain 39: 157-169, 1989.

71. Svensson P, Graven-Nielsen T, Arendt-Nielsen L: Mechanical hyperesthesia of human facial skin induced by tonic painful stimulation of jaw-muscles. Pain 74: 93-100, 1998.

72. Howell JN, Chleboun G, Conatser R: Muscle stiffness, strength loss, swelling and soreness following exercise-induced injury in humans. J Physiol (Lond) 464: 183-196, 1993.

73. Arendt-Nielsen L, Drewes AM, Svendsen L, Brennum J: Quantitative assessment of joint pain following treatment of rheumatoid arthritis with ibuprofen cream. Scand J Rheumatol 23: 334-337, 1994.

74. Whitty CWM, Willison RG: Some aspects of referred pain. Lancet 2: 226-231, 1958.

75. Hockaday JM, Whitty CWM: Patterns of referred pain in the normal subject. Brain 90: 481-496, 1967.

76. Sinclair DC, Wenddell G, Feindel WH: Referred pain and associated phenomena. Brain 71: 184-211, 1948.

77. Klingon GH, Jeffreys WH: Distribution of cutaneous hyperalgesia. Neurol 8: 272-276, 1958.

78. Cook AJ, Woolf CJ, Wall PD, McMahon SB: Dynamic receptive field plasticity in rat spinal cord dorsal horn following C-primary afferent input. Nature 325: 151-153, 1987.

79. Hoheisel U, Mense S, Simons DG, Yu XM: Appearance of new receptive fields in rat dorsal horn neurons following noxious stimulation of skeletal muscle: a model for referral of muscle pain? Neurosci Lett 153: 9-12, 1993.

80. Hu JW, Sessle BJ, Raboisson P, Dallel R, Woda A: Stimulation of craniofacial muscle afferents induces prolonged facilitatory effects in Trigeminal nociceptive brainstem neurons. Pain 48: 53-60, 1992.

81. Mense S: Referral of muscle pain. New aspects. APS 3: 1-9, 1994.

82. Lewis T, Kellgren JH: Observations relating to referred pain, viscero-motor reflexes and other associated phenomena. Clin Sci 4: 47-71, 1939.

83. Simone DA, Baumann TK, LaMotte RH. Dose-dependent pain and mechanical hyperalgesia in humans after intradermal injection of capsaicin. Pain 38: 99-107, 1989.

84. Steinbrocker O, Isenberg SA, Silver M, Neustadt D, Kuhn P, Schittone M: Observations on pain produced by injections of hypertonic saline into muscles and other supportive tissues. J Clin Inv 32: 1045-1051, 1953.

85. Graven-Nielsen T, Arendt-Nielsen L, Svensson P, Jensen TS: Stimulus-response functions in areas with experimentally induced referred muscle pain–A psychophysical study. Brain Res 744: 121-128, 1997.

86. Tuveson B, Lindblom B, Fruhstorfer H: Experimental muscle pain and sensory changes at the site of referred pain. Proceedings of SASP, 22th Annual Meeting, Reykjavik, Iceland 1999, p. 77.

87. Leffler AS, Kosek E, Hansson P: Injection of hypertonic saline into musculus infraspinatus resulted in referred pain and sensory disturbances in the ipsilateral upper arm. Eur J Pain 4: 73-82, 2000.

88. Graven-Nielsen T, Gibson S, Svensson P, Arendt-Nielsen L: Sensitivity to pressure stimuli in capsaicin-induced referred pain areas. European Federation of IASP Chapters (EFIC), Nice, France, 2000, p. 213.

89. Gjerstad J, Tjolsen A, Svendsen F, Hole K: Inhibition of evoked C-fibre responses in the dorsal horn after contralateral intramuscular injection of capsaicin involves activation of descending pathways. Pain 80: 413-418, 1999.

90. Gjerstad J, Tjolsen A, Svendsen F, Hole K: Inhibition of spinal nociceptive responses after intramuscular injection of capsaicin involves activation of noradrenergic and opioid systems. Brain Res 859: 132-136, 2000.

91. Travell JG, Simons DG: Myofascial pain and dysfunction. The trigger point manual. Williams & Williams, Baltimore, USA, 1982.

92. Simons DG: Clinical and etiological update of myofascial pain from trigger points. J Musculoske Pain 4(1/2): 93-121, 1996

93. Mense S, Simons DG, Russell IJ: Muscle Pain. Understanding its nature, diagnosis, and treatment. Lippincott Williams & Wilkins, Baltimore, USA, 2001, pp. 62-83.

94. Sörensen J, Graven-Nielsen T, Henriksson KG, Bengtsson M, Arendt-Nielsen L: Hyperexcitability in fibromyalgia. J Rheumatol 25: 152-155, 1998.

95. Graven-Nielsen T, Kendall SA, Henriksson KG, Bengtsson M, Sörensen J, Johnson A, Gerdle B, Arendt-Nielsen L: Ketamine reduces muscle pain, temporal summation, and referred pain in fibromyalgia patients. Pain 85: 483-491, 2000.

96. Johansen MK, Graven-Nielsen T, Olesen AS, Arendt-Nielsen L: Generalised muscular hyperalgesia in chronic whiplash syndrome. Pain 83: 229-234, 1999.

97. Bajaj P, Bajaj P, Graven-Nielsen T, Arendt-Nielsen L: Osteoarthritis and its association with muscle hyperalgesia: an experimental controlled study. Pain 93: 107-114, 2001.

98. Bajaj P, Bajaj, P, Graven-Nielsen T, Arendt-Nielsen L: Trigger points in patients with lower limb osteoarthritis. J Musculoske Pain 9(3): 17-33, 2001.

Pathophysiology
of Inflammatory Muscle Pain

Dieter Pongratz
Petra Fischer
Michael Späth

SUMMARY. Objectives: Immunogenic inflammatory myopathies represent the most important group of acquired muscular disorders. Based on clinical as well as histopathological criteria they can be divided into interstitial myositis, focal nodular myositis, and polymyositis. Muscle pain is prominent especially in acute myositis, but is missed in chronic cases and especially inclusion body myositis.

Findings: Muscle pain is caused by excitation of intramuscular free nerve endings, so called nociceptors. In skeletal muscle, nociceptors seem to be preferentially localized next to small vessels. The process of nociception is mediated by endogenous substances like bradykinin, serotonin, and histamine, which are released from inflammatory cells and bind to specific receptors in the nociceptor membrane. Furthermore, neuropeptides like substance P, calcitonin-gene related peptide, or nerve growth factor, which are altered in inflammatory myopathies, may be involved in this process.

Conclusion: The concept of nociceptor sensitization by chemical stimuli, which are released during inflammation, is supported by numer-

Dieter Pongratz, MD, Petra Fischer, MD, and Michael Späth, MD, are affiliated with Friedrich-Baur-Insitut, University of Munich, Munich, Germany.

Address correspondence to: Prof. Dr. Dieter Pongratz, Friedrich-Baur-Institut, Ziemssenstr. 1a, D-80336, München, Germany [E-mail: dieter.pongratz@fbs.med.uni-muenchen.de].

[Haworth co-indexing entry note]: "Pathophysiology of Inflammatory Muscle Pain." Pongratz, Dieter, Petra Fischer, and Michael Späth. Co-published simultaneously in *Journal of Musculoskeletal Pain* [The Haworth Medical Press, an imprint of The Haworth Press, Inc.] Vol. 10, No. 1/2, 2002, pp. 121-129; and: *The Clinical Neurobiology of Fibromyalgia and Myofascial Pain: Therapeutic Implications* [ed: Robert M. Bennett] The Haworth Medical Press, an imprint of The Haworth Press, Inc., 2002, pp. 121-129. Single or multiple copies of this article are available for a fee from The Haworth Document Delivery Service [1-800-HAWORTH, 9.00 a.m. - 5.00 p.m. [EST]. E-mail address: getinfo@haworthpressinc.com].

121

ous studies, and may explain the origin of inflammatory muscle pain especially in dermatomyositis with an local effect on the intramuscular vessels. Nevertheless, the absence of muscle pain in chronic myositis and inclusion body myositis is not yet fully understood. *[Article copies available for a fee from The Haworth Document Delivery Service: 1-800-HAWORTH. E-mail address: <getinfo@haworthpressinc.com> Website: <http://www. HaworthPress.com> © 2002 by The Haworth Press, Inc. All rights reserved.]*

KEYWORDS. Pain, dermatomyositis, polymyositis, inclusion body myositis, cytokines, neuropeptides

OBJECTIVES

Inflammatory myopathies represent the most frequent and important group of acquired muscular disorders (1). Pathogenetic aspects separate infectious from immunogenic inflammatory myopathies, which are either idiopathic [i.e., dermatomyositis [DM], polymyositis [PM], and inclusion body myositis [IBM] (2)] or associated with vasculitis, neoplasia, or a connective tissue disorder.

The most prominent clinical symptoms shared by all inflammatory myopathies except very early stages of acute interstitial myositis are muscle weakness and muscular atrophies with acute muscle weakness with only slight atrophies in early stages and increasing muscular atrophies later on. Muscle pain is common, but most prominent in acute DM and less prominent or even missing in chronic forms and IBM, respectively.

Irrespective of pathogenesis, the first stage of inflammatory myopathy is an interstitial infiltration of the connective tissue without damaging the muscle parenchyma. Such forms of acute interstitial myositis are common in viral infections. The next step is a focal nodular myositis with an additional local degeneration of muscle fibers. A focal nodular myositis is found in many especially immunogenic diseases [systemic lupus erythematosus, mixed connective tissue disease, or diffuse scleroderma (3)] as well as in acute forms of PM and DM. Finally, a chronic myositis may develop, particularly in IBM and PM.

Morphology of inflammatory myopathies. A hallmark of all types of inflammatory myopathies is infiltration [B-cells, CD4+- and CD8+-T cells and macrophages] in muscle tissue. In DM, inflammatory infiltrates with B-cells and CD4 T cells are found predominantly in perivascular and perifascicular regions, producing the characteristic picture of a myositis of the perifascicular type [Figure 1a]. There are striking lesions of the small intramuscular blood vessels with endothelial proliferation and so-called tubulovesicular inclusions seen by electron microscopy. In more severe cases, especially in childhood, signs of active vasculitis and microinfarcts within the muscle can be seen. Perifascicular atrophy [Figure 1b] and fiber damage is diagnostic of DM even in the absence of infiltration. It is found in more than 50 percent of adults and in nearly all cases of childhood DM.

Deposits of C5b9 complement components within small blood vessels [Figure 2] and capillaries of muscle are very characteristic, causing destruction of the capillaries and muscle ischemia.

In PM infiltrates are predominantly endomysial, producing the picture of a diffuse myositis [Figure 3a]. Perifascicular atrophy does not develop. There is also no evidence of microangiopathy. Immunohistologically, cytotoxic CD8+ lymphocytes are the predominant cells that invade nonnecrotic muscle fibers [Figure 3b]. The muscle fibers themselves express the major histocompatibility complex class I [MHC I] antigen, which is absent in normal muscle.

Inclusion body myositis is characterized by endomysial inflammation with cluster determinant-8 positive [CD8+] lymphocytes in particular, similar to those seen in PM. In addition, rimmed vacuoles with eosinophilic cytoplasmatic inclusions can be found, as a rule, within many muscle fibers [Figure 4a.] On electronmicroscopy, the vacuoles

FIGURE 1. Polymyositis of the perifasciculare type in dermatomyositis. a. cellular perimysial infiltration [hematoxylin & eosin, original ×100]; b. perifascicular atrophy and fiber damage [adenosine triphosphatase at pH 9.4, original ×100].

a b

FIGURE 2. Complement C5b9 deposits in a small perimysial vessel [alkaline phosphatase-antialkaline phosphatase-immunostaining original ×400].

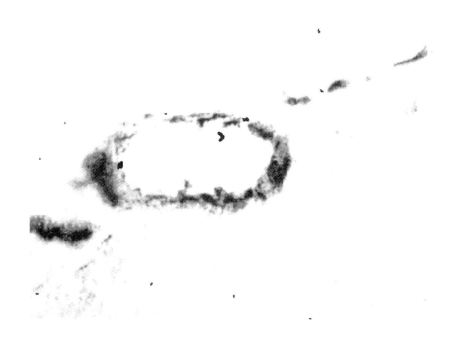

correspond to the so-called autophagic vacuoles. In addition, filamentous inclusions in the cytoplasm and nuclei are prominent but not pathognomonic [Figure 4b].

Clinical aspects. Immunogenic inflammatory myopathies [DM, PM, and IBM] are muscle diseases sharing muscle weakness as the principle clinical symptom, but reveal different clinical entities [Table 1].

Dermatomyositis is mostly an acute illness, which may affect all ages from childhood to the elderly. It is clinically characterized by skin lesions accompanying or, more often, preceding muscle symptoms. The most characteristic skin finding in DM is a heliotrope rash ["lilac disease"], involving especially the eyelids, face, and upper trunk. It can extend to other body surfaces including the elbows, knees, neck, and upper chest. More chronic skin lesions show de- and hyperpigmentations. In the skin near the knuckles violaceous scaly eruptions [sign of Gottron] occur. Dilated painful capillary loops at the base of the fingernails [sign of Keinig] are also typical. Rough and cracked areas with ir-

FIGURE 3. Diffuse polymyositis. a. endomysial infiltrates with diffuse damage of the parenchyma [hematoxylin & eosin, original ×100]; b. Cluster determinant-eight positive [CD8+]-T-cells surrounding non-necrotic muscle fibers [APAAP-technique, original ×400].

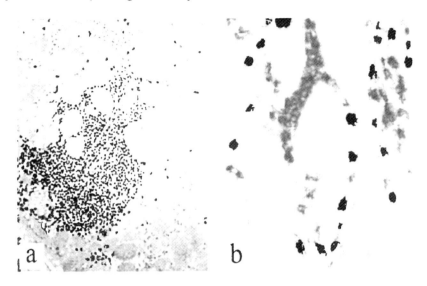

FIGURE 4. Inclusion body myositis. a. so called rimmed vacuoles [hematoxylin & eosin, original ×400]; b. filamentous inclusions in the cytoplasm [electron microscopy, courtesy of J. Müller-Höcker, Munich].

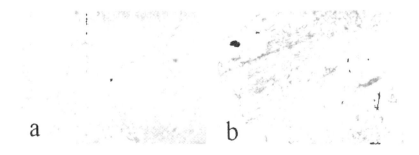

regular, dirty, horizontal lines [mechanic's hands] are also frequently found on the palmar areas of the fingers. As the disease progresses, subcutaneous calcifications occur. Muscle pain is almost always prominent.

Idiopathic PM is mostly seen in adults. The progression may be subacute or more chronic. The most prominent clinical features are weak-

TABLE 1. Classification of Immunogenic Inflammatory Myopathies

	DM	PM	IBM
Age of onset	All ages	Above 18 years	Above 50 years
Development of muscle symptoms	Acute or subacute	Subacute	Slowly
Predominant involvement of muscle weakness	Proximal muscles	Proximal muscles	Proximal and distal muscles
Muscle wasting	Not prominent	Present in chronic forms	Nearly always pronounced in selected muscles [triceps, finger flexors, quadriceps]
Muscle pain	Often [especially in acute cases]	Sometimes	Never

Abbreviations: DM = dermatomyositis, PM = polymyositis, IBM = inclusion body myositis

ness and atrophy of the proximal muscles of the limbs and arms. Cutaneous lesions are never present. Muscle pain is a fluctuating symptom and sometimes missing.

Inclusion body myositis is a disease of the elderly, affecting more men than women (4). Its progression is very slow with a characteristic, asymmetric involvement of proximal as well as distal muscles. Atrophies are prominent, myalgias never occur.

FINDINGS CONCERNING MUSCLE PAIN

The current concept of muscle pain is focusing on nociceptor-excitation (5,6). Nociceptors are free nerve endings of thin myelinated and nonmyelinated afferents. In skeletal muscle, they are preferentially found next to intramuscular capillaries. From immunohistochemical studies primary afferent sensory neurons are known to contain neuropeptides like substance P [SP] or calcitonin-gene related peptide [CGRP]. In rat skeletal muscle and in humans suffering from myositis the number of SP and CGRP positive fibers is significantly higher compared to normal controls [Späth et al., unpublished results and Figure 5]. Substance P and CGRP are both able to cause vasodilatation with a subsequent release of histamine and prostaglandins. Histamine and prostaglandins are effective stimulants of free nerve endings including muscle nociceptors (7), as are other algesic substances like bradykinin, or capsaicin, as well as electrical, mechanical stimuli, and ischemia. At the molecular level muscle nociceptors were found to express receptors for algesic sub-

FIGURE 5. Calcitonin-gene related peptide positive free nerve endings in a case of dermatomyositis [immunofluorescence, original ×400, with S. Mense, Heidelberg].

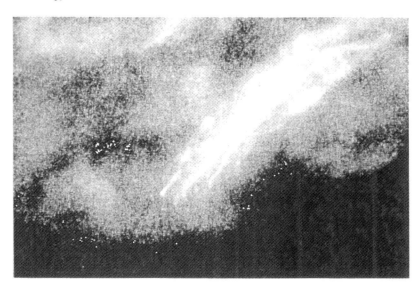

stances, which bind highly specific [like serotonin or bradykinin receptors] or unspecific [like the capsaicin receptor VR1] to their ligand. In particular, binding of algesic molecules result in nociceptor sensitization as it was shown for serotonin, which induces muscle hyperalgesia to chemical stimuli in animals and for serotonin plus bradykinin, which sensitizes muscle nociceptors to pressure in humans (8).

Several of the above mentioned algesics are endogenous substances [serotonin, bradykinin, prostaglandins, and histamine], which are known or supposed to be released from inflammatory cells, such as histamine and bradykinin, which are produced by histiocytes and lymphocytes. Thus, release of endogenous algesic substances may result in nociceptor sensitization with a subsequent increase of neuropeptides followed by SP and/or CGRP mediated vasodilatation and a further increase in endogenous algesics. Additionally, pro- and anti-inflammatory cytokines like tumor necrosis factor-alpha, interleukin [IL]-1, IL-6, and IL-10 are involved in the process of nociception, which was recently shown in rat (9) and human painful neuropathies (10). In this context, our preliminary results show an upregulation of IL-2 receptor in painful inflammatory myopathies [Fischer et al., unpublished results]. It seems to be likely, that anti-inflammatory cytokines like IL-2 may be released from inflammatory cells during inflammation to mediate the process of nociception.

CONCLUSION

Pain in inflammatory myopathies is a local pain and is caused exclusively due to an excitation of muscle nociceptors. The different sites of inflammation may explain the difference in muscle pain in DM versus IBM. Muscle pain is predominant in DM with inflammation at perivasular sites, which means, next to muscle nociceptors, and muscle pain is absent in IBM with a more endomysial distribution of inflammatory cells. On the other hand, there is a remarkable lack of correlation between the amount of inflammation and clinical symptoms in myositis patients, which is particular evident in IBM and DM patients, in whom inflammatory cells may be absent despite clinical symptoms (11).

As known to date, inflammatory muscle pain is mediated by endogenous analgetic substances resulting in sensitization of muscle nociceptors and modulated by neuropeptides, which act together in complex process, which is not yet fully understood.

REFERENCES

1. Pongratz DE and Dalakas M: Inflammatory Myopathies; Neurological Disorders: Course and Treatment. Acad. Press Inc., 1996, pp. 965-969.

2. Dalakas MC: Polymyositis, dermatomyositis, and inclusion body myositis. N Engl J Med 325: 1487-1498, 1991.

3. Genth E, Reininghaus A, and v. Muehlen CA: Serologische Befunde bei entzündlichen Muskelerkrankungen, Aktuelle Myologie. Edited by D Pongratz, CD Reimers and M Schmidt-Achert. Urban & Schwarzenberg, München, 1992, pp. 92-101.

4. Mikol J and Engel AG: Inclusion body myositis, Myology 2nd edition, Edited by AG Engel and C Franzini-Amstrong. McGraw-Hill, New York, 1994, pp. 1384-1398.

5. Graven-Nielsen T and Mense S: The peripheral apparatus of muscle pain: evidence from animal and human studies. Clin J Pain 17:2-10, 2001.

6. Mense S: Pathophysiological basis of muscle pain syndrome, Myofascial Pain. Edited by AA Fischer, Saunders, Philadelphia, 1997, pp. 23-54.

7. Pongratz D, Späth M, and Fischer P: Myositis as a cause of muscle pain. J Musculoske Pain 7(1/2):93-100, 1999.

8. Babenko V, Svensson P, Graven-Nielssen T, Drewes AM, Jensen TS, and Arent-Nielsen L: Duration and distribution of experimental muscle hyperalgesia in hu-

mans following combined infusions of serotonin and bradykinin. Brain Res 853: 275-281, 2000.

9. Okamoto K, Martin DP, Schmelzer JD, Mitsui Y, Low PA: Pro- and anti-inflammatory cytokine gene expression in rat sciatic nerve chronic constriction injury model of neuropathic pain. Exp Neurol 169:386-391, 2001.

10. Empl M, Renaud S, Erne B, Fuhr P, Straube A, Schaeren-Wiemers MAJ: TNF-alpha expression in painful and nonpainful neuropathies. Neurology 56:1371-1377, 2001.

11. Engel AG, Hohlfeld R and Banker BQ: The polymyositis and dermatomyositis syndrome, Myology 2nd edition, Edited by AG Engel and C Franzini-Amstrong. McGraw-Hill, New York, 1994, pp. 1325-1383.

Masticatory Myofascial Pain: An Explanatory Model of Regional Muscle Pain Syndromes

James R. Fricton

SUMMARY. Objectives: To review the current clinical status of masticatory myofascial pain [MMP].

Findings: Masticatory myofascial pain is a regional muscle pain disorder that is consistent with regional muscle pain disorders in other parts of the body. It is characterized by localized muscle tenderness in taut bands of skeletal muscles with associated regional and referred pain. The affected muscles may also display an increased fatigability, stiffness, subjective weakness, pain in movement, and slight restricted range of motion that is unrelated to joint restriction. Understanding these factors that contribute to the development and progression of MMP can help to validate an explanatory model for etiology and treatment of MMP. This model includes peripheral mechanisms from local repetitive biomechanical strain leading to the onset of early cases of MMP while central mechanisms associated with systemic and psychosocial factors lead to increased chronicity of MMP. Management of the syndrome naturally follows

James R. Fricton, DDS, MS, is affiliated with the Department of Diagnostic and Surgical Sciences, University of Minnesota School of Dentistry, Minneapolis, MN 55455.

Address correspondence to: James R. Fricton, DDS, MS, 6-320 Moos Tower, Division of TMD and Orofacial Pain, University of Minnesota School of Dentistry, Minneapolis, MN 55455.

Funding for this project by NIDR R23 DEO746-03 and NIDR R01DE11252 have helped contribute to the development of this paper.

[Haworth co-indexing entry note]: "Masticatory Myofascial Pain: An Explanatory Model of Regional Muscle Pain Syndromes." Fricton, James R. Co-published simultaneously in *Journal of Musculoskeletal Pain* [The Haworth Medical Press, an imprint of The Haworth Press, Inc.] Vol. 10, No. 1/2, 2002, pp. 131-150; and: *The Clinical Neurobiology of Fibromyalgia and Myofascial Pain: Therapeutic Implications* [ed: Robert M. Bennett] The Haworth Medical Press, an imprint of The Haworth Press, Inc., 2002, pp. 131-150. Single or multiple copies of this article are available for a fee from The Haworth Document Delivery Service [1-800-HAWORTH, 9:00 a.m. - 5:00 p.m. [EST]. E-mail address: getinfo@haworthpressinc.com].

131

from this model with therapy to rehabilitate the trigger points while focusing effort on reducing both regional and central contributing factors.

Conclusions: Pain in the masticatory muscle region should be evaluated thoroughly seeking evidence for MMP. The historical and examination features can help to make a prospective diagnosis based on established clinical criteria. Treatment of this condition, based on a painful muscle model, can be very rewarding. *[Article copies available for a fee from The Haworth Document Delivery Service: 1-800-HAWORTH. E-mail address: <getinfo@haworthpressinc.com> Website: <http://www.HaworthPress.com> © 2002 by The Haworth Press, Inc. All rights reserved.]*

KEYWORDS. Myofascial pain, muscles, pain, etiology, mechanisms

The myofascial pain syndrome [MPS] is a regional muscle pain disorder characterized by localized muscle tenderness and pain and is a common cause of persistent regional pain such as back pain, neck pain, shoulder pain, headaches, and orofacial pain. The affected muscles often display an increased fatigability, stiffness, subjective weakness, pain in movement, and slight restricted range of motion that is unrelated to joint restriction. Although the exact etiology of MPS is unclear, recent clinical, epidemiological, and basic research has improved our understanding of the development and underlying peripheral and central mechanisms associated with MPS. The purpose of this paper is to discuss this recent knowledge and implications for an explanatory model of etiology and treatment for MPS.

CLINICAL CHARACTERISTICS

The major characteristics of MPS include tenderness in muscles termed trigger points [TrP] and local and referred pain. However MPS, particularly in the head and neck, have numerous ancillary findings and common associations with joint disorders and other pain disorders that can confuse diagnosis.

Trigger Points

A TrP can be characterized as a 2 to 5 mm diameter point of hypersensitivity to pressure in a palpable taut band of skeletal muscle, tendon, and ligament with decreasing hypersensitivity as one palpates the band further away from the TrP. Active TrPs are hypersensitive and display continuous pain in the zone of reference that can be altered with specific palpation (1). Latent TrPs display only hypersensitivity with no continuous pain. This localized tenderness has been found to be a reliable indicator of the presence and severity of MPS with both manual palpation and pressure algometry (2-4). However, the presence of taut bands appears to be a characteristic of skeletal muscles in all subjects regardless of the presence of MPS (5). Palpating the active TrP with sustained deep single finger pressure on the taut band will elicit an alteration of the pain [intensify or reduce] in the zone of reference [area of pain complaint] or cause radiation of the pain towards the zone of reference. This can occur immediately or be delayed a few seconds. The pattern of referral is both reproducible and consistent with patterns of other patients with similar TrPs [Table 1]. Figure 1 shows three examples of MPS involving different muscles of mastication.

Local and Referred Pain

In examining the basic concept of MPS, namely local and referred pain from TrPs, there must be evidence that supports the concept that the pain is related to and/or generated by the TrP, particularly if it is distant from the TrP. This evidence primarily stems from clinical observation and needs to be studied more rigorously in well controlled scientific studies. First, clinical examination of TrPs demonstrates that in accessible muscles palpation of the active TrPs will alter the referred pain [usually intensification]. In addition, injections of local anesthetic into the

TABLE 1. Clinical Characteristics of Myofascial Pain Syndrome

Trigger Points in Taut Band of Muscle	Pain in Zone of Reference
Tenderness on palpation	Constant dull ache
Consistent points of tenderness	Fluctuates in intensity
Palpation alters pain locally or distant	Consistent patterns of referral
	Alleviation with extinction of trigger point
Associated symptoms	Contributing factors
Otologic	Traumatic and whiplash injuries
Paresthesias	Occupational and repetitive strain injuries
Gastrointestinal distress	Disuse
Visual disturbances	Parafunctional muscle tension producing habits
Dermatographia	Postural and repetitive strains
	Metabolic/Nutritional
	Sleep disturbance
	Psychosocial and emotional stressors

active TrP will reduce or eliminate the referred pain and the tenderness (6,7). Treatment such as spray and stretch, exercises, or massage, directed at the muscle with the TrP will also predictably reduce the referred pain (8). Other evidence to confirm the relationship includes the use of pressure algometry to show a positive correlation between both the scope of tenderness and the severity of pain (9). In addition, the change in scope of tenderness in response to treatment correlates positively with the change in symptom severity [r = .54] (9).

FIGURE 1. Three examples of trigger points [TrP] in masticatory muscles with associated regions of referred pain. Panel A. The TrP syndrome involving the temporalis causes pain in the temple area, frontal area, retro-orbital area, and the anterior teeth of the maxilla. A common symptom associated with this syndrome is sensitivity of the teeth in the affected area. Panel B. The TrP syndrome involving the deep masseter muscle causes pain in the area anterior to the ear, pain that may be interpreted as ear ache, and of the posterior teeth of the maxilla. A common symptom associated with this syndrome is sensitivity of the teeth in the affected area. Panel C. The TrP syndrome involving the splenius capitus muscle causes pain in the frontal, vertex, occipital areas and at the back of the neck. A common syndrome associated with involvement of this muscle is migraine headache.

Panel A:

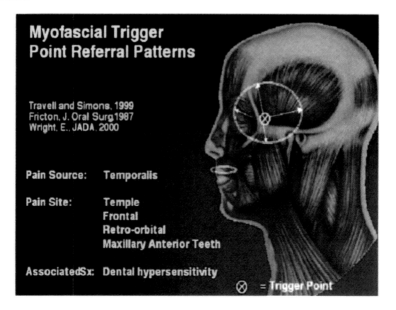

Panel B:

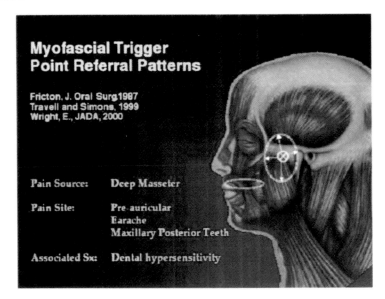

Panel C:

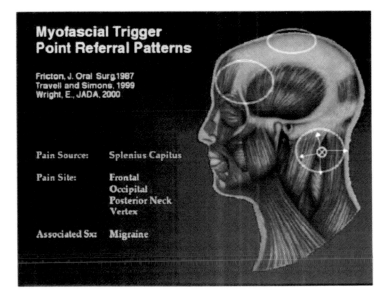

Ancillary Findings and Relationship with Other Disorders

The affected muscles may also display an increased fatigability, stiffness, subjective weakness, pain in movement, and slight restricted range of motion that is unrelated to joint restriction (1,10). The muscles are painful when stretched, causing the patient to protect the muscle through poor posture and sustained contraction (1). Although routine clinical electromyographic [EMG] studies show no significant abnormalities associated with TrPs, some specialized EMG studies such as the local twitch response reveal differences (11,12). The consistency of soft tissues over the TrPs has been found to be more than adjacent muscles (13,14). Skin overlying the TrPs in the masseter muscle appears to be warmer as measured by infrared emission (15,16).

PREVALENCE

Because of this lack of objective findings and clear etiology, MPS is often overlooked as a common cause of persistent pain. Yet numerous studies have suggested that this disorder is a common cause of back pain, headache, neck pain, orofacial pain, and other persistent pain problems. For example, two studies of pain clinic populations have revealed that MPS was cited as the most common cause of pain responsible for 54.6 percent of a chronic head and neck pain population (10) and 85 percent of a back pain population (17). In addition, Skootsky et al. (18) studied MPS in a general internal medicine practice and found that among those patients that present with pain, 29.6 percent were found to have MPS as the cause of the pain. An epidemiological study of orofacial pain in a young female general population [age 20-40] using specific criteria, Schiffman et al. (19) found that MPS in the masticatory muscles occurred in about 50 percent of this general population with six percent having symptoms severe enough to be comparable to patients seeking treatment.

RISK FACTORS FOR DEVELOPMENT AND PROGRESSION OF MASTICATORY MYOFASCIAL PAIN

When symptomatic MPS of the muscles of mastication becomes chronic and intractable, it is referred to as masticatory myofascial pain [MMP]. It is important to review the risk factors related to the full temporal progression of MPS from onset, to acute and mild, to chronic and severe, and finally to those few cases who progress into a chronic, intractable MMP syndrome. Figure 2 illustrates this progression and the associated risk factors classification. Although there have been many studies examining aspects of this progression, a series of studies at the University of Minnesota will illustrate how some of the risk factors associated with each step in the progression were identified.

In one case series study of 164 consecutive patients presenting with head and neck pain that was diagnosed as MPS, onset factors as self reported by the patient was studied (10). Trauma was the most common onset factor at 50.6 percent. Traumatic events included motor vehicle accidents, dental visits, oral surgery, and other. About 30.1 percent had no known onset factors. In these cases of insidious onset, it is possible that the cumulative effects of repetitive strain play a role.

Only longitudinal studies can determine risk factors for progression of MMP. A longitudinal study of 269 young female nursing students at the University of Minnesota was conducted to study of the development

FIGURE 2. All intractable chronic pain syndromes begin as an acute problem and progress into chronic pain in association with specific risk factors that are associated with this progression. Research has suggested that the factors listed in this figure play a role in progression to masticatory myofascial pain.

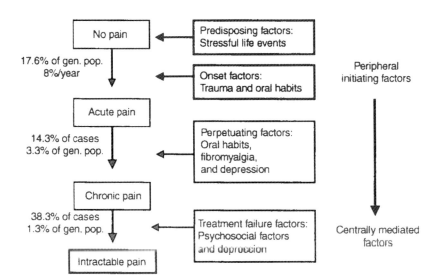

and risk factors associated with temporomandibular disorders [TMD] including MMP (20). At baseline, 31 percent of the subjects met specific criteria for normal [N = 83] and were followed at 18 months and 36 months for the onset and risk factors associated with development of MMP. All subjects were administered a signed consent form, questionnaire, and a clinical examination. The questionnaire included questions regarding the presence of symptoms, initiating events, care seeking, and items to determine the Symptom Severity Index (9), Oral Habit Index (20), and the Social Readjustment Rating Scale (21). The calibrated examination included items assessing the Craniomandibular Index (2,9) and included mandibular movement, temporomandibular joint [TMJ] noise, structural and functional aspects of malocclusion, muscle and joint tenderness, and indicators of parafunctional habits. Stressful life events, oral habits such as clenching and grinding of the teeth, and malocclusion were evaluated for their predictive ability in the process of onset or perpetuation of MMP.

The results demonstrated that 14.9 percent and 16.3 percent of the normal subjects developed MMP either with or without accompanied TMJ problems over 18 months and 36 months, respectively, suggesting an annual incidence of about eight percent in this higher risk young female population. Oral habits and stressful life events were significant factors involved in the development of MMP. Stress was the only factor that was a predictor at baseline showing statistical differences between those who developed MMP at 18 months versus those who did not [P = .01] suggesting this is a predisposing factor. Oral habits were the only factor that significantly differentiated the groups at the 18 months [P = .02], suggesting that this may be an initiating or perpetuating factor. Occlusal disharmony as measured here was not associated with the development of MMP problems at any point for this normal group suggesting that occlusion may only be a cofactor in MMP.

Another longitudinal study examined the risk factors for progression of acute noncomplex TMD patients to chronic complex disorders in 600 subjects using similar methodology as the previous described study (22). This prospective longitudinal observational study design completed identical data collection at baseline and at 18 month follow-up with 232 subjects of 243 [95 percent] at time of analysis. Among the subjects 90.5 percent were females with a mean age of 33.5 ± 11.2 years. An analysis of the relationship of baseline risk factors on progression in Chronic Pain Grade and pain severity was conducted by Von Korff and colleagues (23). Both unadjusted analysis, using Proc Freq

[SAS Institute], and adjusted analysis, controlling for gender and age using Proc Logistic [SAS Institute], were conducted. The preliminary results found that 14.3 percent of subjects progressed to a more severe Chronic Pain Grade [CPG] with increased pain and interference. Depression at baseline was a significant predictor for progression in CPG [P < 0.04]. A subject with depression had a 2.61 times higher odds of progressing in CPG. The presence of a widespread pain disorder, like fibromyalgia, at baseline was a significant predictor for progression in CPG [P < 0.004]. A subject with fibromyalgia had a 4.66 times higher odds of progressing in CPG. Finally, oral habits at baseline was a significant predictor for progression in pain severity [P < 0.05]. A subject with high oral habits had a 2.35 times higher odds of progressing in pain severity.

Another important area of research recently has been efforts to determine which risk factors are important in delaying recovery in patients who develop MPS, and thus, contributing to further development of MPS into chronic intractable pain syndrome. As with all chronic pain conditions, concomitant physical, social, behavioral, and psychological disturbances often precede or follow the development of MMP (24). We conducted a study to determine which factors among physical, demographic, behavioral, and psychosocial factors were significant in delaying the recovery of patients with MMP.

In this study, 94 subjects with MMP were studied using a validated assessment instrument called "Integrated Multi-Dimensional Patient Assessment Tool for Health" [IMPATH:TMJ] prior to their entering an interdisciplinary treatment program to determine which factors were most predictive of outcome (9,24-26). Treatment outcome was determined based on significant decreases in the Craniomandibular Index and the Symptom Severity Index from pre- to post-treatment. The data obtained from IMPATH:TMJ were regressed on treatment outcome for a random sample of half of the subjects [N = 47] to isolate the psychosocial and demographic items most predictive of treatment response. Discriminant analysis was then employed to test the predictive utility of the identified items for these subjects [criterion group], followed by a cross-validation of the items on the remaining 47 subjects [cross-validation group].

Low self-esteem, feel worried, low energy, and sleep activity were identified as useful predictors of treatment outcome for the criterion group. Each are correlates of depression. The discriminant analysis employing these four items accounted for 49 percent of the variance in treatment response, was statistically significant [P < .0001] and correctly predicted treatment, outcome for 41 out of 47 subjects [87 percent] in the criterion group. The predictive utility of the identified items remained statistically significant when applied to the cross-validation group [P < .01], as the discriminant function employing the items correctly predicted treatment outcome for 37 out of 47 subjects [79 percent], and explained for 28 percent of the variance in treatment response. Findings of this study suggest that pretreatment psychosocial information is important in predicting treatment outcome for chronic TMD, and that symptoms of depression mediate treatment response for chronic pain patients. Twenty-nine of 47 [61.7 percent] in the criterion group and 27 of the 47 subjects [57.4 percent] in the cross validation group were classified as "successfully treated" at post-treatment. While this is considerably less than the 70-90 percent success rate which is typically reported for TMD patients (26), it should be noted that the study employed stringent criteria for determining treatment success and all subjects had had chronic temporomandibular pain for at least six months.

Stepwise multiple regression was the statistical procedure used to isolate IMPATH:TMJ items predictive of treatment outcome. Each cluster of IMPATH:TMJ items [i.e., demographics, emotions, behaviors, cognition, and social] was separately regressed on treatment outcome [success or failure to identify items most predictive of treatment response from each of the psychosocial components theorized to contribute to the experience of chronic pain]. This process yielded a total of 10 potential predictors of poor treatment response for chronic temporomandibular subjects. These items included poor attitude about success of treatment, low self-esteem, low energy, feeling worried, low level of sexual activity, poor eating habits, poor sleep, feeling confused, unrealistic expectations on reducing problem, and frequent use of the problem as an excuse to avoid activities.

MECHANISMS OF MYOFASCIAL PAIN

The results of this research suggest that an explanatory model can account for the mechanisms in the development of MMP from its onset to increasing severity found with clinical and chronic cases. It is apparent that both central and peripheral mechanisms are associated with this process. However, the nature of the peripheral neuropathological and/or dysfunctional processes of MPS TrPs and the central nervous changes associated with the regional pain are still not fully understood. A number of histologic and biochemical studies have been completed on biopsies of tender points in patients with both generalized and regional muscle complaints. These studies suggest that there is localized progressive increases in oxidative metabolism particularly in muscle fiber type I with depleted energy supply, increase in metabolic by-products or inflammatory mediators and resultant muscle nociception at the periphery. This results in local and referred pain in the central nervous system that can be altered by a central biasing mechanism that either amplifies or suppresses the pain.

Injury to Muscle Fiber Type I

Each skeletal muscle has different proportions of muscle fiber types that group into three broad categories, type I, type IIA, and type IIB [Table 2] (27) [type IIC and IIM are involved in development and are not frequently seen in the adult masticatory muscles]. Type I muscle fiber are functionally associated with static muscle tone and posture. They are slow twitch, fatigue resistant fibers with a high number of mitochondria needed for oxidative phosphorylation used in energy metabolism. Type II fibers are functionally associated with increased velocity and force of contraction over brief periods. They are fast twitch fibers that fatigue easily, are rich in glycogen, and use anaerobic glycolysis for energy metabolism. These fiber types can transform from one type to another depending on the demands placed on a muscle. For example, Uhlig and colleagues found signs of fiber transformation from type I to type IIc fibers in cervical muscles associated with pain and dysfunction after spondylodesis (28). This is consistent with transformation associated with prolonged inactivity due to the injury. Furthermore, Mayo and colleagues found decreases in the cross sectional diameter of muscle fiber type I and II in the masticatory system in rhesus monkeys undergoing maxillomandibular fixation (29).

Thus, transformation due to inactivity and pain can decrease both the percent and size of type I fibers available to maintain normal postural and resting muscle activity. On the other hand, an increase in demands of postural muscle activity may result in an increase in type I fibers and a decrease in type II fibers as found by Bengsston and colleagues in muscle pain patients (30,31). If the increased demand placed on the type I fiber types due to repetitive strain from activities such as clenching or gum chewing is beyond normal physiologic parameters, the intracellular components of these fibers will be damaged. This will result in hyper-polarization outside the muscle due to high levels of potassium ion from sustained motor unit activity and K^+ pump damage, damage to the actin and myosin myofilaments, disruption of the sarcoplasmic re-

TABLE 2. Characteristics of Muscle Fiber Types I, IIA, and IIB in Masticatory Muscles. Type IIC and IIM Are Primarily Involved in Growth and Development and Not Often Seen in Skeletal Muscles of the Masticatory System. Adapted from Miller A (54)

| | Major Fiber Types | | |
	Type I [red]	Type IIA [pink]	Type IIB [white]
Staining	Weak–ATPase [light pink] Strong NADH-TR [dark pink]	Strong–ATPase [light pink] Strong NADH-TR [dark pink]	Strong–ATPase [light pink) Weak NADH-TR [dark pink]
Contraction speed and fatigue	Slow twitch Without fatigue Gradual recruitment to maximal force	Fast twitch Fatigue resistant Higher threshold to recruitment	Slow twitch Fatigue resistant Develops highest muscle tension
Cellular characteristics	Low glycogen High # of mitochondria High oxidative enzymes Slow myosin	Low glycogen Low # of mitochondria Low oxidative enzymes Fast myosin	Rich in glycogen Low # of mitochondria Low oxidative enzymes Fast myosin
Morphology	1. Less in deep masseter with short face 2. More with loss of teeth	1. More in deep masseter with short face 2. Less with loss of teeth	1. Hypertrophy with long face 2. Less with loss of teeth
Function	Posture Sustained low force contraction Increase muscle length does not alter function or morphology	Long-term use Sustained high force contraction Increase muscle length does not alter function or morphology	Strength Brief high force contraction Increase muscle length does not alter function or morphology
Response to electrical stimulation	At 50 Hz: Type I to II Increase glycogen Decreased mitochondria	At 10 Hz: Type II to I Decrease glycogen Increased mitochondria	At 10 Hz: Type II to I Decrease glycogen Increased mitochondria
Metabolism	Oxidative phosphorylation	Glycolytic	Glycolytic

ticulum and the calcium pump, and decrease in local blood flow. Specific factors that were important in initiating this process included both direct macrotrauma and indirect microtrauma from repetitive strain factors such as clenching and grinding of the teeth.

Metabolic Distress at the Motor End Plates

In explaining the local nature of MPS TrPs, Simons (32) suggests that the damage to the muscle occurs primarily at the motor endplates creating an energy crisis at the TrP (32). He suggests that this crisis occurs from grossly abnormal increase in acetylcholine release at the endplate and generation of numerous miniature endplate potentials, resulting in an increase in energy demand, sustained depolarization of the post-junction membrane, and mitochondrial changes. Other studies support this mechanism (12,33-35). For example, Hubbard and Berkoff found spontaneous EMG activity at the TrP (12). Hong and Torigoe found that the EMG characteristics of the local twitch response are generated locally without input from the central nervous system [CNS] (34). Also, botulinum A toxin injections that act on the neuromuscular junction only have also been shown to be effective in MPS TrPs (33).

Histologic studies also provide some support to this mechanism. They have shown myofibrillar lysis, moth eaten fibers, and ragged red type I fibers with deposition of glycogen and abnormal mitochondria but little evidence of cellular inflammation hypothesis (31,36). Studies of muscle energy metabolism found a decrease in the levels of adenosine triphosphate, adenosine diphosphate, phosphoryl creatine, and abnormal tissue oxygenation in muscles with TrPs (30). El-Labban and colleagues (37) demonstrated histological that TMJ ankylosis will result in degenerative changes in masseter and temporalis muscles. It has been hypothesized that these changes represent localized progressive increases in oxidative metabolism and depleted energy supply in type I fibers [Table 3]. This may result in progressive abnormal muscle changes that initially include reactive dysfunctional changes occurring within the muscle, particularly muscle fiber type I and surrounding connective tissue (36).

Activation of Muscle Nociceptors

The resulting metabolic by-products of this damage, whether it be inflammatory mediators such as bradykinin from tissue damage or meta-

TABLE 3. The Percent of Each Muscle Fiber Type in Masticatory Muscles. Type I Muscles Are Slow Twitch Fatigue Resistant and Are Involved in Postural Muscle Tone and Sustained Contraction While Type II Are Fast Twitch Fatigue Prone and Are Involved in Activities Involving High Force and Velocity. Adapted from Miller A (54)

Percent of Each Muscle Fiber Type in Masticatory Muscles

Masticatory Muscle	I	IM	IIA	IIB	IIC
Masseter	63	6	2	27	3
Medial Pterygoid	54	8	0	6	2
Temporalis	53	5	0	39	2
Lateral Pterygoid	70	14	0	11	5
Digastric	34	0	27	38	0

bolic by-products such as high adenosine triphosphate or potassium from damage to the cellular structures, the result can be peripheral sensitization of nociceptors in the muscle, fatigue, and disuse (38). Localized tenderness and pain in the muscle involve type III and IV muscle nociceptors [Table 4] and has shown to be activated by noxious substances including potassium, bradykinin, histamine, or prostaglandins that can be released locally from the damage and trigger tenderness (39-44). It is important to note the potassium activated a higher percent of type IV muscle nociceptors than other agents supporting the concept that localized increases in potassium at the neuromuscular junction may be responsible for sensitization of nociceptors. This peripheral sensitization is thought to play a major role in local tenderness and pain together with central sensitization to produce hyperalgesia in patients with persistent muscle pain.

Transmission of Pain to the Central Nervous System

The afferent inputs from type III and IV muscle nociceptors in the body are transmitted to the CNS through cells such as those of the lamina I, V, and possibly IV of the dorsal horn on the way to the cortex,

TABLE 4. The Percent of Nociceptor Stimulated by Different Noxious Substances in the Cat. Adapted from Kniffki et al. and Mense S (39,55). It Is Suggested That Sensitization of Type III Muscle Afferents Is Responsible for Increased Resting Spontaneous Pain While Sensitization of Type IV Muscle Afferents Is Responsible for Transmitting Increased Tenderness of the Tissues

Noxious Stimulant	Muscle Afferent Type	Percent of Afferent Activated
Potassium	IV	63
Bradykinin	IV	53
Local pressure	IV	45
Repetitive contraction	IV	19
Sustained stretch	IV	17
Lactate	IV	12
Phosphate	IV	10
Algesic chemicals [K+, bradykinin, histamine]	IA	0
Algesic chemicals	IB	0
Algesic chemicals	III	67
Algesic chemicals	IV	50

resulting in perception of local pain (45,46) [Figure 3]. However, in the trigeminal system, these afferent inputs project to the second order neurons in the brain stem regions including the superficial lamina of trigeminal subnucleus caudalis as well as its more rostral lamina such as interpolaris and oralis (47,48). These neurons can then project to neurons in higher levels of the CNS such as the thalamus, cranial motor nuclei, or the reticular formation (49). In the thalamus, the ventrobasal

FIGURE 3. This figure shows the major trigeminal pathways transmitting sensory information from the mouth, temporomandibular joint, jaw muscles, and face (48). Primary afferents from the muscles project through the trigeminal ganglion [Gasserian] to second order neurons in the brain stem complex. These will project to neurons in higher levels of the central nervous system including the thalamus, the cranial nerve motor nuclei, or reticular formation. (Printed with permission of Lippincott Williams & Wilkins from *Advances in Pain Research and Therapy* 22:413-421, 1995.)

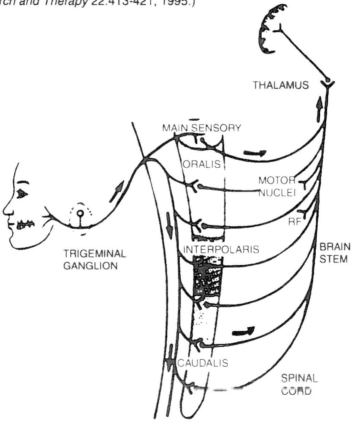

complex, the posterior group of nuclei, and parts of the medial thalamus are involved in receiving and relaying somatosensory information (50). These inputs can also converge with other visceral and somatic inputs from tissues such as the joint or skin and be responsible for referred pain perception (49).

Modification of Central Nociceptive Input

Nociceptive inputs have been shown to be modified by multiple factors in their transmission to the CNS. For example, low- and high-intensity electrical stimulation of sensory nerves or noxious stimulation of sites remote from site of pain will suppress nociceptive responses of trigeminal brain stem neurons and related reflexes (48). This provides support that afferent inputs can be *inhibited* by multiple peripherally or centrally initiated alterations in neural input to the brain stem through various treatment modalities such as cold, heat, analgesic medications, massage, muscular injections, and transcutaneous electrical stimulation (44).

Likewise, persistent peripheral or central nociceptive activity can result in an increase in abnormal neuroplastic changes in cutaneous and deep neurons. These neuroplastic changes may included prolonged responsiveness to afferent inputs, increased receptive field size, and spontaneous bursts of activity (51-53). Thus, peripheral inputs from muscles may also be *facilitated or accentuated* by multiple peripherally or centrally initiated alterations in neural input with further sustained neural activity such as persistent joint pain, sustained muscle activity from clenching or postural tension, or CNS alterations such as depression and anxiety that can support the central sensitization further perpetuating the problem.

These alterations constitute an integrated "central biasing mechanism" in the CNS that will dampen or accentuate peripheral input (44). This mechanism may explain many of the characteristics of MPS including the broad regions of pain referral, the recruitment of additional muscles in chronic cases, the interrelationship between muscle and joint pain, and the ability of many treatments including medication, spray and stretch, massage, and TrP injections to reduce the pain for longer than the duration of action.

CONCLUSION

Masticatory myofascial pain is a regional muscle pain disorder of the muscles of mastication characterized by localized muscle tenderness and pain and the most common causes of persistent regional pain in the jaw, temples, and head. Both peripheral neuropathological and central pathological processes are active in the development and perpetuation of MMP. Factors that perpetuate MMP include sustained contraction of the muscle, coincidental pathology conditions, such as temporomandibular joint disorders, and behavioral and psychosocial problems. As MMP persists, chronic pain characteristics often precede or follow its development and further complicate treatment. Early treatment of MMP and its contributing factors is recommended.

REFERENCES

1. Travell J, Simons DG: Myofascial Pain and Dysfunction: The Trigger Point Manual. Baltimore, Williams & Wilkins Co., 1998.

2. Fricton JR, Schiffman EL: Reliability of a craniomandibular index. J Dent Res 65(11):1359, 1986.

3. Schiffman E, Fricton JR, Haley D, Tylka D: A pressure algometer for MPS: reliability and validity. Pain 4(supp):S291, 1987.

4. Reeves J, Jaeger, B, Graff-Radford, SB: Reliability of the pressure algometer as a measure of myofascial trigger point sensitivity. Pain 24(3):313, 1986.

5. Fricton J: Myofascial pain: clinical characteristics and diagnostic criteria. J Muskuloske Pain 1(3/4):37, 1993.

6. Jaeger B, Skootsky SA: Double blind, controlled study of different myofascial trigger point injection techniques. Pain 4(supp):S292, 1987.

7. Cifala J: Myofascial (trigger point pain) injection: theory and treatment. Osteopath Med April:31, 1979.

8. Jaeger B, Reeves JL: Quantification of changes in myofascial trigger point sensitivity with the pressure algometer following passive stretch. Pain 27(2):203, 1986.

9. Fricton JR, Schiffman EL: The craniomandibular index: validity. J Prosthetic Dent 58(2):222, 1987.

10. Fricton J, Kroening R, Haley D, Siegert R: Myofascial pain syndrome of the head and neck: a review of clinical characteristics of 164 patients. Oral Surgery, Oral Med Oral Path 60(6):615, 1985.

11. Fricton J, Auvinen MD, Dykstra D, Schiffman E: Myofascial pain syndrome: electromyographic changes associated with local twitch response. Arch Phys Med Rehabil 66(5):314, 1985.

12. Hubbard DR, Berkoff GM: Myofascial trigger points show spontaneous needle EMG activity. Spine 18:1803, 1993.

13. Fischer AA: Tissue compliance meter for objective, quantitative documentation of soft tissue consistency and pathology. Arch Phys Med Rehabil 68(2):122, 1987.

14. Fischer A: Documentation of myofascial trigger points. [Review]. Arch Phys Med Rehabil 69(4):286, 1988.

15. Berry DC, Yemm R: Variations in skin temperature of the face in normal subjects and in patients with mandibular dysfunction. Brit J Oral Surg 8(3):242, 1971.

16. Berry DC, Yemm R: A further study of facial skin temperature in patients with mandibular dysfunction. J Oral Rehabil 1(3):255, 1974.

17. Fishbain D, Goldberg M, Meagher BR, Steele R, Rosomoff H: Male and female chronic pain patients categorized by DSM-III psychiatric diagnostic criteria. Pain 26(2):181, 1986.

18. Skootsky S, Jaeger B, Oye RK: Prevalence of myofascial pain in general internal medicine practice. West J Med 151(2):157, 1989.

19. Schiffman E, Fricton JR, Haley DP, Shapiro BL: The prevalence and treatment needs of subjects with temporomandibular disorders. J Am Dent Assoc 120(3): 295, 1990.

20. Schiffman E, Fricton JR, Haley D: The relationship of occlusion, parafunctional habits and recent life events to mandibular dysfunction in a non-patient population. J Oral Rehabil 19(3):201, 1992.

21. Holmes TH, Rahe RH: The Social Readjustment Rating Scale. J Psyc Res 11(2):213, 1967.

22. Fricton JR, Look JO, Jackson AK, Carlson PL, Lenton PA, Hodges JS: Depression: a risk factor for progression of TMD chronic pain grade. J Dent Res 80 (special issue) 154, 2001, (abst).

23. Von Korff M, Ormel J, Keefe FJ, Dworkin SF: Grading the severity of chronic pain. Pain 50(2):133-149, 1992.

24. Fricton JR, Olsen T: Predictors of outcome for treatment of temporomandibular disorders. J Orofacial Pain 10(1):54, 1996.

25. Fricton JR, Nelson A, Monsein M: IMPATH: microcomputer assessment of behavioral and psychosocial factors in craniomandibular disorders. Cranio 5(4): 372-381, 1987.

26. Fricton JR: Measuring outcome of treatment for temporomandibular disorders. In Fricton JR, Dubner R (eds): Orofacial Pain and Temporomandibular Disorders, vol 21. New York, Raven Press, 1995, p. 165.

27. Eriksson PO, Thornell LE: Histochemical and morphological mucscle-fiber charateristics of the human masseter, the medial pterygoid, and the temporal muscles. Arch Oral Biol 28:781, 1983.

28. Uhlig Y, Weber BR, Grob D, Muntener M: Fiber composition and fiber transformation in neck muscles of patients with dysfunction of the cervical spine. J Ortho Res 13:240, 1995.

29. Mayo KH, Ellis III E, Carlson DS: Histochemical characteristics of masseter and temporalis muscles after 5 weeks of maxillomandibular fixation–An investigation in Macaca mulatta. Oral Surg Oral Med Oral Pathol 66:421, 1988.

30. Bengtsson A, Henriksson KG, Larsson J: Reduced high-energy phosphate levels in the painful muscles of patients with primary fibromyalgia. Arthritis Rheum 29(7):817, 1986.

31. Bengtsson A, Henriksson KG, Jorfeldt L, Kagedal B, Lennmarken C, Lindstrom F: Primary fibromyalgia. A clinical and laboratory study of 55 patients. Scand J Rheumatol 15(3):340, 1986.

32. Simons DG: Myofascial trigger points: the critical experiment. J Musculoske Pain 5(4):113, 1997.

33. Cheshire WP, Abashian SW, Mann JD: Botulinum toxin in the treatment of myofascial pain syndrome. Pain (59):65, 1994.

34. Hong C-Z, Torigoe Y: Electrophysiological charateristics of localized twitch responses in responsive taut bands of rabbit skeletal muscle. J Musculoske Pain 2(2):17, 1994.

35. Hong C-Z: Persistence of local twitch response with loss of conduction to and from the spinal cord. Arch Phys Med Rehabilil 75:12, 1994.

36. Yunus M, Kalyan-Raman UP, Kalyan-Raman K, Masi AT: Pathologic changes in muscle in primary fibromyalgia syndrome. Am J Med 81(3A):38, 1986.

37. El-Labban NG, Harris M, Hopper C, Barber P: Degenerative changes in masseter and temporalis muscles in limited mouth opening and TMJ ankylosis. Oral Pathol Med 19:423, 1990.

38. Mao J, Stein RB, Osborn JW: Fatigue in human jaw muscles: a review. J Orofacial Pain 7:135, 1993.

39. Kniffki K, Mense S, Schmidt RF: Responses of group IV afferent units from skeletal muscle to stretch, contraction and chemical stimulation. Exp Brain Res 31(4):511, 1978.

40. Lim R, Guzman F, Rodgers DW: Note on the muscle receptors concerned with pain. In Barker D (ed): Symposium on Muscle Receptors. Hong Kong, Hong Kong University Press, 1962, p. 215.

41. Mense S, Schmidt RF: Muscle pain: which receptors are responsible for the transmission of noxious stimuli? pp. 265-78. In: Rose FC, ed. Physiological Aspects of Clinical Neurology. Oxford, Blackwell Scientific Publications 102:575, 1977.

42. Pomeranz B, Wall PD, Weber WV: Cord cells responding to fine myelinated afferents from viscera, muscle and skin. J Physiol 199(3):511, 1968.

43. Selzer M, Spencer WA: Convergence of visceral and cutaneous afferent pathways in the lumbar spinal cord. Brain Res 14(2):331, 1969.

44. Melzack R: Myofascial trigger points: relation to acupuncture and mechanisms of pain. Arch Phys Med Rehabil 62(3):114, 1981.

45. Dubner R, Bennett GJ: Spinal and trigeminal mechanisms of nociception. [Review]. Ann Rev Neurosci 6:381, 1983.

46. Dubner R: Hyperalgesia in response to injury to cutaneous and deep tissues. In: Fricton J, Dubner R (eds): Orofacial Pain and Temporomandibular Disorders. New York, Raven Press, Ltd., 1995, p. 61.

47. Sessle BJ, Bryant PS, Dionne RA: Temporomandibular disorders and related pain conditions. Progress in Pain Research and Management, vol 4. Seattle, IASP Press, 1995, p. 492.

48. Sessle B: Brainstem mechanisms of orofacial pain. In: Fricton J, Dubner R (eds): Orofacial Pain and Temporomandibular Disorders. New York, Raven Press, Ltd., 1995, p. 43.

49. Sessle BJ: Masticatory muscle disorders: basic science perspectives. In: Sessle BJ, Bryant PS, Dionne RA (eds.): Temporomandibular Disorders and Related Pain Conditions: Progr Pain Res Ther, vol 4. Seattle, IASP Press, 1995, p. 47.

50. Willis WD: The Pain System. Basel, Karger, 1985.

51. Mense S: Nociception from skeletal muscle in relation to clinical muscle pain. Pain 54:241, 1993.

52. Guilbaud G: Central neurophysiological processing of joint pain on the basis of studies performed in normal animals and in models of experimental arthritis. Can J Physiol Pharmacol 69:637, 1991.

53. Dubner R: Neuronal plasticity in the spinal dorsal horn following tissue inflammation. In: Inoki R, Shigenaga Y, Tohyama M (eds.): Processing and Inhibition of Nociceptive Information. Tokyo, Excerpta Medica, 1992, p. 35.

54. Miller A: Craniomandibular Muscles: Their Role in Function and Form. Boca Raton, Florida, CRC Press, 1991.

55. Mense S: Nervous outflow from skeletal muscle following chemical noxious stimulation. J Physiol 267(1):75, 1977.

Neurophysiological Basis of Visceral Pain

Maria Adele Giamberardino
Giannapia Affaitati
Rosanna Lerza
Silvana De Laurentis

SUMMARY. Objectives: In spite of visceral pain being a prominent symptom in the clinical setting, its mechanisms have been less explored than those underlying somatic pain. The objectives of this article are to review the current knowledge on pathophysiology of the most prominent phenomena related to visceral nociception, i.e., *true visceral pain, referred pain without and with hyperalgesia, visceral hyperalgesia,* and *viscero-visceral hyperalgesia.*

Findings: The poor localization and diffuse nature of *true visceral pain* results from the low density of sensory innervation of the viscera and the extensive functional divergence of the visceral input within the central nervous system [CNS]. *Referred pain without hyperalgesia* is explained by the phenomenon of "convergence-projection," i.e., convergence of visceral and somatic afferent fibers onto the same sensory neurons at various CNS levels. *Referred pain with hyperalgesia* is partly due to central sensitization of viscero-somatic convergent neurons [triggered by the massive afferent visceral barrage]. The muscle hyperalgesia also probably results from a reflex arc activation; the visceral input

Maria Adele Giamberardino, MD, Giannapia Affaitati, MD, Rosanna Lerza, MD, and Silvana De Laurentis, MD, are affiliated with the Pathophysiology of Pain Laboratory, Department of Medicine and Science of Aging, "G. D'Annunzio" University of Chieti, Italy.

Address correspondence to: Maria Adele Giamberardino, MD, via Carlo de Tocco n. 3, 66100 Chieti, Italy [E-mail: mag@unich.it].

[Haworth co-indexing entry note]: "Neurophysiological Basis of Visceral Pain." Giamberardino, Maria Adele et al. Co-published simultaneously in *Journal of Musculoskeletal Pain* [The Haworth Medical Press, an imprint of The Haworth Press, Inc.] Vol. 10, No. 1/2, 2002, pp. 151-163; and: *The Clinical Neurobiology of Fibromyalgia and Myofascial Pain: Therapeutic Implications* [ed: Robert M. Bennett] The Haworth Medical Press, an imprint of The Haworth Press, Inc., 2002, pp. 151-163. Single or multiple copies of this article are available for a fee from The Haworth Document Delivery Service [1-800-HAWORTH, 9:00 a.m. - 5:00 p.m. [EST]. E-mail address: getinfo@haworthpressinc.com].

151

would trigger reflex muscle contraction in turn responsible for sensitization of muscle nociceptors in the area of referral. Recent experimental studies by this group in a rat model of ureteric calculosis support this hypothesis by documenting: a. positivity of a number of morphofunctional indices of skeletal muscle contraction in specimens of the oblique musculature ipsilateral to the stone [site of referred hyperalgesia] and b. c-Fos labeled motoneurons in the spinal cord segments of sensory projection from the ureter. *Visceral hyperalgesia*, e.g., hypersensitivity of an internal organ due to inflammation, has been attributed to phenomena of both peripheral and central sensitization. *Viscero-visceral hyperalgesia*, i.e., the enhancement of painful symptoms because of algogenic conditions of two visceral districts sharing part of their sensory innervation [e.g., urinary tract and female reproductive organs] is probably explained, at least in part, by sensitization of viscero-visceral convergent neurons in the CNS.

Conclusions: Some aspects of visceral nociception have been fully elucidated, while the pathophysiology of other phenomena–mostly referred hyperalgesia from viscera and viscero-visceral hyperalgesia–still needs clarification. Experimental studies on adequate animal models will hopefully provide a better understanding of these phenomena, leading ultimately to an improvement of diagnostic tools and management of visceral pain in the clinical setting. *[Article copies available for a fee from The Haworth Document Delivery Service: 1-800-HAWORTH. E-mail address: <getinfo@haworthpressinc.com> Website: <http://www.HaworthPress.com>* © 2002 by The Haworth Press, Inc. All rights reserved.]

KEYWORDS. Visceral pain/hyperalgesia, referred pain/hyperalgesia, muscle contraction, viscero-visceral hyperalgesia, mechanisms

INTRODUCTION

Mechanisms of pain from internal organs have been poorly understood for a long time, mainly due to the greater difficulty of access to visceral than superficial structures, which has limited the number of clinical and experimental investigations in the field (1,3). Thanks to notable advancements in technology–allowing the testing of sensory function at various levels both in humans and animals (4)–in the past few decades the situation has partly reverted, with the gaining of significant new pieces of knowledge about the pathophysiology of this important form of pain (5).

After an indispensable premise on the clinical presentation of pain from internal organs, this manuscript reviews the current interpretation of the most relevant phenomena related to visceral nociception.

VISCERAL PAIN PHENOMENA IN CLINICS

Visceral pain is a major symptom in internal medicine and one of the most frequent reasons for hospitalization and/or seeking medical care (6,7). The features of the symptom are very typical in the first phases of an algogenic process involving internal organs [*true visceral pain*] but tend to modify with time in the course of the same episode or on the occasion of subsequent painful attacks [*referred pain*] (5). The phase of true visceral pain, experienced in the early stages, consists of a vague, poorly defined, and scarcely localized sensation, always perceived in the same site whatever the viscus in question [usually the midline of the thorax or abdomen, mostly the lowest sternal or epigastric regions, anteriorly or posteriorly], and accompanied by marked neurovegetative signs [nausea, vomiting, pallor, sweating, changes in heart rate and blood pressure, alvus disturbances, etc.] and emotional reactions [anxiety, anguish, sense of impending death]. Additional stimuli applied onto the painful area do not modify the perception of the symptom. True visceral pain can vary in intensity from slight to unbearable; characteristically the intensity has no relationship with the extent of the internal damage. A typical example is coronary heart disease; extensive damage to the myocardium can, in fact, be only mildly painful or even painless [silent myocardial infarction] while some forms of angina [involving only ischemia, without any permanent damage] can be the cause of intense suffering (8).

True visceral pain is always transitory; it lasts from a few minutes to a few hours, after which it either ceases or becomes referred to somatic structures usually included in the same metameric field as the viscus in question. Thus referred visceral pain is no longer perceived in a site common to all viscera, but in areas which differ depending on the specific organ involved. Referred pain is sharper, better localized, and defined than true visceral pain, qualitatively more similar to pain of deep somatic origin, no longer accompanied by emotional reactions and marked neurovegetative signs. At this stage, the symptom may or may not be associated with a condition of secondary hyperalgesia [increased sensitivity to painful stimuli, decreased pain threshold] of the tissues in the painful area, so that two types of referred pain from viscera can be distinguished: a *referred pain without hyperalgesia* and a *referred pain with hyperalgesia*. The hyperalgesia most frequently involves the muscle layer, where it is often accompanied by a state of sustained contraction, but can often extend upwards to also involve the subcutaneous tissue and the skin, in the case of repeated and/or longlasting algogenic processes (9).

The muscle hyperalgesia was documented in the areas of referred pain from viscera in terms of a significant decrease in pain thresholds to both mechanical and electrical muscle stimuli in a number of clinical studies on patients affected with different visceral pathologies [e.g., renal colics, biliary colics, primary dysmenorrhea] (10-14). This hyperalgesia appeared to be an early process, as it tended to manifest as early as the first visceral episodes, was accentuated in extent by the repetition of the visceral pains and lasted for a long time, i.e., it not only outlasted the spontaneous pain from the internal organ, but sometimes also the presence itself of the primary focus in the viscus. In patients affected with urinary calculosis it was in fact often detectable even a long time after the stone had been expelled. In addition to the sensory changes–hyperalgesia–the somatic tissues in the areas of referred pain from viscera are also often the site of trophic changes, mostly in terms of increased thickness and consistency of the subcutaneous tissue and decreased thickness and section area of muscles [tendency to muscle atrophy] (7). These phenomena were documented via clinical procedures but also precisely quantified through ultrasound evaluation in patients (15).

In the context of algogenic conditions affecting internal organs, phenomena of hyperalgesia are very frequent, not only involving the somatic areas of referral, as just described, but also affecting the visceral structures themselves (2,5). A given internal organ can, in fact, become hyperalgesic due to local inflammation and/or excess [repetitive-prolonged] stimulation [*visceral hyperalgesia*]. This is a form of primary hyperalgesia, i.e., involving the site of injury. In the clinical setting, hypersensitivity from inflammation indeed appears one of the most common and best known forms of visceral hyperalgesia. Typical examples are pain upon ingestion of food or liquids in the esophagus or stomach when the mucosa is inflamed or by pain upon bladder distension from inflammatory processes of the lower urinary tract, such as, for instance, those accompanying common infections like cystitis (15).

Phenomena of hyperalgesia can also occur as a result of an algogenic interaction between different visceral domains. This is the case of hyperalgesia of one visceral organ which becomes clinically manifest because of an algogenic condition of another viscus whose segmental afferent innervation is partially overlapping [*viscero-visceral hyperalgesia*] (2,5). An example is provided by patients with ischemic heart disease who are also affected with gallbladder calculosis. They are frequently observed to complain of a higher number of anginal attacks than patients with ischemic heart disease and a normal gallbladder [gallbladder and heart have a partially overlapping central projection at T5 level]. Another example is the interaction between pathologies of the urinary tract and female reproductive organs, e.g., urinary calculosis and pelvic inflammatory conditions, such as dysmenorrhea–primary or secondary to endometriosis [for female reproductive organs and urinary tract, common segments: T10-L1]. A recent study by our group was indeed devoted to exploring this interaction (16). The first part of this study examined the influence of dysmenorrhea on pain reactivity of the urinary tract via an epidemiologic and sensory investigation. A five-year survey was conducted among 69 fertile women with calculosis of one upper urinary tract via an ad-hoc questionnaire. At both retrospective [three years] and prospective [two years] investigation, dysmenorrheic women reported significantly more colics than nondysmenorrheic women and women with previous dysmenorrhea treated with estroprogestins. In addition, a specific temporal pattern of the episodes was observed as a function of the menstrual cycle, with colics being significantly more numerous perimenstrually in nondysmenorrheic women and perimenstrually and periovulatorily in dysmenorrheic women.

Pain thresholds to electrical stimulation of the oblique musculature ipsilateral to the stone [L1] were significantly lower in dysmenorrheic than nondysmenorrheic women and women with previous dysmenorrhea treated with estroprogestins, even for a comparable number of colics experienced by the different groups. Thus, in addition to a higher number of urinary colics, dysmenorrheic women with respect to nondysmenorrheic women also presented a much greater degree of referred muscle hyperalgesia at lumbar level, that is the typical site of referred pain from the upper urinary tract.

The second part of the study explored the influence of asymptomatic pathologic conditions of the reproductive organs on pain reactivity of the urinary tract. In a six-month prospective evaluation, calculosis women with asymptomatic endometriosis/ovarian cysts reported significantly more colics and greater threshold lowering at lumbar level than women with calculosis alone, similarly to what was observed in the case of dysmenorrhea plus urinary calculosis.

Thus the results of the reported study indicate that both manifest [dysmenorrhea] and latent [pelvic congestion at ovulation/menstruation; asymptomatic endometriosis, ovarian cysts] algogenic conditions of the female reproductive organs enhance pain and hyperalgesia from the urinary tract. The interdependence of these phenomena is indirectly confirmed by the finding that effective treatment of the painful pelvic condition [i.e., dysmenorrhea treated with estroprogestins] results in pain reactivity from the urinary tract which does not differ significantly from that of women without any pelvic pathology.

MECHANISMS OF VISCERAL PAIN PHENOMENA

True visceral pain is usually felt around the midline because visceral organs are supplied with afferents bilaterally; exceptions are the cecum, ascending colon, descending and sigmoid colon, kidneys, and ureters, whose innervation is unilateral or predominantly so (6). The poor localization and diffuse nature of the pain results from the low density of sensory innervation of the viscera, together with the extensive functional divergence of the visceral input within the central nervous system. The relative aspecificity of the visceral sensation in this phase [i.e., the difficulty in identifying its source] is also contributed to by the phenomenon of viscero-visceral convergence on the same sensory neurons that has been documented at various levels in the central nervous system [CNS] (5,9).

Referred pain without hyperalgesia is easily accounted for by the theory of the "convergence-projection," based on the extensive experimental evidence of the convergence at central level [spinal and supraspinal centers] of visceral and somatic afferent fibers onto the same neurons (17,18). The message from the viscera would thus be interpreted by higher brain centers as coming from the somatic structure because of mnemonic traces of previous experiences of somatic pain (3,7).

Referred pain with hyperalgesia, by far more common than the corresponding form without hyperalgesia, is more difficult to interpret and the simple convergence-projection theory does not appear adequate to account for it. There is at present an increasing body of evidence, in experimental studies, for the contribution of central mechanisms to the generation of the hyperalgesia (5). The massive afferent barrage from the visceral domain would trigger a number of neuroplastic changes in the CNS, involving hyperactivity and hyperexcitability of sensory neurons [convergent viscero-somatic], so that the normal input from the somatic periphery of pain referral would have an enhanced effect at central level [convergence-facilitation]. This phenomenon of central sensitization involving viscero-somatic convergent neurons has indeed been documented in electrophysiological studies on animal models of referred muscle hyperalgesia from viscera. It is the case of the rat model of experimental ureteric calculosis originally set up by our group (19-21) and subsequently employed by other laboratories (22,23), where rats with an artificial stone in one ureter show behavioral signs indicative of both direct visceral pain [multiple complex "ureteral crises" over four days postoperatively] and referred hyperalgesia of the ipsilateral oblique musculature [decrease in vocalization thresholds to electrical muscle stimulation for over a week postoperatively] whose extent is proportional to the number of visceral episodes displayed, as happens in patients.

While the process of central sensitization has received substantial experimental support, no clear evidence has existed so far for the so-called "reflex arc theory," which has also been postulated to explain the phenomenon of referred pain with hyperalgesia. According to this theory, the visceral algogenic input would activate a number of reflex arcs whose afferent branch is represented by the afferent fibers from the viscus and efferent branch by sympathetic [for skin and subcutis] and/or somatic [for muscle] efferences towards the tissues of the peripheral area of referral (7,9). Regarding the muscle, in particular, the "reflex arc activation" would promote reflex muscle contraction, in turn possibly responsible for sensitization of nociceptors locally, which would account for the hyperalgesia (7).

This theory had originally been put forward on the basis of the clinical observation of the sustained muscle contraction that so often accompanies the states of prolonged visceral pain in the area of referral (6,7). Recent studies by our group have provided some experimental evidence for this so far theoretic mechanism, by employing the previously described animal model of artificial ureteric calulosis. In stone rats, we investigated the possible correlations between the condition of hyperalgesia of the ipsilateral oblique musculature and some morphofunctional indices of skeletal muscle contraction (24). Specimens from the obliquus externus muscle of both sides were obtained from stone-implanted [left ureter] and from sham-operated rats [2, 4 or 8 days postoperatively]. In these specimens, the following parameters were measured: a. I band length/sarcomere length ratio [as ultrastructural contracture index]; b. muscle cell membrane fluidity; c. sarcoplasmic reticulum calcium [Ca^{2+}]-uptake capacity [measured as Ca^{2+}-adenosine triphosphatase activity]; and d. sarcoplasmic reticulum–Ca^{2+} release capacity [measured as ryanodine binding].

In sham-controls, all parameters were not significantly different on the two sides. In stone rats, parameters of the right obliquus externus muscle [i.e., contralateral to the implanted ureter] did not differ significantly from those of sham controls. On the left [ipsilateral] versus right obliquus externus muscle of stone rats, the following significant changes were found: a. decreased I band length/sarcomere length ratio; b. increased muscle cell membrane fluidity; c. increased Ca^{2+}-uptake capacity [correlated linearly to the number of ureteral "crises"]; and d. decreased ryanodine binding. These results suggest the presence, proportional in degree to the activity of the ureteral pain focus, of a state of skeletal muscle contraction in the oblique musculature ipsilateral to the stone, an event which could contribute to the generation of the local hyperalgesia via sensitization of muscle nociceptors. In a parallel study we explored c-Fos expression in the spinal cord of calculosis rats versus sham controls (25). Stone rats were sacrificed two hours after the first ureteral "crisis" and sham controls [no crisis] were suppressed after matching time lapses. All were perfused intracardially; the T9-L3 thoracolumbar spinal cord segment was removed and post-fixed. Frontal frozen sections [40 µm thick] were cut and immunostained for c-Fos-like protein. Four-five sections/level/rat were examined under lightfield microscopy to evaluate Fos-positive cell number.

Fos-labeled cells were never observed in sham controls. In stone rats, they were found throughout the dorsal horn [laminae I-VI] bilaterally, but significantly more on the side ipsilateral to the implanted ureter. As expected, most of the Fos expression was in the superficial dorsal horn. Fos-labeled cells, however, were also found in the ventral gray [laminae VII-X], mostly in lamina VII [containing preganglionic sympathetic neurons of the intermediolateral nucleus in segments T1-L3] but also in lamina IX [motoneurons]. These results thus suggest that nociceptive input from the ureter in this model activates not only sensory neurons but also efferent neurons in the spinal cord, supporting the notion that reflex arcs are triggered by the visceral focus and that the muscle contraction in the referred site results from a reflex mechanism.

Though further studies will be needed to test this hypothesis more thoroughly, the data so far reported are strongly indicative that referred phenomena from viscera cannot be merely due to central mechanisms but should be also explained on the basis of real changes taking place at the periphery. This seems all the more probable in the light of the clinical evidence that the areas of referred pain from viscera are the site of trophic alterations in addition to the hyperalgesia; these objective changes cannot, in fact, be the result of purely central processes.

Visceral hyperalgesia. Hyperalgesia from inflammation and/or excess stimulation is among the most extensively investigated phenomena of hypersensitivity from a visceral domain. To account for this form of hyperalgesia, mechanisms have been advocated which are similar to those involved in primary cutaneous hyperalgesia [at the site of an injury], i.e., mechanisms of both peripheral and central sensitization (5,26).

Peripheral sensitization involves a lowering in threshold of nociceptors. In internal organs, based on the present knowledge about the nature and characteristics of visceral sensory receptors, peripheral sensitization due to inflammation and/or repetitive-prolonged stimulation is likely to involve both a lowering in threshold of "high threshold receptors" and the bringing into play of previously unresponsive units ["silent nociceptors"] (27).

The increased input to the CNS would then trigger neuroplastic changes which amplify the effects of every further signal coming from the affected viscus (28). This process, known as central sensitization, involves phenomena of increased spontaneous activity of neurons, enlarged receptive field areas and an increase in response evoked by large and small caliber primary afferent fibers (29).

The results of a number of experimental studies on animal models of visceral hyperalgesia point to a pivotal role played by N-methyl-D-aspartate receptors in mediating the state of central hyperexcitability. N-methyl-D-aspartate receptor agonists, in fact, have been shown to enhance visceral nociceptive responses and antagonists to prevent or inhibit these same responses due to experimental visceral inflammation in the rat produced via intracolonic instillation of zymosan or turpentine application in the urinary bladder (30-32).

Viscero-visceral hyperalgesia. Viscero-visceral hyperalgesia is a complex form of hypersensitivity which is likely to be explained by more than one mechanism (5). Since this phenomenon takes place preferentially between visceral organs which share, at least in part, their central projection, it is plausible that phenomena of central sensitization play an important role. Hyperactivity and hyperexcitability could involve viscero-visceral convergent neurons at the central level. As already mentioned, in fact, viscero-visceral convergences have been documented in electrophysiological studies in animals, for instance between gallbladder and heart (33)–which would explain the frequent interaction between pathologies of these two organs–and between colon/

rectum, urinary bladder, vagina, and uterine cervix–which would explain the clinical interaction between female reproductive organs and urinary tract (34-36). The increased input from one visceral domain could trigger changes in the excitability of these neurons and thus enhance the central effect of the input from the second visceral domain (5).

This hypothesis, however, needs to be verified experimentally, and other possible mechanisms could also be implicated. In this perspective, it would be of great importance to have available a reliable animal model of the condition of viscero-visceral interaction observed in patients. One such kind of model has recently been set up which reproduces the characteristics of the viscero-visceral interaction between the female reproductive organs and the urinary tract. Our group combined the model of urinary calculosis in rats with a model of experimental endometriosis (37). Endometriosis was chosen because it is a very frequent cause of secondary dysmenorrhea in women (6). Experiments in this model have shown that rats with endometriosis plus urinary stones display a significantly higher number and duration of typical ureteral crises than rats with sham endometriosis plus urinary stones. In addition, they also show a much higher degree of referred muscle hyperalgesia than sham endometriosis rats (38,39). The enhanced poststone pain behavior is a function of the degree of activity of the endometriotic cysts as it is the more pronounced the greater the diameter of the cysts, which are known to contain algogenic substances (37). Preventive treatment of the endomtriotic condition via a classic nonsteroidal anti-inflammatory drug results in both a reduction of the dimensions of the cysts and in a prevention of the pain enhancement subsequent to stone formation (Giamberardino et al., unpublished data). This appears as the experimental counterpart of the clinical condition just described, and this model may be a useful tool for further investigation of underlying mechanisms of viscero-visceral hyperalgesia.

CONCLUSION

Visceral pain phenomena are numerous and complex and their pathophysiological mechanisms have been clarified only in part. While true visceral pain, referred pain without hyperalgesia and visceral hyperalgesia have been provided with clear explanations, knowledge is still incomplete on the exact origin of the phenomena of referred pain with hyperalgesia and of viscero-visceral hyperalgesia. This global picture is also complicated by the fact that the various expressions of visceral nociception are often intermingled, so that several of the described phenomena can coexist in the same patient affected with painful diseases of internal organs. As a result, the clinical reality of visceral pain can still be complex in many circumstances, creating both diagnostic and therapeutic problems.

Full elucidation of the mechanisms underlying the described phenomena is thus of crucial importance for improving modalities of approach to and management of the symptom in the clinical setting. Further studies on experimental models which adequately reproduce the different clinical conditions will hopefully lead to a better understanding of visceral pain pathophysiology and, consequently, to the development of treatment strategies which are not merely symptomatic.

REFERENCES

1. Cervero F, Laird JM: Visceral pain. Lancet 353:2145-2148, 1999.

2. Giamberardino MA: Recent and forgotten aspects of visceral pain. Eur J Pain 3:77-92, 2000.

3. Joshi SK, Gebhart GF: Visceral pain. Curr Rev Pain 4:499-506, 2000.

4. Arendt-Nielsen L: Induction and assessment of experimental pain from human skin, muscle and viscera, Progress in Pain Research and Management. Edited by TS Jensen, JA Turner, Z Wiesenfeld-Hallin. IASP Press, Seattle, 1997, pp. 393-425.

5. Giamberardino MA: Visceral hyperalgesia, Progress in Pain Research and Management. Edited by M Devor, MC Rowbotham, Z Wiesenfeld-Halin. IASP Press, Seattle, 2000, pp. 523-550.

6. Bonica JJ: The Management of Pain. Lea & Febiger, Philadephia, 1990.

7. Procacci P, Zoppi M, Maresca M: Clinical approach to visceral sensation, Visceral Sensation, Progress in Brain Research. Edited by F Cervero, JFB Morrison JFB. Elsevier, Amsterdam, 1986, pp. 21-28.

8. Foreman RD: Mechanisms of cardiac pain. Ann Rev Physiol 61:143-147, 1999.

9. Giamberardino MA, Vecchiet L: Pathophysiology of visceral pain. Curr Rev Pain 1:23-33, 1996.

10. Vecchiet L, Giamberardino MA, Dragani L, Albe-Fessard D: Pain from renal/ureteral calculosis: evaluation of sensory thresholds in the lumbar area. Pain 36:289-295, 1989.

11. Vecchiet L, Giamberardino MA, Dragani L, Galletti R, Albe-Fessard D: Referred muscular hyperalgesia from viscera: clinical approach. Adv Pain Res Ther 13: 175-182, 1990.

12. Vecchiet L, Giamberardino MA, de Bigontina P: Referred pain from viscera: when the symptom persists despite the extinction of the visceral focus. Adv Pain Res Ther 20:101-110, 1992.

13. Giamberardino MA, de Bigontina P, Martegiani C, Vecchiet L: Effects of extracorporeal shock-wave lithotripsy on referred hyperalgesia from renal/ureteral calculosis. Pain 56:77-83, 1994.

14. Giamberardino MA, Berkley KJ, Iezzi S, de Bigontina P, Vecchiet L: Pain threshold variations in somatic wall tissues as a function of menstrual cycle, segmental site and tissue depth in non-dysmenorrheic women, dysmenorrheic women and men. Pain 71:187-197, 1997.

15. Giamberardino MA, Vecchiet J, Affaitati G, Vecchiet L: Visceral pain mechanisms, Topics in Anaesthesia and Critical Care, Neuroscience: Focus on Acute and Chronic Pain. Edited by MA Tiengo. Springer, Milan, 2000, pp. 59-70.

16. Giamberardino MA, De Laurentis S, Affaitati G, Lerza R, Lapenna D, Vecchiet L: Modulation of pain and hyperalgesia from the urinary tract by algogenic conditions of the reproductive organs in women. Neurosci Lett 304:61-64, 2001.

17. Cervero F: Sensory innervation of the viscera: peripheral basis of visceral pain. Physiol Rev 74(1):95-138, 1994.

18. Foreman RD: Integration of viscerosomatic sensory input at the spinal level, Progress in Brain Research. Edited by EA Mayer, CB Saper. Elsevier, Amsterdam, 2000, pp. 209-221.

19. Giamberardino MA, Valente R, de Bigontina P, Vecchiet L: Artificial ureteral calculosis in rats: behavioural characterization of visceral pain episodes and their relationship with referred lumbar muscle hyperalgesia. Pain 61:459-469, 1995.

20. Giamberardino MA, Dalal A, Valente R, Vecchiet L: Changes in activity of spinal cells with muscular input in rats with referred muscular hyperalgesia from ureteral calculosis. Neurosci Lett 203:89-92, 1996.

21. Giamberardino MA, Valente R, Affaitati G, Vecchiet L: Central neuronal changes in recurrent visceral pain. Int J Clin Pharmacol Res 17(2/3):63-66, 1997.

22. Laird JMA, Roza C, Cervero F: Effects of artificial calculosis on rat ureter motility: peripheral contribution to the pain of ureteric colic. Am J Physiol 272:1409-1416, 1997.

23. Roza C, Laird JMA, Cervero F: Spinal mechanisms underlying persistent pain and referred hyperalgesia in rats with an experimental ureteric stone. J Neurophysiol 79:1603-1612, 1998.

24. Giamberardino MA, Affaitati G, Lerza R, Fanò G, Fulle S, Belia S, Vecchiet L: Relationship between referred hyperalgesia and skeletal muscle contracture in rats with an artificial ureteric stone. Soc Neurosci Abstr, 2001, in press.

25. Aloisi AM, Scaramuzzino A, Affaitati G, Lerza R, Vecchiet L, Giamberardino MA: C-fos expression in the spinal cord of female rats with artificial ureteric calculosis. Soc Neurosci Abstr, 2001, in press.

26. Gebhart GF: Pathobiology of visceral pain: molecular mechanisms and therapeutic implications IV. Visceral afferent contributions to the pathobiology of visceral pain. Am J Physiol Gastrointest Liver Physiol 278:834-838, 2000.

27. Cervero F: Visceral Pain: mechanisms of peripheral and central sensitization. Ann Med 2:235-239, 1995.

28. Westlund KN: Visceral nociception. Curr Rev Pain 4:478-487, 2000.

29. Li J, Simone DA, Larson AA: Windup leads to characteristics of central sensitization. Pain 79:75-82, 1999.

30. Kolhekar R, Gebhart GF: Modulation of spinal nociceptive transmission by NMDA receptor activation in the rat. J Neurophysiol 75:2344-2351, 1996.

31. Coutinho SV, Meller ST, Gebhart GF: Intracolonic zymosan produces visceral hyperalgesia in the rat that is mediated by spinal NMDA and non-NMDA receptors. Brain Res 736:7-15, 1996.

32. Rice ASC, McMahon SB: Pre-emptive intrathecal administration of an NMDA receptor antagonist [AP-5] prevents hyper-reflexia in a model of persistent visceral pain. Pain 57:335-340, 1994.

33. Foreman RD: Organization of the spinothalamic tract as a relay for cardio-pulmonary sympathetic afferent fiber activity. Progr Sens Physiol 9:1-51, 1989.

34. Berkley KJ, Guilbaud G, Benoist JM, Gautron M: Responses of neurons in and near the thalamic ventrobasal complex of the rat to stimulation of uterus, cervix, vagina, colon and skin. J Neurophysiol 69:557-568, 1993.

35. Berkley KJ, Hubscher CH, Wall PD: Neuronal responses to stimulation of the cervix, uterus, colon and skin in the rat spinal cord. J Neurophysiol 69: 533-544, 1993.

36. Ness TJ, Gebhart GF: Visceral pain: a review of experimental studies. Pain 41:167-234, 1990.

37. Berkley KJ, Cason A, Jacobs H, Bradshaw H, Wood E: Vaginal hyperalgesia in a rat model of endometriosis. Neurosci Lett 306:185-188, 2001.

38. Giamberardino MA, Affaitati G, Vecchiet L, Berkley KJ: Effects of endo-metriosis on pain behaviours induced by ureteral calculosis in female rats. J Musculoske Pain 6(2):172,1998.

39. Giamberardino MA, Berkley KJ, Affaitati G, Lerza R, Vecchiet L: The influence of endometriosis on pain behaviors induced by ureteral calculosis in female rats. Abstracts 9th IASP Congress, IASP Press, Seattle, 1999, p. 392.

Myofascial and Visceral Pain Syndromes: Visceral-Somatic Pain Representations

Robert D. Gerwin

SUMMARY. Objective: To describe the relationship between viscero-somatic pain syndromes and myofascial pain syndromes [MPS].

Findings: Myofascial pain syndromes can be primary conditions or secondary. When they are secondary, they occur as a manifestation of another disorder. A regional pain referral from a visceral disorder can induce secondary MPS. Visceral disorders induce central sensitization with hypersensitivity and expansion in the number and size of receptive fields. Central sensitization is topographically organized in the spinal cord, being segmentally predominant at the level of the affected viscera. The associated MPS tend to be regional, but are related to the segmental innervation of the affected viscera. Regional MPS in turn can mimic visceral disease, or be the diagnostic sign of visceral disease. Cardiac disease, gastrointestinal disorders, hepatic and biliary disorders, irritable bowel syndrome and interstitial cystitis are some of the conditions in which MPS can occur secondarily or mimic.

Conclusion: Myofascial pain syndromes can occur as a result of visceral disorders, but can also mimic visceral disease. Visceral disease must be considered in the differential diagnosis of regional MPS. *[Article copies available for a fee from The Haworth Document Delivery Service: 1-800-HAWORTH. E-mail address: <getinfo@haworthpressinc.com> Website: <http://www.HaworthPress.com> © 2002 by The Haworth Press, Inc. All rights reserved.]*

Robert D. Gerwin, MD, is Assistant professor of Neurology, Johns Hopkins University School of Medicine, Baltimore, MD and Medical Director, Pain and Rehabilitation Medicine, Ltd., Bethesda, MD.

Address correspondance to: Robert D. Gerwin, MD, 7830 Old Georgetown Road, Suite C15, Bethesda, MD 20814-2432 USA [E-mail: gerwin@painpoints.com].

[Haworth co-indexing entry note]: "Myofascial and Visceral Pain Syndromes: Visceral-Somatic Pain Representations." Gerwin, Robert D. Co-published simultaneously in *Journal of Musculoskeletal Pain* [The Haworth Medical Press, an imprint of The Haworth Press, Inc.] Vol. 10, No. 1/2, 2002, pp. 165-175; and: *The Clinical Neurobiology of Fibromyalgia and Myofascial Pain: Therapeutic Implications* [ed: Robert M. Bennett] The Haworth Medical Press, an imprint of The Haworth Press, Inc., 2002, pp. 165-175. Single or multiple copies of this article are available for a fee from The Haworth Document Delivery Service [1-800-HAWORTH, 9.00 a.m. - 5.00 p.m. (EST). E-mail address: getinfo@haworthpressinc.com].

KEYWORDS. Myofascial pain syndrome, visceral disease, referred pain, pain, muscle

INTRODUCTION

Visceral pain is one of the most common forms of disease-induced pain. Referred pain from viscera is likewise common, occurring in both pathologic conditions such as ureteral colic or myocardial infarction, and in nonpathologic conditions such as bowel or bladder distention. Any visceral disease can be manifest by referred pain [renal stone, gastroenteritis, appendicitis, myocardial infarction, pleurisy, pulmonary embolism, cystitis, gallbladder colic, prostatitis, etc.], and referred pain can be an important diagnostic feature. Pain can be referred from viscera to the skin or to muscle, or regionally, as to the low back where both skin and muscle are involved. An early description of a muscle or somatic component of pain that both resulted from visceral organ injury and mimicked the pain from such an injury were left pectoral muscle trigger points [TrPs] that occurred with acute myocardial infarction, and which were relieved by procaine injection into the trigger areas reported by Travell and Rinzler in 1952 (1). The clinical importance of referred pain syndromes associated with visceral disease relates to the diagnostic value of such syndromes, to the awareness that similar pain syndromes may mimic visceral disease, and to the therapeutic benefit of treating the myofascial component of pain in providing clinical relief. The same myofascial pain syndromes [MPS] that result from visceral disease, can also mimic visceral disease when they occur from other causes.

Visceral and somatic pain mechanisms share many common features. Visceral pain, for example, can be referred to the body wall. An initial response to visceral disease can be muscle tightness that is not necessarily painful, but can be a tight band or a muscle spasm (2, pp. 142-143). As in other pain-producing conditions, the referred pain may outlast the inciting pain, and remain a problem long after the original pain resolved. The referred pain syndrome may then be the only sign of a previous visceral disorder. When that is the case, it usually can be differentiated from an acute visceral condition by its persistent, dull quality. However, not all visceral pathology is acute or causes acute pain, and sometimes the residual chronic myofascial component can be sharp and severe, and appear acute, as if there is a flare-up of the underlying condition.

VISCERAL PAIN PHYSIOLOGY

Visceral referred pain shares the same central mechanisms as pain input from other structures in the development of neuroplastic changes that lead to hypersensitivity, allodynia, and expansion of receptive fields.

Hypersensitivity. Irritable bowel syndrome [IBS] is accompanied by altered visceral perception (3,4). Although studies through the mid-1990's failed to show an increase in general pain sensitivity, recent studies have shown that patients with IBS have both visceral and cutaneous hyperalgesia that is at least partly dependent on topographically organized spinal mechanisms [more pronounced in the lower extremities than the upper extremities] (5). This is reflected in the predominant localization of pain in the low back and pelvic region in persons with IBS.

Visceral pain or hyperalgesia is caused by mechanisms that are both shared with somatic pain mechanisms and that are unique to viscera (6). Tissue injury is not necessary in order to produce visceral pain. Non-damaging mechanical causes of visceral hyperalgesia include excessive distention or abnormal contraction of a hollow visceral organ, rapid stretching of the capsule of a solid organ such as the liver, and traction on ligaments and vessels. Visceral hypersensitivity to stimulation such as distention or traction is seen in visceral pain syndromes, and has been particularly well studied in IBS. Anoxia, ischemia or the accumulation of nociceptive substances, chemical irritants, and inflammatory conditions that release potassium, kinins, 5-hydroxytryptamine, histamine, or prostaglandins and that can cause tissue injury are biochemical initiators of visceral hyperalgesia. The referred pain is generally the same in both cases.

Central mechanisms of referred pain involving viscera. Central sensitization occurs at the level of the dorsal horn cell in the posterior horns of the spinal cord. Modulation of nociceptive dorsal horn cell activation occurs as a result of supraspinal facilitatory and inhibitory ascending and descending impulses.

The majority of dorsal horn cells that receive input from the viscera also receive input from receptors in the skin and/or deep tissues [viscerosomatic neurons] (7,8). Viscerosomatic convergence is the rule in visceral pain (6,9). Almost all dorsal horn cells driven by visceral input have additional somatic input (10,11). In the rat experimental model of artificial stone-induced ureteral colic, referred muscle hyperalgesia occurred early, was accentuated by repeated episodes of colic, and outlasted the presence of the irritant (12). Thus, muscle pain is commonly felt with visceral nociceptive activation of dorsal horn neurons.

The dorsal columns of the spinal cord transmit visceral pain information. Information carried in the dorsal columns affects pain awareness in humans. For example, midline dorsal column lesions are effective treatment for the relief of pelvic visceral pain (13). This has also been shown to be the case in animals for pain arising from colorectal distention, the duodenum, and the pancreas (14). The dorsal midline of the rat spinal cord contains both ascending tracts to the gracile and cuneate nucleus and descending corticospinal pathways. Ventrolateral cordotomies alone do not abolish visceral stimulation-evoked responses. Both the ventrolateral quadrants and dorsolateral funiculi are important for the transmission of visceral nociceptive information. Dorsal midline structures are important for input into the ventrobasal thalamus, whereas lateral spinothalamic pathways are more important for input into the ventrolateral medullary structures (15). The ventrolateral medulla is greatly involved in autonomic regulation. Visceral input through the lateral spinothalamic tracts to the ventrolateral medulla therefore plays an important role in autonomic reflex activity [such as change in heart rate], and is attenuated by lesions of the lateral column of the spinal cord, but not by midline dorsal lesions. However, the spinal cord dorsal column does not only transmit visceral nociceptive information. The dorsal columns have a more general function in pain, and, for example, have been shown to transmit information in peripheral nerve injuries like experimental mononeuropathy (16).

Sex and gender effects. Chronic visceral pain syndromes are more common in women than in men, and reflect the influence of hormonal factors on the algesic response both peripherally and centrally, the direct effect of estrogen, progesterone, and testosterone on organ function, and psychological and social factors [e.g., abuse history and gender role differences] (17,18). The effect of sex and gender on pain states is not simple, however, and changes with age as well as with sex and gender, but occurrence of pain states remains higher in women than in men in such conditions as abdominal pain, migraine, temperomandibular joint syndrome, and fibromyalgia syndrome [FMS] (19). Thus, IBS and interstitial cystitis [IC] are more common in women, and therefore, associated low back pain syndromes and pelvic floor MPS are more common in women than in men.

REFERRED PAIN AND REFERRED HYPERALGESIA FROM VISCERA

In areas of referred pain from viscera, hypersensitivity often occurs. Visceral pain referred to the body wall is associated with muscle tenderness in the referred pain zone (6,20). Proposed mechanisms are dichotomizing or split sensory fibers, afferent-afferent interactions with orthodromic and antidromic impulses, and sympathetic reflexes to the skin causing fluid extravasation and edema. Sustained muscle contraction can occur as a result (21). Examples are hyperalgesia in the pectoralis major, the interscapular region and the forearm in myocardial infarction, lumbar muscle pain, groin pain, and flank pain in patients with ureteral colic, right upper abdominal quadrant muscle tenderness in patients with biliary colic, and lower abdominal and pelvic muscle tenderness in women with ovarian or uterine pain. The overlying cutaneous and subcutaneous tissues may also be hypersensitive. Trophic changes in the cutaneous zone of referred pain have been reported for experimental uterine inflammation in the rat (22), emphasizing the fact that functional changes also occur in the referred pain zone, from skin edema to TrP formation.

Noncardiac chest pain is a psychophysical disorder that has an organic cause like gastroesophageal reflux disease or a psychological disorder like anxiety and depression. Patients with noncardiac chest pain have a lower pain threshold to forearm ischemia and electrical skin stimulation than coronary artery patients, similar to other types of visceral pain syndromes (23).

Pain from liver and gallbladder disease is often referred to the right shoulder. The referral pattern from diaphragmatic irritation is mediated via the phrenic nerve that provides motor and sensory innervation to the diaphragm as well as to mediastinal and pleural tissues. The phrenic nerve is derived from C3-C5, so that pain referral to the shoulder in a C4-C5 distribution is really a segmental pain referral. Trigger points and a regional MPS affecting the shoulder that looks like an impingement syndrome or frozen shoulder can occur in persons with hepatic or gallbladder disorders. In addition, a local abdominal muscle wall myofascial syndrome can occur. In one instance, a 60-year-old woman presented with shoulder pain and restricted abduction and internal rotation of the arm of several weeks duration, seemingly the result of heavy household cleaning. Treatment of TrPs points in the shoulder muscles, including the infraspinatus, the subscapularis, the latissimus dorsi, and the trapezius muscles relieved her pain. There was no abdominal or right upper quadrant [RUQ] pain or tenderness. Within two weeks she developed right abdominal wall pain following further heavy physical household cleaning, again with no RUQ tenderness or evidence of hepatic enlargement. Local treatment of abdominal oblique muscle TrPs again eliminated her pain. The shoulder and flank pain recurred within two weeks, and this time she had RUQ tenderness made worse with deep breathing and an enlarged liver. Initial investigation showed normal gallbladder and pancreatic function and appearance. She had massively enlarged congenital hepatic cysts, one of which contained 1.5 liters of fluid. Drainage of the cysts resolved her regional MPS.

Irritable Bowel Syndrome. The IBS and FMS are both common hyperalgesic syndromes, and overlap to a considerable degree. Patients with IBS show visceral hyperalgesia and cutaneous allodynia/hyperalgesia indicative of a widely distributed yet topographically organized central hypersensitivity, being more pronounced in the lower than in the upper extremities (5). The overlap between FMS and IBS is considerable, with 70 percent of FMS patients reporting chronic visceral pain and 65 percent of IBS patients having primary FMS in one study (24). The FMS is associated with hypervigilence, or hypersensitivity to stimuli of different types (25-27). Patients with IBS show hypervigilence similar to FMS patients, but show somatic hyperalgesia only when there is comorbid FMS (28). Patients with IBS show an increased vigilance towards expected aversive events, and a decreased tolerance for such stimulation, as well as hyperalgesia following a series of painful sigmoid colon distentions in contrast to controls. One postulated mechanism to explain these observations is that the pain modulatory system is altered. In support of this finding is the greater efficacy of fentanyl in attenuating the perception of phasic rectal distention and discomfort ratings to rectal fixed stimuli in IBS patients compared to controls, suggesting that IBS patients have a diminished release of endogenous opioids in response to visceral aversive stimulation (29).

Chronic pelvic pain and urologic disease. Vecchiet and Giamberardino have studied hyperalgesia in referred pain zones from urinary colic extensively (21,30). Hypersensitivity was found to be greatest in muscle in the referred pain zone. There was persistent hypersensitivity in one of three layers of the body wall in 90 percent, most predominantly in muscle, but also in skin or subcutaneous layers, and in all three layers in 25 percent of subjects. This is also true in biliary colic and dysmenorrhea. Persistent abdominal wall pain after ureteral colic can be relieved by TrP injections. Likewise, lateral abdominal wall MPS looks like ureteral colic.

Chronic pelvic pain [CPP] and IC remain enigmas and are frustrating conditions to treat (31). Interstitial cystitis is only one of a group of painful bladder-related conditions that include a variety of bladder infectious diseases, including chlamydia, drug-induced cystitis [e.g., cyclophosphamide], and sarcoid, that can cause low back and pelvic region MPS. When an organic cause for CPP is not readily found, surgery may be done to find a cause. The pain of IC is usually a moderate to severe, constant pain that is dull and aching in character. There may also be a sharper, stabbing like pain and spasm. The pain is worsened by voiding, intercourse, exercise, and by tight clothing. Pain is experienced in the perineal region [vagina, urethra] and in the supra pubic region. Fifty percent of persons with IC report having been abused as a child. In these persons, the learned behavior of voluntary sphincter control is not learned properly, causing pelvic floor muscle dysfunction. This can result in the development of TrPs that can in turn induce bladder pain, and sphincter spasm. In males, intra pelvic TrPs can cause pain like prostatitis (31). Treatment of the TrPs can decrease pain and improve bladder function. Medullary sponge kidney [MSK] is a possible cause for costo-vertebral angle [CVA] MPS. Little is written about pain from this condition, but it is associated with hematuria, red blood cell casts, and recurrent stone formation. We do not know if a patient with MSK and CVA pain and no other cause for musculoskeletal pain has MSK unrelated to MPS, or a renal-origin pain referred to the CVA.

The urogenital [pelvic] floor is innervated by the sympathetic, parasympathetic, and somatic nervous systems. The sympathetic and parasympathetic [pelvic splanchnic nerve] nervous system input is through the inferior hypogastric plexus. Somatic innervation is through the sacral spinal cord. The pudendal nerve receives sympathetic fibers in addition to somatic nerves. It innervates the penis or clitoris, the anal canal, the urethral sphincter, and anterior perineal muscles. The posterior pelvic floor musculature is innervated by the coccygeal plexus. There is an overlap of pelvic splanchnic nerve and pudendal nerve afferent input in the spinal cord, such that stimulation of one area of the urogenital floor can influence the output to another area (32). Thus, persons with urogenital pain syndromes complain about bowel and bladder dysfunction, sexual dysfunction, and show increased pelvic floor muscle tone or develop pelvic floor TrPs, and a global dysfunction of the pelvic region is often seen clinically [IBS, IC, dyspareunia]. The urogenital pain syndromes that are commonly seen include vulvodynia [which is associated with a profound hyperalgesia as shown by the stabbing neuropathic-like pain associated with touching the vulva with a moist cotton swab], testicular pain [orchialgia], urethral syndrome [urgency, frequency, dysuria, and regional pain, similar to IC], and prostatodynia [accounting for 30 percent of patients with prostatitis, often associated with pelvic floor muscle pain] (32).

Referred pain from experimental bladder distention in female volunteers is to the suprapubic region. Repeated urinary bladder distention results in an increase in perceived painful sensations [hypersensitivity], a decrease in the intravesicular pressure required to produce discomfort [a lowering of pain threshold], and a progressive increase in cardiovascular responses [pseudo-affective reflex] (33). This correlates with the reports of urgency and discomfort reported in persons with IC in response to low intensity bladder distention. The study showed a progressive sensitization for perception of pain and for autonomic responses, although somatic [muscle wall] sensitivity was not measured. A similar finding of progressive sensitization was seen in studies of colorectal distention. It would be interesting to know if repeated bladder distention or persistent IC would lead to progressive somatic sensitivity and a lowered threshold for muscle tenderness. Could there be a reciprocal role for IC and IBS in the production of muscle wall tenderness in FMS and MPS, each leading to central sensitization that makes both the visceral symptoms worse and the muscle tenderness greater?

These questions were addressed in part in a study of sensory changes during the ovulatory phase of the menstrual cycle in healthy women (34). Pressure pain threshold, heat pain threshold, and tactile threshold were all reduced in the referred pain zones of the abdomen and low back in females during all phases of the menstrual cycle. The thresholds were also further reduced during the ovulatory phase of the cycle. A lowered threshold to pressure pain over referred pain zones in the abdominal wall and the back, but not to regions outside of the referred pain zone, supports the general notion that MPS are induced by visceral pain, but does not indicate that the visceral pain can be made worse by the TrP.

The complexity of the relationship between the pelvic floor musculature and visceral function in visceral CPPs is illustrated by a patient with a history of sexual abuse as a child, and chronic urinary dysfunction with impaired control of voiding [pressure, pain, urgency, retention] and chronic rectal and anal pain with poorly formed stools. The patient had severe pelvic floor MPS with active TrPs in all of the pelvic-related muscles [gluteal muscles, piriformis, hamstrings, psoas, quadratus lumborum, abdominal obliques, and levator ani]. Treatment was directed towards the inactivation of the TrPs in the muscles that could be reached externally, and also towards the levator ani treated internally. Biofeedback was used to improve the patient's awareness of muscle tension. Voiding changed to become more controlled, with a more predictable stream, complete emptying, and less urgency, and decreased frequency. The stool became better formed and less painful to evacuate. The presence of TrPs contributed to the visceral dysfunction that improved when the TrPs were inactivated.

CONCLUSION

Visceral pain states commonly refer pain to the axial or extremity muscle, creating a regional MPS. Similar regional MPS resulting from other causes can look identical to visceral pain-induced MPS. Therefore, visceral disorders are part of the differential diagnosis of regional MPS. A thorough history, physical examination, and a high degree of suspicion are required to distinguish a primary MPS from a secondary one.

REFERENCES

1. Travell JG, Rinzler SH: The myofascial genesis of pain. Postgrad Med, 11: 452-434, 1952.

2. Mense S, Simons DG, Russell IJ: Muscle Pain. Baltimore: Lippincott Williams & Wilkins, 2001, p. 385.

3. Accarino A, Azpiroz F, Malagelada JR: Selective dysfunction of mechano-sensitive intestinal afferents in the irritable bowel syndrome. Gastroenterology, 108: 636-643, 1995.

4. Zighelboim J, Talley NJ, Phillips SF, Harmsen WS, Zinsmeister AR: Visceral perception in irritable bowel syndrome. Digestive Dis Sci, 40: 819-827, 1995.

5. Verne GN, Robinson ME, Price DD: Hypersensitivity to visceral and cutaneous pain in the irritable bowel syndrome. Pain, 93: 7-14, 2001.

6. Giamberardino MA: Visceral hyperalgesia, in Proceedings of the 9th World Congress on Pain, Edited by M Devor, MC Rowbotham, Z Wiesenfeld-Hallin, 2000, IASP Press, Seattle, pp. 523-550.

7. Foreman RD: Viscerosomatic convergence onto spinal neurons responding to afferent fibers located in the inferior cardiac nerve. Brain Res, 137: 164-168, 1977.

8. Tattersall JEH, Cervero F, Lumb BM: Effects of reversible spinalization on the visceral input to viscerosomatic neurons in the lower thoracic spinal cord of the cat. J Neurophys, 56: 785-796, 1986.

9. Ito SI: Possible representation of somatic pain in the rat insular visceral sensory cortex: a field potential study. Neurosci Letters, 24: 171-174, 1998.

10. Cervero F: Somatic and visceral inputs to the thoracic spinal cord of the cat: effectss of noxious stimulation of the biliary system. J Physiol, 337: 51-67, 1983.

11. Foreman RD, Blair RW, Weber RN: Viscerosomatic convergence onto T2-T4 spinoreticular, spinoreticular-spinothalamic, and spinothalamic tract neurons in the cat. Exp Neurol, 85: 597-619, 1984.

12. Giamberardino MA, Valente R, de Bigontina P, Vecchiet L: Articficial ureteral calculosis in rats: behavioral characterization of visceral pain episodes and their relationship with referred lumbar muscle hypyeralgesia. Pain, 61: 459-469, 1995.

13. Houghton AK, Wang C-C, Westlund KN: Do nociceptive signals from the pancreas travel in the dorsal column? Pain, 89: 207-220, 2001.

14. Willis WDJ, Westlulnd KN : The role of the dorsal column pathway in visceral nociception. Curr Pain Headache Reports, 5(1): 20-26, 2001.

15. Ness TJ: Evidence for ascending visceral nociceptive information in the dorsal midline and lateral spinal cord. Pain, 87: 83-88, 2000.

16. Miki K, Iwata K, Tsuboi Y, Morimoto T, Kondo E, Dai Y, Ren K, Noguchi K: Dorsal column-thalamic pathway is involved in thalamic hyperexcitability following peripheral nerve injury: a lesion study in rats with experimental mononeuropathy. Pain, 85: 263-271, 2000.

17. Heitkemper MM, Jarrett M: Gender differences and hormonal modulation in visceral pain. Curr Pain Headache Reports, 5: 35-43, 2001.

18. Giamberardino MA: Sex-related and hormonal modulation of visceral pain, in Sex, Gender, and Pain. Edited by RB Fillingim, 2000, IASP Press: Seattle. pp.135-163.

19. LeResche L: Epidemiological perspectives on sex differences in pain, in Sex, Gender, and Pain, Edited by RB Fillingim, 2000, IASP Press: Seattle. pp. 233-249.

20. Giamberardino MA: Recent and forgotten aspects of visceral pain. Eur J Pain, 3: 77-92, 1999.

21. Giamberardino, MA, Affaitati G, Iezzi S, Vecchiet L: Referred muscle pain and hyperalgesia from viscera. J Musculoske Pain, 7(1/2): 61-69, 1999.

22. Wesselman U, Lai J: Mechanisms of referred visceral pain: uterine inflammation in the adult virgin rat results in neurogenic plasma extravasation in the skin. Pain, 73: 309-317, 1997.

23. Thurston RC, Keefe FJ, Bradley L, Rama Krishnan KR, Caldwell DS: Chest pain in the absence of coronary artery disease: a biophysical perspective. Pain, 93: 95-100, 2001.

24. Veale D, Kavanagh G, Fielding JF, Fitzgerald O: Primary fibromyalgia and the irritable bowel syndrome: different expressions of a common pathogenic process. Brit J Rheumatol, 30: 220-222, 1991.

25. Granges G, Littlejohn G: Pressure pain thresholds in pain-free subjects, in patients with chronic regional pain syndromes, and in patients with fibromyalgia syndrome. Arthritis Rheum, 36: 642-646, 1993.

26. Lautenbacher S, Rollman GB, McCain GA: Multi-method assessment of experimental and clinical pain in patients with fibromyalgia. Pain, 59: 45-53, 1994.

27. Norregaard J, Bendtsen L, Lykkegaard J, Jenson R: Pressure and heat pain thresholds and tolerances in patients with fibromyalgia. J Musculoske Pain, 5(2): 43-53, 1997.

28. Chang L, Mayer EA, Johnson T, FitzGerald LZ, Naliboff B: Differences in somatic perception in female patients with irritable bowel syndrome with and without fibromyalgia. Pain, 84: 297-307, 2000.

29. Lembo T, Naliboff BD, Matin K, Munakata J, Parker RA, Gracely RH, Mayer EA: Irritable bowel syndrome patients show altered sensitivity to exogenous opioids. Pain, 87: 137-147, 2000.

30. Vecchiet L, Giamberardino MA: Referred pain: clinical significance, pathophysiology and treatment, in Myofascial Pain: Update in Diagnosis and Treatment, Edited by AA Fischer, 1997, WB Saunders Company, Philadelphia. pp. 119-136.

31. Doggweiler-Wiygul R, Blankenship J, MacDiarmid SA: Review on chronic pelvic pain from a urologic point of view. World J Urology, 19(3):160-165, 2001.

32. Wesselman U: Urogenital pain syndromes in men and women, in Proceedings of the 9th World Congress on Pain, Edited by M Devor, MC Rowbotham, Z Weisenfeld-Hallin, 2000, IASP Press: Seattle.

33. Ness TJ, Richter HE, Varner RE, Fillingim RB: A psychophysical study of discomfort produced by repeated filling of the urinary bladder. Pain, 76: 61-69, 1998.

34. Bajaj P, Arendt-Nielsen L, Bajaj P, Madsen H: Sensory changes during the ovulatory phase of the menstrual cycle in healthy women. Eur J Pain, 5(2): 135-144, 2001.

Physical Therapy Approach to Fibromyalgia with Myofascial Trigger Points: A Case Report

Joseph M. Donnelly

SUMMARY. Background: Fibromyalgia and myofascial pain syndrome are clearly distinguishable, different clinical conditions and can interact strongly. Each condition can be managed when it is clearly identified as such and the appropriate management corrections are applied.

Findings: 1. The patient learned how to manage this combination of syndromes effectively. 2. The patient learned to gain control of FMS symptoms. 3. Gaining control of symptoms from myofascial trigger points required help from a skilled physical therapist.

Conclusion: The management of patients with fibromyalgia and myofascial pain syndromes is often a very complicated process. Neuro-mobilization techniques and treatment of trigger points were quite effective in finally achieving a good functional outcome for this patient with both conditions. *[Article copies available for a fee from The Haworth Document Delivery Service: 1-800-HAWORTH. E-mail address: <getinfo@haworthpressinc.com> Website: <http://www.HaworthPress.com> © 2002 by The Haworth Press, Inc. All rights reserved.]*

Joseph M. Donnelly, PT, MS, Board Certified Specialist in Orthopedic Physical Therapy, Part Time Instructor, Department of Physical Therapy, Georgia State University, Clinical Specialist, The Sports Rehabilitation Center, Atlanta, GA.

Address correspondence to: Joseph M. Donnelly, PT, MS, The Sports Rehabilitatioon Center at Georgia Tech, Georgia Tech Athletic Association, 150 Bobby Dodd Way, N. W., Atlanta, GA 30332-0455.

[Haworth co-indexing entry note]: "Physical Therapy Approach to Fibromyalgia with Myofascial Trigger Points: A Case Report." Donnelly, Joseph M. Co-published simultaneously in *Journal of Musculoskeletal Pain* [The Haworth Medical Press, an imprint of The Haworth Press, Inc.] Vol. 10, No. 1/2, 2002, pp. 177-190; and: *The Clinical Neurobiology of Fibromyalgia and Myofascial Pain: Therapeutic Implications* [ed: Robert M. Bennett] The Haworth Medical Press, an imprint of The Haworth Press, Inc., 2002, pp. 177-190. Single or multiple copies of this article are available for a fee from The Haworth Document Delivery Service [1-800-HAWORTH, 9:00 a.m. - 5:00 p.m. (EST). E-mail address: getinfo@haworthpressinc.com].

KEYWORDS. Myofascial trigger points, fibromyalgia, neuromobilization, manual physical therapy

INTRODUCTION

Rehabilitation of patients diagnosed with fibromyalgia syndrome [FMS] and myofascial pain syndrome [MPS] presents a unique challenge for the physical therapist [PT]. These patients usually present with a great complexity of common enigmatic neuromusculoskeletal pain problems. Fibromyalgia syndrome and MPS are clearly distinguishable, different clinical conditions (1) and can interact strongly. Each can be managed when it is clearly identified as such and the appropriate management corrections are applied. Fibromyalgia syndrome can be effectively treated if the treatment also includes effective management of the concurrent myofascial trigger point [TrP] problem.

This case report identifies three remarkable findings and observations: 1. This patient learned how to manage this combination of syndromes effectively for herself because she learned how to identify which was causing her pain, FMS or MPS, 2. The patient got control of her symptoms from FMS by breaking into the positive feedback loop: disturbed sleep-increased pain from FMS-more disturbed sleep, 3. At first she failed to get control of the other positive feedback loop: TrP pain-aggravation of FMS pain and dysfunctions producing increased TrP activation, and became disheartened. A previous attempt at physical therapy failed clearly because the PT had limited knowledge of the identification and treatment TrPs. Skilled clinical examination with an open clinical decision making mind without preconceived assumptions and treatment (2,3), which incorporated neuromusculoskeletal principles proved to be very successful. Identification of specific TrPs and instruction in self-management was paramount to the successful outcome of this patient's physical therapy experience.

CASE REPORT

A 29-year-old female was referred to physical therapy with a diagnosis of FMS and MPS. The patient is a veterinarian responsible for accounts in South America but had become unable to travel due to severe pain. She started this job in January 1997. For two and one-half years she traveled 210 days per year, taking a trip two or three times per week.

She experienced increasing frequency and severity of symptom flares that were present since childhood. By October 1999, the patient was experiencing bilateral upper extremity pain so severe that she was unable to lift her arms over head. She was seen by her primary care physician and was diagnosed with cervical radiculopathy. By the end of October the patient was unable to work or perform activities of daily living, walk for more than 10 minutes and was unable to climb stairs due to intense body pain and what she described as "flu-like symptoms." The patient was referred to a rheumatologist, diagnosed with FMS, told that there was no cure, and referred to physical therapy. The patient searched the Internet and obtained a self-help book (4) and found valuable information regarding sleep deprivation and management strategies for FMS. A caring and knowledgeable sleep specialist did an extensive sleep study and identified a loss of both alpha and delta sleep levels. The patient was placed on popular sleep medications to assist with restoring delta level sleep, which initially failed. She worked with the sleep specialist for three months until they found diphenylhydramine that helped greatly to restore a normal delta pattern and an effective sleep routine. Once she started sleeping through the night uninterrupted she began to notice a significant difference in her FMS symptoms, however, the localized pain from the TrPs persisted.

The difference reported by the patient between symptoms from FMS and MPS were that in the former "every cell hurt equally" and with the latter "a distinct pattern of pain in a more localized area was noted" which responded favorably to moist heat. The patient had established what she referred to as "a perfect sleep hygiene" which has kept the symptoms of FMS such as overwhelming fatigue, lack of concentration, global body pain, allodynia, and hyperactive TrPs to a minimum. When sleep was disturbed by travel the patient did note an increase in generalized pain where "every cell hurt," difficulty arousing herself in the morning with overwhelming fatigue, and TrP hyperactivity. The patient discerned clearly that, when the FMS was active, normal activity seemed to overload her muscles and to activate her TrPs.

In October 1999 the patient started physical therapy and by this time was experiencing total body symptoms, headache and was only able to work four hours a day in a home office. The patient reported, following physical therapy sessions in the first three to four weeks that she got physically ill with nausea and vomiting and had to lie on the floor for five to six hours waiting for symptoms to decrease. The patient attended physical therapy sessions three times weekly from October 1999 through July 2000, which included numerous manual therapy techniques and an attempt of exercise regimes. The patient continued her physical therapy sessions in spite of its ill effects expecting that it would eventually help her return to "a functioning human being." The patient also received treatments from a neuromuscular therapist who was trained in craniosacral techniques and myofascial release and this intervention seemed very helpful, but temporary in nature.

Upon completion of physical therapy the patient continued to have pain from TrPs which were not going away and preventing her from carrying out activities of daily living and returning to work. The patient obtained a copy of The Trigger Point Manual (5) and began to map out TrPs that she thought were causing her the most difficulty by locating the taut bands and pressing on the TrP. She tried to find a clinician who was trained in identifying and treating TrPs. The patient was unable to find a clinician close to home that had knowledge of TrPs and had to drive 75 miles for treatment of her symptoms from MPS.

The patient was seen by this PT in September 2000 approximately one year following the diagnosis of FMS and MPS. The patient presented with a thorough understanding of her symptoms that were generated from FMS and those that were generated from MPS as cited above and recognized the interaction between the two. The past medical history was significant for spinal meningitis and temporomandibular joint dysfunction. A familial history was significant for a sister and mother with FMS. The patient reported that she had achieved "a perfect sleep hygiene" and was resting six to eight hours nightly. The patient was able to work full time from a home office but was unable to travel and carry out her assigned duties without an acute exacerbation of her symptoms for one year now. The patient's goals of therapy were self-management of TrPs and progression to an exercise program so she could function as close to that of a "normal 30 year old person as possible" and to return to her prior position at work.

The patient's primary complaints included pain 8/10 in the left upper extremity, head pain localized to the right side, pain with cervical left rotation and right side bending. The patient also complained of generalized tightness throughout the body especially in the lower extremities with a description of "tight flesh." The patient also described a "feeling of chaos" in her nervous system and a constant "buzzing feeling." She used the analogy of snow on the television screen after the late night news to describe the central nervous system [CNS] "chaos." Functionally the patient was unable to do household chores, walk for more than 20 minutes, lift groceries out of the cart, or reach into cabinets overhead and felt very disabled. The patient's anxiety level was very high and she was seeking guidance for rehabilitation of her condition as she was beginning to feel hopeless.

A skilled examination was carried out over two one hour treatment sessions due to the complexity of the patient's history and presentation. The subjective examination of this patient lead me to believe there was a high level of CNS input and that the threshold control from the CNS needed to be addressed via explanation, understanding, and validation of symptoms followed by a skilled physical examination. The influence of the autonomic system, neuroendocrine system, immune system, and the motor system would also have to be considered as output control mechanisms of the CNS in maintenance of this patient's painful complaints (6). The patients global reports of pain, prevalence of TrPs, FMS, and level of anxiety lead me to believe there is a high component of CNS sensitivity maintaining TrP activity, altered movement patterns, and related dysfunctions.

The physical exam considered specific physical dysfunctions including TrPs, articular dysfunctions, changes in movement patterns, muscle imbalances, changes in fascia as well as identification of hyperalgesic zones in the skin. The specific physical dysfunctions identified during the examination were only clinical findings that helped to forge links to the general physical dysfunctions such as not being able to lift overhead, carry groceries, walk for more than twenty minutes, or carry out household chores [vacuuming, sweeping, dusting]. The key issue with this patient was limitation of function, regardless of cause, which is what the patient wanted changed.

Postural examination of this patient revealed a flattened cervical lordosis, increased thoracic kyphosis and lumbar lordosis, a moderate forward head position with anterior rounded shoulders. A facial scoliosis was noted with the mandible deviated to the right. *Active cervical movements* were limited and painful with left rotation and side bending right. There was a loss of thoracic extension and lumbar flexion and all movements were painful. Limited and painful ankle dorsi flexion was noted bilaterally. Painful *limited stretch range of motion* was noted with passive hip extension, ankle dorsi flexion, hip abduction and adduction. Painful limited stretch range of motion was noted in cervical side bending, rotation, flexion, and upper extremity horizontal abduction, shoulder external and internal rotation. *Palpation* revealed a significant number of active and latent TrPs throughout the body, which are listed in Table 1. An active TrP causes a clinical pain complaint, is always tender, prevents full lengthening of the muscle, weakens the muscle, and refers a patient recognized pain pattern on direct compression. A latent

TABLE 1. Identified Myofascial Trigger Points

Trigger Points	Upper Body	Lower Body
Active	Scalenes Pectoralis minor Subscapularis Upper trapezius Levator scapulae	Piriformis Gluteus minimus Gastrocnemius
Latent	Strenocleidomastoid Sub occipitals Splenius capitus Masseter Temporalis Digastric Infraspinatus Sternalis Pectoralis major Deltoid Brachioradialis Wrist extensors	Erector spinae Gluteus maximus Piriformis Hamstrings Psoas Iliacus Adductor longus Quadriceps Tibialis anterior Peroneal muscles Foot intrinsics

TrP is only painful when it is palpated and may have all the other clinical characteristics of an active TrP and always has a taut band that increases muscle tension and restricts stretch range of motion. Assessment of *skin drag* revealed hyperalgesia and increased resistance throughout both lower extremities. The patient was unable to tolerate grasping the skin to produce a *skin fold* due to fascial changes and extreme pain. Assessment of *movement patterns* as described by Janda (7), including hip abduction, hip extension, trunk curl, and upper extremity elevation were found to be quite impaired with excessive activation of phasic muscles. The abdominal obliques, transverse abdominus, gluteus maximus and medius, and scapula stabilizers were *weak and inhibited. Neurodynamic* testing revealed a positive slump test reproducing lower extremity, middle and low back symptoms. The *straight-leg raise test* [SLR] was positive bilaterally with significant pain in the posterior knee, which increased with cervical flexion. *Upper limb tension tests* for the median, ulnar, and radial nerve were positive in the left upper extremity (8). *Proprioceptive testing* revealed an inability to perform unilateral stance on the left with a poor balance strategy. Unilateral stance on the right was performed with a good strategy for 30 seconds.

In this case there appeared to be a high level of CNS sensitivity possibly maintaining activity of the TrPs. The muscle imbalances, proprioceptive deficits, and hyperalgesia in the lower extremities along with the TrP chains were considered by the author as an expression of CNS sensitivity. It was apparent that the left upper extremity pain was being caused by TrPs in the scalene, pectoralis minor, and wrist extensor muscles (5) and by altered neurodynamics (8). There were many unhealthy tissues identified in this patient most likely being maintained by the enhanced CNS responsiveness. This proposed a significant challenge in the management and prognosis of this patient.

The prognosis was probably the most difficult decision for the author and required consideration of recovery of function and relief from pain, which can be quite different. The prognosis for return to function was very good for this patient as she was educated well and was highly motivated to return to a "normal" lifestyle. The patient had extensive knowledge of FMS and MPS and had a remarkable understanding of the symptoms that were caused by each syndrome. She also had a clear understanding of the effect her FMS had on the MPS. The prognosis for resolution of pain was fair as this was a chronic problem that was not only being maintained by peripheral nociceptive and neurogenic mechanism but also by increased CNS sensitivity. The prognosis for exacerbation of symptoms was high following completion of her physical therapy program due to FMS and central sensitivity. The patient would likely need intermittent therapy sessions for the rest of her life to maintain an acceptable level of function.

It was important to identify the TrP chains through a well-trained examination and to find the "key" whether it be an articular dysfunction, TrP, altered neurodynamics, or biomechanical fault. Lewit (9) feels it is important to identify the key and reassess the effect on the identified chain. The chains needed to be identified in order to find relevant links for treatment and rehabilitation.

A decision was made to treat the altered neurodynamics specifically the dural restrictions that were identified. The patient responded favorably to myofascial release in the past which had been done by her neuromuscular massage therapist and a general technique [leg pull and arm pull] were performed on the lower extremities and upper extremities. Myofascial release is a whole-body hands on approach for the evaluation and treatment of the human structure (10). The patient was given a gentle dural stretch to be performed bilaterally three times daily, 10 repetitions only, introducing a gentle stretch throughout the thoracic spine and lower extremity. The patient was advised to use extreme caution during stretching and only to approach the pain and not to push into the pain. The patient demonstrated a thorough understanding of the technique and was able to reproduce the technique independently.

Posttreatment the patient reported decreased pain level of 4/10 throughout the upper half of the body. Left upper extremity pain persisted in a referral pattern of the scalene muscles. The patient was instructed in postisometric relaxation techniques (11) for the scalene muscles and this significantly decreased her left upper extremity symptoms to being barely noticeable. Her home exercise program following this visit is listed in Table 2.

FIRST TREATMENT VISIT

The patient returned for treatment five days later and reported a significant relief in her nervous system "chaos" and "buzzing" which she related to the dural stretches. The nervous system "chaos" was easily aggravated with prolonged standing [more than 15 minutes] and with walking more than 15 minutes. The left upper extremity pain was eliminated with the postisometric relaxation exercises of the scalene muscles. The patient now complained of pain 7/10 in the right pectoral region secondary to sweeping the kitchen floor along with increased pain in the left buttocks and posterior thigh. Physical examination revealed two TrP chains, one in the upper half of the body on the right and one on the lower half of the body on the left as seen in Table 3. Neurodynamic testing was improved with increased range of motion in trunk flexion, hip flexion, knee extension, and ankle dorsiflexion, however, reproduced subjective painful complaints with the slump position, SLR, and upper limb tension testing. The patient reported less discomfort in the test position than the last time these test positions were assumed. Treatment included postisometric relaxation of the right pectoralis major and minor, left hip adductors, piriformis, and manual release of the foot intrinsic musculature utilizing a vibratory technique. Myofascial release techniques [arm pull, leg pull] from the last treatment were performed along with manual dural stretches. Posttreatment, the patient rated the pain 2/10 in the right pectoral region no residual lower extremity pain or headache. Latent TrPs were identified in the right pec-

TABLE 2. Home Exercise Prescription Following the Examination

Exercise	Frequency
1. Dural stretch	Three times daily; 10 repetitions
2. Post isometric relaxation scalenii	Hold five seconds repeat three times

toralis major and piriformis. The two TrP chains could not be identified posttreatment. The patients home program was updated as outlined in Table 4.

SECOND TREATMENT VISIT

The patient returned in one week and reported an elimination of her nervous system "chaos" and "buzzing" at rest and she was now able to walk for 40 minutes and stand for 30 minutes until her symptoms were activated. Activities that involve repetitive movements activated TrPs very easily and if the activity was stopped and postisometric relaxation techniques were performed the TrP pain would go away. If she continued the activity too long, the TrP would not go away with postisometric relaxation but would begin to activate other TrPs. She reports being able to control activity of recurring TrPs very effectively with the

TABLE 3. Trigger Point Chains Found on the First Treatment Visit

Lower body left side trigger point chain	Upper body right side trigger point chain
Piriformis	Sub occipital muscles
Gluteus medius	Sternocleidomastoid
Gluteus minimus	Upper trapezius
Medial hamstring	Levator scapulae
Gastrocnemius	Pectoralis minor
Foot intrinsics	Pectoralis major
Adductor longus	Diaphragm
Psoas	Abdominal obliques
Iliacus	Thoracic paraspinals
Rectus femoris	
Vastus medialis	

TABLE 4. Home Exercise Prescription Following the First Treatment Visit

Exercise	Frequency
1. Dural stretch	Three times daily; 10 repetitions
2. Post isometric relaxation	
Scalenes	Hold five seconds repeat three times
Pectoral muscles	
Hip adductors	
Piriformis	
3. Single leg stance	Perform for five minutes or onset of trigger point pain [right side then left side]

postisometric relaxation exercises that were performed soon after onset of TrP symptoms. Today her main complaint was pain rated 5/10 in the left upper trapezius and levator scapulae area, which she was unable to relieve with postisometric relaxation and had a very restricted or "tight fleshy feeling" in the lower extremities. Physical exam revealed painful limited left cervical rotation and right side bending. Passive movement revealed painful limited right side bending coupled with right side bending and right side bending with left rotation incriminating possible TrPs in the levator scapulae and upper trapezius. Mobility assessment of the cervical spine was unremarkable. There were moderate muscle length deficits noted in the left and right lower extremities that were not painful at end range. No TrP chains were identified on this day. Neurodynamic testing was positive, however, a full slump position could be achieved. The SLR was positive with the addition of medial rotation and adduction at the hip. Upper limb tension testing was unremarkable. Trunk and lower extremity range of motion were significantly improved. Altered muscle activation patterns were still noted with the trunk curl, hip abduction, and hip extension. Proprioception was significantly impaired on the left with an inability to perform unilateral stance for greater than 20 seconds on the left as compared to 60 seconds on the right.

Treatment consisted of manual dural stretching, myofascial release [arm and leg pull], pressure release with contract relax, spray and gentle stretch of the left upper trapezius and levator scapulae. Postisometric relaxation techniques were reviewed and pressure release techniques were introduced for control of TrPs that recurred. Posttreatment the patient had 0/10 pain for the first time in fourteen months and an overwhelming tearful emotional response. The patient would continue her home exercise prescription as outlined in Table 4. The patient felt confident that she could manage her symptoms with her home exercise prescription and she would gradually increase functional activities utilizing energy conservation techniques.

THIRD TREATMENT VISIT

The patient returned in two weeks and reported that she was pain free. She had a complaint of tightness in both calves, which she attributed to her menstrual cycle. The patient reported a dissipation in her nervous system "chaos" or "buzzing" and could prevent recurrence of these symptoms with her dural stretches. She did note that the dural restrictions changed from day to day and some days noted a significant difficulty performing the stretches due to painful limitation in her thoracic spine and lower extremities. She was unable to correlate these findings of painful stretch with the amount of functional activities she was performing.

The TrPs were being treated with postisometric relaxation techniques and it was very effective when the technique was performed at the immediate recognition of the specific muscle in "trouble." Functionally she was able to grocery shop, perform intermittent household chores, walk for one hour, and for the first time in a year enjoy shopping at the mall. The patient felt she was in control of her life again and would return to her prior position at work in two weeks. Physical exam revealed a negative TrP exam. Cervical and lumbar range of motion was in a functional range and pain-free. Fascial restrictions were evident in the lower extremities, however, no hyperalgesic zones were noted with skin drag and skin rolling techniques. Altered movement patterns were noted in hip extension and hip abduction with over-activation of trunk musculature. Impaired proprioception was evident in the left lower extremity with unilateral stance limited to twenty seconds with a poor balance strategy.

The patient was instructed in gluteus medius and maximus retraining exercises to be performed daily in addition to her dural stretches, TrP self-treatment and walking program as outlined in Table 5. The patient was discharged from a formal physical therapy program and was instructed to contact our office with any questions or exacerbations of symptoms.

The patient returned in six weeks with an acute exacerbation of oral facial TrPs and general pain complaints rated 6/10. Patient reports that she had to travel to South America and her sleep pattern had been interrupted due to time zones and was not able to get her symptoms under control. She also reports not performing her home exercise regularly and had noticed recurrence of nervous system "chaos" and "buzzing." Patient reports that her sleeping hygiene has been restored for one week now and this has helped decrease the FMS complaints. Physical examination revealed altered neurodynamics with positive slump, SLR, and upper limb tension tests similar to the initial examination. A TrP chain was noted in the right upper body including sternocleidomastoid, upper trapezius, levator scapulae, masseter, temporalis, medial pterygoid, pectoralis minor, triceps, and wrist extensors. Hyperalgesic zones were noted in both lower extremities with palpation. Treatment of the masseter

TABLE 5. Final Home Exercise Prescription

Exercise	Frequency
1. Dural stretch	Three times daily; 10 repetitions
2. Post isometric relaxation Muscle in trouble	Hold five seconds repeat three times
4. Single leg stance	Perform for five minutes or onset of trigger point pain [right side then left side]
5. Scapular retraction	Yellow Theraband 15-20 repetitions or until fatigue. Daily
5. Gluteal retraining	15-20 repetitions or until fatigue. Daily
6. Self leg pull stretching	Daily each leg
7. Pep walking	20 minutes daily

and pterygoid muscle eliminated the upper extremity TrP chain. Myofascial release and dural stretching techniques reduced resting pain levels to 2/10 and eliminated reported nervous system "chaos" and "buzzing." The patient was seen in two weeks for a follow-up visit and was discharged from physical therapy.

Over the past eight months of 2001, I have seen this patient on eight different occasions for exacerbations of MPS. In this time the patient has had two exacerbations of her FMS, once due to the flu and once due to extensive travel. In my last consultation with this patient she specifically noted dramatic changes in trunk range of motion and dorsi flexion with the dural stretches and self-stretching techniques which were keeping her nervous system "chaos" and "buzzing" under control. The postisometric relaxation techniques are very effective in eliminating a specific TrP pain pattern. The patients awakening to the importance of performing her home exercise prescription was when she had an acute exacerbation of symptoms in January 2001. It became very clear that dural stretching which would keep her nervous system clear of "chaos" and "buzzing," and postisometric relaxation at onset of activation of a TrP would allow her muscles and body to function more normally. The patient has progressed to a regular exercise program including light resistance and can now perform all activities of daily living, household chores, and work activities at will.

DISCUSSION

Identifying the anatomical sources of the patient's symptoms through a skilled examination is quite easy when there is pain from an injury or acute overload of a muscle. In the patient with chronic MPS with perpetuating factors such as FMS it is more difficult to pinpoint the exact source of the patients symptoms. The management of patients with FMS or MPS or a combination of both is often a very complicated process. The PT must have extensive training with an experienced clinician to become proficient in the identification and management techniques of TrPs, which usually takes a period of two years. Neurodynamic testing and management also require extensive hands-on training to become proficient in the testing and management of these dysfunctions. Syndromal diagnoses such as MPS are said to exist in "The Grey Zone of Practice" (12) where all is not black and white. This zone where neither the pathobiology of the syndrome nor the risk benefit ratio of treatment are fully understood set up a unique opportunity for investigating new treatments and technologies and for professions to identify answers. The exact pathoanatomy and pathophysiology of TrPs now has a credible working hypothesis (13) but the benefits and risk to treatment are poorly documented in the literature. Neuromobilization techniques along with self-treatment of TrPs were quite effective in achieving a good functional outcome for this patient. We must continue attempts to build a bridge between scientific research and the clinical application of these concepts and principles to improve the management strategies for patients suffering with MPS or FMS.

REFERENCES

1. Harden RN, Bruehl SP, Gass S, Niemiec C, Barbick B: Signs and symptoms of the myofascial pain syndrome: a national survey of pain management providers. Clin J Pain 16(1):64-72, 2000.

2. Jones MA: Clinical reasoning in manual therapy. Physical Therapy 72(12): 875-883, 1992.

3. Butler DS: The Sensitive Nervous System, 1st edition, Noigroup Publications, Adelaide, South Australia; 2000.

4. Starlanyl D, Copeland ME: Fibromyalgia & Chronic Myofascial Pain Syndrome: A Survival Manual. New Harbinger Publications, Oakland, 1996.

5. Simone DG, Travell JG, Simons I S: Travell & Simons' Myofascial Pain and Dysfunction: The Trigger Point Manual, Vol. 1, Ed. 2. Williams & Wilkins, Baltimore, 1999.

6. Gifford LS: Pain: the tissues and the nervous system. Physiotherapy 84: 27-33, 1998.

7. Janda V: Muscle weakness and inhibition in back pain syndromes, in Grieve GP (Ed.) Modern Manual Therapy of the Vertebral Column. Churchill-Livingston, NY, NY 1987; 197-201.

8. Butler DS: Mobilization of the Nervous System, Churchill-Livingston, Melbourne, Australia; 1991.

9. Lewit K: Chain reactions in the locomotor system in the light of co-activation patterns based on developmental neurology. J Orthopedic Med. 21(1):52-56, 1999.

10. Barnes JF: Myofascial release, in Hammer WI (Ed.) Functional Soft Tissue Examination and Treatment by Manual Methods. Aspen Publishers, Gaithersburg, MD, 1999; 533-547.

11. Lewit K: Manipulative Therapy in Rehabilitation of the Locomotor System; ed. 3, Butterworth, London; 1999.

12. Naylor CD: Grey zones of clinical practice: some limits to evidence-based medicine. The Lancet 345: 840-842, 1995.

13. Mense S, Simons DG, Russell IJ: Muscle Pain: Its Nature, Diagnosis, and Treatment. Lippincott, Williams & Wilkins, Philadelphia, 2001.

The Epidemiology
of Chronic Widespread Pain

Peter Croft

SUMMARY. Objectives: To discuss some aspects of the epidemiology of widespread pain: case definition, occurrence, and associated characteristics.

Findings: The fibromyalgia definition of chronic widespread pain is useful from an epidemiological standpoint because it facilitates comparison between studies. In studies of widespread pain sufferers, back pain and osteoarthritis represent important subgroups. The overall prevalence of widespread pain remains fairly stable but is dynamic with influx from no pain and regional pain groups as efflux to those same groups occurs. The prevalence of widespread musculoskeletal pain is somewhat higher among women than men in the community, but the very high female-to-male ratio among sufferers with fibromyalgia is unexplained. Distress, fatigue, and frequent consultations for disruptive symptoms appear to be risk factors for the development of chronic widespread pain.

Peter Croft, MD, MSc, is Professor of Primary Care Epidemiology, Keele University, Keele, Staffordshire, ST5 5BG, England [E-mail: p.r.croft@cphc.keele.ac.uk].

[Haworth co-indexing entry note]: "The Epidemiology of Chronic Widespread Pain." Croft, Peter. Co-published simultaneously in *Journal of Musculoskeletal Pain* [The Haworth Medical Press, an imprint of The Haworth Press, Inc.] Vol. 10, No. 1/2, 2002, pp. 191-199; and: *The Clinical Neurobiology of Fibromyalgia and Myofascial Pain: Therapeutic Implications* [ed: Robert M. Bennett] The Haworth Medical Press, an imprint of The Haworth Press, Inc., 2002, pp. 191-199. Single or multiple copies of this article are available for a fee from The Haworth Document Delivery Service [1-800-HAWORTH, 9:00 a.m. - 5:00 p.m. [EST]. E-mail address: getinfo@haworthpressinc.com].

191

Conclusions: It may be that "widespreadness" is our best epidemiological measure of the extent of involvement of central pain processes. *[Article copies available for a fee from The Haworth Document Delivery Service: 1-800-HAWORTH. E-mail address: <getinfo@haworthpressinc.com> Website: <http://www.HaworthPress.com>* © 2002 by The Haworth Press, Inc. All rights reserved.]*

KEYWORDS. Chronic widespread pain, fibromyalgia, epidemiology, occurrence

CASE DEFINITION

Chronic widespread pain is the cardinal symptom of the fibromyalgia syndrome [FMS]. It was given a useful, but arbitrary, standard definition by an American College of Rheumatology [ACR] Committee (1). This definition emphasised that axial pain was a constant feature, and that pain had to be present in the upper and lower quadrants, and the right and left sides, of the body. This definition can incorporate a wide range of pain distribution but, from an epidemiological point-of-view, it is useful because it provides a standard of comparison for different studies.

One major revision has been proposed for epidemiological purposes. The Manchester [United Kingdom] group has proposed a definition which is more restrictive than the ACR criteria (2). This requires that any limb pain needs to have a minimum distribution before it contributes to widespread pain. The latter is then classified as per the ACR description.

There are certain implications in the widespread pain concept that need to be drawn out when interpreting epidemiological studies. Firstly chronic widespread pain need not denote a diagnosis, or even a clinical concept, on its own. The term can simply be used epidemiologically to describe a symptom, at one end of a spectrum of pain complaints, characterized by the extent of its spread in the body. If we plucked any one patient from the epidemiological pool represented by this symptom, the clinician might be faced with a case which he or she would recognize as, for example, polymyalgia, osteoarthritis, osteomalacia, or cancer.

However "widespread pain" is a useful clinical concept for epidemiological studies for three reasons. First, clinicians report an entity of "widespread pain" which is more than the simultaneous presence of two or three pain complaints, with more diffuse pain accompanied by fatigue and poor sleep for example. This is the context for the FMS. Second, serious pathologies may underlie widespread pain, but these are only present in a small minority of those with chronic widespread pain in the population. Wolfe and his colleagues, for example, estimated from their population survey that cancer and recent trauma were reported by about one percent of the population compared with the 10.6 percent who reported chronic widespread pain (3). So in population studies, chronic widespread pain is taken to mean "widespread musculoskeletal pain which has no obvious underlying pathology." Third, there are still common diagnoses which may have widespread features. Osteoarthritis and low back pain are the commonest causes of pain in the population, but the pain cannot simply be explained by local underlying damage or disease (4). They are syndromes of chronic pain, not discrete pathologies, and the pain can spread beyond the confines of a single joint or of the spine. In back pain studies, the occurrence and influence of such "widespreadness" is important. In widespread pain studies, back pain and osteoarthritis sufferers will be important subgroups.

So, in chronic pain epidemiology, the spread or extent of pain should be measured as a separate variable. If epidemiological studies can demonstrate the usefulness of classifying chronic pain sufferers according to the extent of their pain [for prognosis or for treatment selection, for example], then the concept has clinical applicability. At the end of the spectrum lies the widespread pain which extends beyond multiple focal problems [such as osteoarthritis in multiple joints] and incorporates the FMS.

OCCURRENCE

Prevalence is the proportion of the population who have a problem at a certain point in time. Population studies have produced estimates of prevalence ranging from zero to 13 percent (3,5-11) [Table 1]. There is more consistency, however, than first seems apparent:

1. Studies in adult general population samples from Europe, Israel, and America which have used the ACR definition of chronic widespread pain, using postal questionnaires, have prevalence estimates between 9.9 and 12.9 percent (3,5,7,9). The lower estimate from the London, Ontario study [7.3 percent] may be related to their use of telephone interviews as the means to obtain pain in-

formation (8). The Manchester restrictive definition [ACR-M] produced, as expected, a lower prevalence [4.7 percent] (9).

2. Two studies (10,11), including one in children, were based on a simpler concept of multiple pains but produced similar estimates [10.7 and 12.5] to the ACR-based studies.

3. One exception is a small study of Pima Indians (6), which suggests that some populations may have radically different reported chronic widespread pain frequency.

Incidence is the proportion of the population who develop a condition over a specified period of time. It can be calculated separately for population groups with no pain or with regional pain. McBeth and his colleagues from Manchester have specifically studied incidence in the general population (12). They identified 1,480 adults aged 18-65 years who had either no pain at all [N = 825] or who had regional but not widespread pain [N = 833] and who responded one year later to a further questionnaire. The follow-up figures are shown in Table 2A. The cumulative annual incidence of new cases of chronic widespread pain in an initially widespread pain-free population was 5.5 percent [two percent per year in those free of pain; eight percent per year in those with regional pain].

Outcome studies in the general population add to the picture of occurrence by investigating the likelihood of chronic widespread pain

TABLE 1. Prevalence Studies of Chronic Widespread Pain

Reference number	Study setting	Age range [years]	Total number surveyed	Prevalence [Percent]		
				ACR	ACR-M	Multiple pains
5.	England	18-plus	1340	11.2		
3.	USA	18-plus	3006	10.6		
6.	USA [Pima]		105	0		
7.	Israel		2210	9.9		
8.	Canada	18-plus	3395	7.3		
9.	England	18-65	1953	12.9	4.7	
10.	Sweden	25-74	1609			10.7
11.	Netherlands	0-18	5424			12.5

ACR = American College of Rheumatology
ACR-M = Manchester Restrictive ACR criteria

persisting or improving. McBeth et al. followed up the 225 adults with chronic widespread pain in their population survey (13). Table 2B summarizes the one year outcome: 56 percent still had chronic widespread pain, 33 percent regional pain, and 11 percent were pain-free.

Tables 2A and 2B also show the expected pattern at two years if the 12 month figures were to continue into the next year [shown as "expected numbers"]. These projections can then be compared with the results of an earlier study of chronic widespread pain carried out by the same group in another population sample (14). In this earlier study 141

TABLE 2

A. What Happens to Those Who Have Chronic Widespread Pain in the Community?

Groups	Numbers in a population of 1000 people	One year later	Two years later	
			Expected	Observed
No pain		14	22	20
Regional pain		43	67	65
Chronic widespread pain	130	73	41	46

Reference Sources: (13,14)

B. What Happens to Those Without Chronic Widespread Pain in the Community?

Groups	Numbers in a population of 1000 people	One year later	Two years later	
			Expected	Observed
No pain	430	421	412	
Regional pain	440	405	373	
Chronic widespread pain		44	88	84

Reference Sources: (12,14)

C. What Happens Overall?

Groups	Numbers in a population of 1000 people	One year later	Two years later
No pain	430	435	434
Regional pain	440	440	407
Chronic widespread pain	130	117	129

people with chronic, regional, or no pain were followed up after an average of two years [shown as "observed numbers"]. The observed and projected figures from the two studies are very similar.

Table 2C completes the picture by combining the incidence data from Table 2A and the outcome data from Table 2B. This shows the total prevalence of chronic widespread pain is constant over time. There is a small exchange annually with the "no pain population," and a rather larger exchange with the "regional pain population." The numbers of people whose pain becomes widespread is matched by those whose pain becomes less extensive.

ASSOCIATED CHARACTERISTICS

Gender

The very high female-to-male ratio among sufferers from the FMS observed in clinics is not mirrored in population studies of chronic widespread pain. However, the prevalence of musculoskeletal pain generally is higher among women than men in the community and chronic widespread pain is no exception to this. For example, a survey of 2,664 women aged 25 to 55 years from the general population in Oslo, Norway, estimated the prevalence of chronic widespread pain to be 22 percent (15). In most of the population studies quoted in Table 1, the prevalence is approximately twice as high in women compared with men. This female excess remains unexplained.

Age

Chronic widespread pain is found in the young (11) and the old, as well as the middle years. The pattern does change with age, however, and self-reported widespread pain according to the ACR definition does appear to decline in prevalence at those older ages (3,5).

Psychological Distress

Population studies of chronic widespread pain illustrate that anxiety and depression, fatigue, other somatic complaints, anxieties about health, features of somatization, and dissatisfaction with health care and with work, are all more common in sufferers with chronic widespread pain than in those with regional or no pain (3,5). Furthermore the tighter the criterion for chronic widespread pain [for example the Manchester definition], the stronger these associations become (9).

However, most studies are cross-sectional and the direction of cause and effect is not established. Furthermore, an association may not necessarily mean a high absolute difference. In one United Kingdom study, interviewer-confirmed mental illness was common in chronic widespread pain sufferers compared to those without (16). However, the absolute figures showed that 16.9 percent of those with chronic widespread pain had a psychiatric diagnosis compared to 11.9% in the whole of the population sample.

In the same study (13), 1,658 adults free of pain or with regional pain were followed up one year later. Other somatic symptoms and features of somatization predicted the development of widespread pain during the follow-up period. In a Norwegian study of 214 women from the general population followed for five years, extent of baseline pain in regional pain sufferers was a strong predictor of developing subsequent chronic widespread pain (17).

These and other studies have investigated predictors of persistence of chronic widespread pain. In one study, psychological distress, fatigue, and frequent consultations with the family doctor for disruptive symptoms were risks for widespread pain which persisted throughout the subsequent 12 months.

THE REGIONAL PAIN MODEL

Raspe has pointed out that persistence of low back pain is associated with "amplification" of symptoms beyond the confines of the back (18). Part of this amplification involves pain experienced elsewhere in the body. In prospective studies of population samples free of neck pain or free of low back pain, the presence of pain elsewhere is an important predictor of the subsequent development of neck or low back pain. Furthermore, among patients who consult in primary care about low back pain, widespread pain is a major predictor of whether low back pain will persist or not [odds ratio in one study (19) for persistence after adjusting for psychosocial factors = 3.4].

So, widespread pain is an important dimension of regional pain. The "widespreadness" of the pain is a measure of the likelihood that regional pain syndromes will develop or persist. In the epidemiology of pain, both for the clinic and for population studies, the extent of pain should be measured, independent of pain location and psychosocial factors, as a predictor of persistence and progression. Why should this be? It may be that, although crude, "widespreadness" is our best epidemiological measure of the extent of involvement of central pain processes.

FURTHER READING

There have been two excellent reviews of the epidemiology of chronic widespread pain published in recent years (20,21). These cover issues of the health and societal impact of this symptom and its relationship to the FMS, as well as being comprehensive overviews of the descriptive and etiological literature.

REFERENCES

1. Wolfe F, Smythe HA, Yunus MB, Bennett RM, Bombardier C, Goldenberg DL, Tugwell P, Campbell SM, Abeles M, Clark P, Fam AG, Farber SJ, Fiechtner JJ, Franklin CM, Gatter RA, Hamaty D, Lessard J, Lichtbraun AS, Masi AT, McCain GA, Reynolds WJ, Romano TJ, Russell IJ, Sheon RP: The American College of Rheumatology 1990 criteria for the classification of fibromyalgia: report of the Multicenter Criteria Committee. Arthritis Rheum 33: 160-172, 1990.

2. Macfarlane GJ, Croft PR, Schollum J, Silman AJ: Widespread pain: Is an improved classification possible? J Rheumatol 23: 1628-1632, 1996.

3. Wolfe F, Ross K, Anderson J, Russell IJ, Hebert L: The prevalence and characteristics of fibromyalgia in the general population. Arthritis Rheum 38: 19-28, 1995.

4. McAlindon TE, Cooper C, Kirwan JR, Dieppe PA: Knee pain and disability in the community. Br J Rheumatol 31: 189-192, 1992.

5. Croft PR, Rigby AS, Boswell R, Schollum J, Silman AJ: The prevalence of chronic widespread pain in the general population. J Rheum 14: 41-45, 1993.

6. Jacobsson LT, Nagi DK, Pillemer SR, Knowler WC, Hanson RL, Pettitt DJ, Bennett PH: Low prevalences of chronic widespread pain and shoulder disorders among the Pima Indians. J Rheumatol 23: 907-909, 1996.

7. Buskila D, Abramov G, Biton A, Neumann L: The prevalence of pain complaints in a general population in Israel and its implications for utilisation of health services. J Rheumatol 27: 1521-1525, 2000.

8. White KP, Speechley M, Harth M, Ostbye T: The London Fibromyalgia Epidemiology Study: comparing the demographic and clinical characteristics in 100 random community cases of fibromyalgia versus controls. J Rheumatol 26: 1577-1585, 1999.

9. Hunt IM, Silman AJ, Benjamin S, McBeth J, Macfarlane GJ: The prevalence and associated features of chronic widespread pain in the community using the 'Manchester' definition of chronic widespread pain. Rheumatology 38: 275-279, 1999.

10. Andersson HI, Eljertsson E, Leden I, Rosenberg C: Characteristics of subjects with chronic pain in relation to local and widespread pain report. Scand J Rheumatol 25: 146-154, 1996.

11. Perquin CW, Hazebroek-Kampschreur AA, Hunfield JA, Bohnen AM, van Suijlekom-Smit LW, Passchier J, van der Wouden JC: Pain in children and adolescents: a common experience. Pain 87: 51-58. 2000.

12. McBeth J, Macfarlane GJ, Benjamin S, Silman AJ: Features of somatisation predict the onset of chronic widespread pain: results of a large population-based study. Arthritis Rheum 44: 751-753, 2001.

13. McBeth J, Macfarlane GJ, Hunt IM, Silman AJ: Risk factors for persistent chronic widespread pain: a community-based study. Rheumatology 40: 95-101, 2001.

14. Macfarlane GJ, Thomas E, Papageorgiou AC, Schollum J, Croft PR, Silman AJ: Natural history of chronic widespread pain in the community: a better prognosis than in the clinic? J Rheumatol 23: 1617-1620, 1996.

15. Abusdal UG, Hagen KB, Bjorndal A: Self-reported chronic muscle pain among women in Oslo. Tidsskrift for Den Norske Laegeforening 117(11): 1606-1610, 1997.

16. Benjamin S, Morris S, McBeth J, Macfarlane GJ, Silman AJ: The association between chronic widespread pain and mental disorder: a population-based study. Arthritis Rheum 43: 561-567, 2000.

17. Forseth KO, Forre O, Gran JT: A 5.5 year prospective study of self-reported musculoskeletal pain and of fibromyalgia in a female population: significance and natural history. Clinical Rheumatology 18: 114-121, 1999.

18. Raspe H, Kohlmann T: Disorders characterised by pain: a methodological review of population surveys. J Epid Comm Hlth 48: 531-537, 1994.

19. Thomas E, Silman AJ, Croft P, Papageorgiou AC: Predicting who develops chronic low back pain in primary care: a prospective study. British Medical Journal 318: 1662-1667, 1999.

20. Macfarlane GJ: Fibromyalgia and chronic widespread pain, Epidemiology of Pain. Edited by IK Crombie, PR Croft, SJ Linton, L LeResche, M von Korff. International Association for the Study of Pain Press, Seattle, 1999, pp. 113-123.

21. White KP, Horvath M: The Occurrence and Impact of Generalised Pain, Edited by P Croft and AJ Silman. Bailliere Tindall, London, 1999, pp. 379-389.

Fibromyalgia Associated Syndromes

Daniel Clauw

SUMMARY. Objectives: To describe the syndromes that share overlapping clinical features with fibromyalgia [FMS].

Findings: There are a number of semantic terms currently used to described systemic syndromes that share overlapping features with FMS. These include chronic fatigue syndrome, multiple chemical sensitivity, somatoform disorders, and Gulf War Illnesses. There are also a number of regional or "organ-specific" syndromes that overlap with these conditions that have as their common features regional pain, with and without dysfunction of internal organs.

Conclusions: In aggregate, chronic multisymptom illnesses such as FMS are extremely common. Hallmarks of these syndromes include non-nociceptive pain, fatigue, memory difficulties, and dysfunction of visceral organs. *[Article copies available for a fee from The Haworth Document Delivery Service: 1-800-HAWORTH. E-mail address: <getinfo@haworthpressinc. com> Website: <http://www.HaworthPress.com> © 2002 by The Haworth Press, Inc. All rights reserved.]*

KEYWORDS. Fibromyalgia, pain, fatigue, syndromes

INTRODUCTION

As defined by the 1990 American College of Rheumatology [ACR] criteria, fibromyalgia [FMS] is a discrete disorder, characterized by

Daniel Clauw, MD, is Scientific Director, Georgetown Chronic Pain and Fatigue Research Center; Chief, Division of Rheumatology, Immunology and Allergy, Georgetown University Medical Center, Washington, DC 20007.

[Haworth co-indexing entry note]: "Fibromyalgia Associated Syndromes." Clauw, Daniel. Co-published simultaneously in *Journal of Musculoskeletal Pain* [The Haworth Medical Press, an imprint of The Haworth Press, Inc.] Vol. 10, No. 1/2, 2002, pp. 201-214; and: *The Clinical Neurobiology of Fibromyalgia and Myofascial Pain: Therapeutic Implications* [ed: Robert M. Bennett] The Haworth Medical Press, an imprint of The Haworth Press, Inc., 2002, pp. 201-214. Single or multiple copies of this article are available for a fee from The Haworth Document Delivery Service [1-800-HAWORTH, 9:00 a.m. - 5:00 p.m. [EST]. E-mail address: getinfo@haworthpressinc.com].

widespread pain and tenderness on physical examination (1). However, early work by a number of investigators, including Yunus, Goldenberg, and Hudson, suggested that individuals who met these or other criteria for FMS typically had a number of other nondefining clinical features (2-4). A number of terms have been used to describe these overlapping features.

In this manuscript, the term Chronic Multisymptom Illnesses [CMI] will be used to describe these overlapping illnesses and clinical features. This term was coined by Centers for Disease Control and Prevention to describe individuals in the population with multiple chronic somatic symptoms (5). In a series of population-based studies using factor analytic techniques, the "core" symptoms [see Figure 1] that define CMI in the population are multifocal musculoskeletal pain, fatigue, and memory and/or mood difficulties (6,7). Many patients with CMI will meet criteria for one or more systemic conditions such as FMS or chronic fatigue syndrome [CFS], whereas others will not quite meet the diagnostic criteria required for these systemic entities, but will have "regional" syndromes such as irritable bowel syndrome [IBS], migraine, or tension headaches, etc.

Definition and Clinical Features of Systemic Chronic Multisymptom Illnesses. The most commonly recognized systemic conditions that fall within this spectrum include FMS, CFS, somatoform disorders, and multiple chemical sensitivity [MCS]. There are also a variety of less frequent conditions that share considerable homology with these illnesses. Some of these conditions are referred to as "exposure syndromes," since the illness is defined on the basis of an exposure suspected to cause the symptom complex [e.g., "Gulf War Illnesses," sick building syndrome]. Other illnesses within this spectrum affect only one organ system or portion of the body, with the seminal features being pain and/or dysfunction in this region [e.g., migraine headaches, IBS, temporomandibular joint dysfunction]. A Venn diagram outlining this overlap is shown in Figure 2.

Fibromyalgia. To fulfill the criteria for FMS established in 1990, an individual must have *both* chronic widespread pain *and* the presence of 11 of 18 "tender points" [TePs] on examination (1). In contrast to the other systemic CMI illnesses, which are defined entirely on the basis of symptoms, the diagnostic criteria for FMS require a physical finding on examination. This requirement has likely helped FMS research because it identifies individuals with hyperalgesia/allodynia, and has allowed the mechanism[s] for this finding to be explored. But since the ACR cri-

FIGURE 1. Overlap between systemic disorders characterized by chronic pain and fatigue.

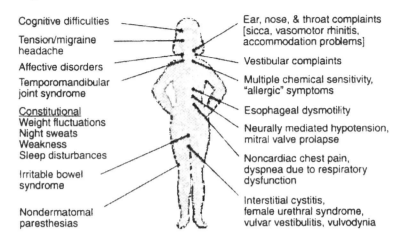

Cognitive difficulties

Tension/migraine headache

Affective disorders

Temporomandibular joint syndrome

Constitutional
Weight fluctuations
Night sweats
Weakness
Sleep disturbances

Irritable bowel syndrome

Nondermatomal paresthesias

Ear, nose, & throat complaints [sicca, vasomotor rhinitis, accommodation problems]

Vestibular complaints

Multiple chemical sensitivity, "allergic" symptoms

Esophageal dysmotility

Neurally mediated hypotension, mitral valve prolapse

Noncardiac chest pain, dyspnea due to respiratory dysfunction

Interstitial cystitis, female urethral syndrome, vulvar vestibulitis, vulvodynia

teria were adopted in 1990, subsequent studies have pointed out potential problems with TePs as well.

Although early studies suggested that FMS patients experienced tenderness only in TePs, it is now very clear that individuals with FMS display increased sensitivity to pain throughout the body (8). There is nothing inherently abnormal about TePs, since many people have some TePs, with the mean value in the general population ranging from one to four, depending on the methodologies employed. Thus, TePs [e.g., the mid-trapezius region, epicondyles, etc.] appear to merely represent regions of the body where everyone is more tender.

More importantly, though, TePs are probably not a good "pure" measure of tenderness. For example, several population-based studies have demonstrated that the number of TePs an individual has is highly correlated with a number of measures of distress (9). But distress is not an inherent feature of persons who are tender, since when a pressure pain threshold is performed concurrently with both a TeP determination and dolorimetry/algometry, the TeP count correlates with measures of distress, whereas this is much less so with the dolorimeter value.

There are several other problems with TePs. For example, the requirement for having 11 of 18 TePs in order to fulfill the ACR FMS criteria is largely responsible for FMS being a condition that is exceedingly more prevalent in females. The other component of the ACR definition, chronic pain in all four quadrants of the body plus the axial skeleton,

FIGURE 2. Localized or organ-specific syndromes.

FIBROMYALGIA
two to four percent of population;
defined by widespread
pain and tenderness

MULTIPLE CHEMICAL
SENSITIVITY–symptoms in
multiple organ systems in
response to multiple
substances

CHRONIC FATIGUE
SYNDROME one percent
of population; fatigue
and four to eight "minor
criteria"

EXPOSURE
SYNDROMES, e.g.,
Silicone, Gulf War
Illnesses, breast implants,
sick building syndrome

SOMATOFORM
DISORDES four percent
of population; multiple
unexplained symptoms
–no "organic" findings

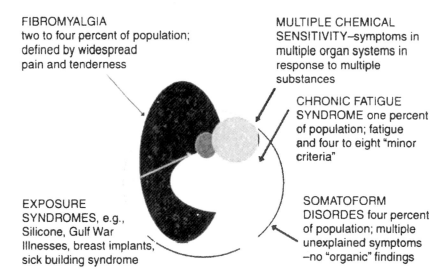

only occurs in approximately 1.5 times as many females as males in the population. Population-based studies using the ACR criteria for FMS have been very instructive. These studies have shown that pain and tenderness occur as a continuum in the general population; thus, some individuals rarely experience pain, some experience continuous widespread pain, and others have occasional pain. There is no bimodal distribution, with a group of patients who are very tender. These same characteristics are seen when examining the frequency or severity of nearly any somatic symptom in the population, and create difficulty with defining this spectrum of illness. Furthermore, these aggregate in the population, with individuals with chronic pain much more likely to experience chronic fatigue, and vice versa. This illustrates the difficulty in using the severity of one or more of these subjective symptoms in an illness definition. Also, this suggests that common mechanisms may be responsible for the development of chronic pain, fatigue, and other somatic symptoms, and perhaps even that these mechanisms may be variations on normal physiology responsible for these symptoms in the general population.

Although chronic widespread pain is the defining feature of FMS, a number of nonmusculoskeletal symptoms occur in increased frequency in patients with this disorder. These features have been reviewed in detail (4,10,11). There is also considerable overlap between patients who fulfill criteria for FMS, and those who fulfill criteria for other systemic disorders such as CFS, somatoform disorders, and "exposure" syndromes. This challenges the notion that any of these illnesses are discrete or unique diseases.

Chronic Fatigue Syndrome. The CFS is another disorder that has attracted increasing attention in recent years. Although the symptom of chronic fatigue affects 5-10 percent of the general population, CFS as currently defined is much less common (12,13). The current definition for CFS requires that the affected individual display severe chronic fatigue without a defined cause, as well as the presence of four of eight of the following symptoms: myalgias, arthralgias, sore throat, tender nodes, cognitive difficulty, headache, postexertional malaise, or sleep disturbance (14). This definition was only recently adopted. The definition used before 1994 was more restrictive, and excluded individuals with concurrent psychological conditions [the new definition only excludes individuals with more severe forms of psychiatric disorders].

There were several perceived reasons for a need for a new definition, including the fact that some objective findings required in previous criteria [e.g., pharyngitis, lymphadenopathy] were actually uncommonly noted in CFS. More frequently, the patient with CFS experiences a sore throat rather than inflammation of the pharynx, and tender nodes rather than enlargement of the lymph nodes. In the new CFS definition, it is of note that five of the eight minor criteria are pain-based, reinforcing the fact that diffuse pain [without accompanying abnormalities in the peripheral tissues] is common in this condition. Besides the "defining symptoms" noted in the criteria, there are a variety of other symptoms seen with increased frequency in CFS. These are very similar to those noted for FMS (15,16). The demographics of CFS are also similar to FMS, with a strong female predominance (14).

Somatoform Disorders. Somatoform disorders are a group of classified psychiatric disorders defined by the presence of physical symptoms that are not fully explained by a known medical condition. These disorders include somatization disorder, hypochondriasis, conversion disorder, and pain disorder (17). Somatization disorder, formerly called Briquet's syndrome, is diagnosed when an individual has multiple somatic complaints that begin before age 30, for which medical attention has been sought but the complaints are not due to a known physical disorder. To meet criteria for this disorder the individual must have at least eight unexplained symptoms over a lifetime. As defined, this condition is quite uncommon [0.1 to 1.0 percent of the population].

However, a less severe form of somatization is diagnosed when an individual displays one or more unexplained symptoms for greater than six months, and is much more common [affecting approximately four percent of the population]. This illness has been variously termed "sub-syndromal somatization disorder" and "undifferentiated somatoform disorder" [DSM-IV] (18). Therefore, if the symptoms of FMS or CFS are considered *unexplained*, most individuals who meet criteria for one of these illnesses will also meet criteria for a somatoform disorder.

Just as with FMS and CFS, there is considerable controversy regarding somatoform disorders. This controversy generally takes a different form than that surrounding FMS and CFS. For example, there has been little "burden of proof" placed on proponents of the concept of somatoform disorders, since by definition these conditions are acknowledged to have a "psychiatric" rather than "physical" basis. This is problematic, since there are multiple objective physiologic abnormalities noted in individuals with FMS and CFS that might explain symptomatology. Thus, it becomes difficult to characterize these symptoms as "physiologically unexplained" (19,20). Moreover, even undeniably psychiatric disorders, such as schizophrenia and major depression, are characterized by symptoms that are no longer considered biologically unexplained, as we learn that these illnesses are likely to be mediated in large part by central neurochemical imbalances.

However, just as with FMS and CFS, there have been research findings in the investigation of somatoform disorders that are of irrefutable value. Perhaps the most important are that somatic symptoms are very common, cluster in the population, and exert a tremendous cost in terms of both health care and related disability (21). For example, it is estimated that about 25 percent of patients attending a primary care clinic will meet criteria for subsyndromal somatization disorder, and up to 50 percent of primary care visits are for somatic complaints within this spectrum (22). Patients with somatization disorder [the most severe form of somatoform disorders] use 10 times the mean outpatient and inpatient medical services as those in the general population (23). Given the high percentage of outpatient and inpatient visits that are due to symptoms within this spectrum, the economic costs of somatoform disorders–or any other semantic term which is chosen–are substantial.

Other "Miscellaneous" Systemic Disorders. There are a number of other systemic conditions that fall within this spectrum. The MCS, and the closely related symptom of chemical intolerance, are examples. Furthermore, the clinical overlap between this condition, and CFS and FMS, has been well established (24). Although there is no accepted definition of this entity, most use some variation of the criteria proposed by Cullen, and require: 1. symptoms in multiple organ systems in response to multiple substances, and 2. a change in behavior in response to these symptoms. It is of particular note that the requirement that an individual change their behavior in order to meet diagnostic criteria. Although this requirement for behavior change was likely felt to be important to judge the severity of the chemical intolerance, there are probably significant implications of this requirement. Since studies suggest that nearly 20 percent of individuals in the population experience occasional chemical intolerance, and only a small percentage of these change their behavior in response to this symptom, those who change their behavior are not likely to be representative of the larger group (25). It is possible if not likely that this accounts for the very high rate of psychiatric comorbidity in individuals who meet criteria for MCS, even in population-based samples (26).

Other CMI are not defined on the basis of symptoms or signs, but instead by an environmental exposure which is alleged to cause the illness. We have previously referred to these conditions as "exposure syndromes" (27), and these include Gulf War Illnesses, sick building syndrome, and illnesses seen in women with silicone breast implants, just to name a few. Usually, the clinical features and laboratory abnormalities described for these illnesses are difficult to distinguish from those of FMS, CFS, MCS, and somatoform disorders.

The epidemic of "Gulf War Illnesses" that occurred in troops deployed to the Persian Gulf in 1990 and 1991 affords an excellent example of how CMI may be triggered. To review, in 1990 and 1991 the United States deployed approximately 700,000 troops to the Persian Gulf to liberate Kuwait from Iraqi occupation. Fortunately, there were relatively few combat-related injuries and diseases during this conflict, but up to 45 percent of deployed veterans [as compared to 15 percent of nondeployed veterans] developed a constellation of symptoms and syndromes including muscle and joint pain, fatigue, memory problems, headaches, and gastrointestinal complaints (6). This experience was not unique to United States troops, since veterans of this conflict from the United Kingdom experienced a similar increase in this spectrum of illness (28). Several expert panels have been convened to examine these illnesses. There is agreement that this is not a single illness, but rather a constellation of symptoms and syndromes very similar to that seen in FMS and CFS. Only a single population-based study has identified an environmental exposure associated with a higher risk of developing CMI [a series of vaccinations given to United Kingdom troops], whereas numerous other studies have demonstrated no link between single exposures, and the development of illness. Given that similar symptom complexes have recently been retrospectively noted after nearly every war, many believe that it is not any single "stressor" that leads to the increase in CMI after war, but instead the exposure to a large number of different types of stressors over a relatively short period of time (29,30).

Regional or Organ-Specific Syndromes Within the Same Spectrum. Irrespective of the defining features of illnesses such as FMS and CFS, most individuals who meet criteria for these conditions also experience a high lifetime and current prevalence of nondefining symptoms. Fibromyalgia has long been considered to be characterized by a high frequency of nonmusculoskeletal conditions, and the clinical features of this illness have been more completely characterized than those of the other systemic conditions within this spectrum (2-4).

Most patients with FMS, and all patients with CFS, complain of fatigue. Similarly, insomnia and a variety of different sleep abnormalities are seen frequently in individuals with both FMS and CFS (31,32).

Other constitutional symptoms which may be seen in these individuals include large fluctuations in weight, heat and cold intolerance, and the subjective sensation of weakness. Individuals with this spectrum of illness also experience a variety of neurologic symptoms. Patients with both FMS and CFS have a higher than expected prevalence of both tension and migraine headaches. Numbness or tingling, typically fleeting in nature and in a nondermatomal distribution, is also a common complaint. Cognitive complaints, especially difficulty with attention and short-term memory, are seen frequently in patients with these entities, and in some may be the most debilitating aspect of their illness. Objective abnormalities on neuropsychological testing have also been noted, although these findings are not consistent.

Patients with these illnesses also display a wide array of "allergic" symptoms, ranging from adverse reactions to drugs and environmental stimuli [as seen in MCS], to higher than expected incidences of rhinitis, nasal congestion, and lower respiratory symptoms (24,33). Although some of these individuals may truly be atopic, there are likely nonallergic mechanisms that contribute substantially to these symptoms (34). Hearing, ocular, and vestibular abnormalities have also been noted, including a high incidence of a decreased painful sound threshold, nystagmus, ocular dysmotility, and asymptomatic low frequency sensorineural hearing loss. Other accompanying symptoms include sicca symptoms and temporomandibular joint dysfunction.

Individuals with FMS likewise suffer from a number of symptoms of "functional" disorders of visceral organs, including a high incidence of recurrent noncardiac chest pain, heartburn, palpitations, and IBS (1,35). However, prospective studies of randomly selected individuals with FMS have detected *objective* evidence of dysfunction of several visceral organs, including up to a 75 percent incidence of echocardiographic evidence of mitral valve prolapse, a 40 percent incidence of esophageal dysmotility, and diminished static inspiratory and expiratory pressures on pulmonary function testing (36-38). Neurally mediated hypotension and syncope also appear to occur more frequently in individuals with both FMS and CFS (39). Similar syndromes characterized by visceral pain and/or smooth muscle dysmotility are also seen in the pelvis. Well-established examples of such symptoms are the association with dysmenorrhea, as well as with urinary frequency and urgency (40). There may also be an association between FMS and other genitourinary conditions such as interstitial cystitis, endometriosis, and vulvar vestibulitis or vulvodynia [the latter of which are characterized by dyspareunia and sensitivity of the vulvar region] (41,42).

A discussion of the localized conditions within this spectrum must include the fact that conditions such as FMS are commonly identified in individuals with chronic regional musculoskeletal pain, such as low back pain (43). It is also common for any type of regional pain syndrome [e.g., temporomandibular joint dysfunction, vulvodynia, myofascial pain or costochondritis] to eventually "spread" to become more systemic and involve the entire body, i.e., transform into FMS. Animal studies of allodynia and of phenomena such as central sensitization may provide clues about why this may occur.

Relationship with Psychiatric Disorders. The symptoms of chronic multisymptom illnesses, and those of psychiatric disorders, overlap significantly. Although some contend that *all* of these symptoms are "supra-tentorial" in origin, others counter that the rate of psychiatric comorbidities in these conditions is similar to any chronic disease. A review of the accumulated data in these conditions supports a few consistent observations:

Approximately 20-40 percent of individuals with FMS seen in tertiary care centers have an identifiable current mood disorder such as depression or anxiety disorder (44). The lifetime incidence of psychiatric co-morbidities in tertiary care patients may be as high as 40-70 percent over several studies (44,45). These data are among those used by Hudson and colleagues to posit that there is a spectrum of disorders including FMS, migraines, IBS, and affective disorders which may share a common genetic predisposition, and underlying pathogenic mechanisms. However, some of these differences in the current and lifetime history of mood disorders are likely due to health care seeking behaviors, since lower lifetime incidences of affective disorders are typically noted in individuals with FMS who are identified in the general population (46). This same relationship between the setting of care, and the rate of comorbid psychiatric conditions, has been consistently noted in IBS.

There are a myriad of complex psychosocial factors which play a significant role in some individuals with FMS, as with nearly any chronic medical illness. These include behavioral pathways, such as sick role behavior and maladaptive coping mechanisms, cognitive pathways such as victimization and loss of control, and social pathways, such as interference with role functioning and deterioration of social or other support networks. Psychosocial factors are known to play a particularly prominent role in the transition form acute pain to chronic pain and disability. As pain progresses from the acute phase into chronicity, problems emerge for the individual such as job loss, financial constraints, distancing of friends, etc. If patients' responses to these problems are maladaptive such as avoidance of work, friends, financial responsibilities, and physical activity, the patient may become distressed and overwhelmed by the pain and its negative impact on life. Increased stress, learned helplessness, depression, increased anxiety, anger, distrust, and entitlement can all emerge and worsen symptoms, probably by interrelated physiological and psychological mechanisms. All of these factors can be important in dictating how individuals report symptoms, how and when they seek health care, and how they respond to therapy. This may also explain why cognitive-behavioral therapy, which addresses many of these issues, has generally been effective in the treatment of individuals with FMS, as well as nearly any other chronic medical condition (47).

Figure 3 summarizes the relationship between physiologic factors, and psychobehavioral factors, in this spectrum of illness. At the far left of the graph, perhaps when individuals first develop symptoms, there may be primarily physiologic factors that are responsible. Such factors are discussed in more detail below. With chronicity of illness, some individuals may develop psychological and behavioral cofactors that exacerbate or perpetuate the illness. These factors, in combination with the physiologic factors, are likely to be the biggest determinants of disability in this spectrum of illness. These latter factors are seen much more commonly in individuals who attend tertiary care clinics, and con-

FIGURE 3. Relationship between physiologic and psychobehavioral factors in chronic multisymptom illnesses.

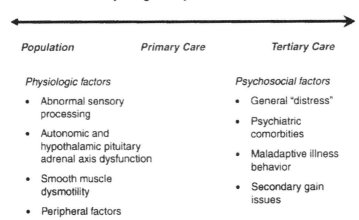

The Physiological/Psychosocial Continuum

Population	*Primary Care*	*Tertiary Care*

Physiologic factors

- Abnormal sensory processing
- Autonomic and hypothalamic pituitary adrenal axis dysfunction
- Smooth muscle dysmotility
- Peripheral factors

Psychosocial factors

- General "distress"
- Psychiatric comorbities
- Maladaptive illness behavior
- Secondary gain issues

versely, individuals who are found with these syndromes in the general population, or in primary care, are less likely to have such factors, and are likely to respond much better to purely physiologic [e.g., pharmacologic] interventions.

REFERENCES

1. Wolfe F, Smythe HA, Yunus MB, Bennett RM, Bombardier C, Goldenberg DL, Tugwell P, Campbell SM, Abeles M, Clark P, et al: The American College of Rheumatology 1990 Criteria for the Classification of Fibromyalgia. Report of the Multicenter Criteria Committee [see comments]. Arthritis Rheum 33:160-172, 1990.

2. Hudson JI, Goldenberg DL, Pope HG, Jr., Keck PE, Jr., Schlesinger L: Comorbidity of fibromyalgia with medical and psychiatric disorders. Am J Med 92:363-367, 1992.

3. Yunus MB: Towards a model of pathophysiology of fibromyalgia: aberrant central pain mechanisms with peripheral modulation [editorial]. J Rheumatol 19:846-850, 1992.

4. Clauw DJ: Fibromyalgia: more than just a musculoskeletal disease. Am Fam Phys 52:843-851, 1995.

5. Nisenbaum R, Barrett DH, Reyes M, Reeves WC: Deployment stressors and a chronic multisymptom illness among Gulf War veterans. J Nerv Ment Dis 188:259-266, 2000.

6. Fukuda K, Nisenbaum R, Stewart G, Thompson WT, Robin L, Washko RM, Noah DL, Barrett DH, Randall B, Herwaldt BL, Mawle AC, Reeves WC: Chronic

mutlisymptom illness affecting air force veterans of the gulf war. JAMA 280(11): 981-988, 1999.

7. Doebbeling BN, Clarke WR, Watson D, Torner JC, Woolson RF, Voelker MD, Barrett DH, Schwartz DA: Is there a Persian Gulf War syndrome? Evidence from a large population-based survey of veterans and nondeployed controls. Am J Med 108:695-704, 2000.

8. Granges G, Littlejohn G: Pressure pain threshold in pain-free subjects, in patients with chronic regional pain syndromes, and in patients with fibromyalgia syndrome. Arthritis Rheum 36:642-646, 1993.

9. Wolfe F: The relation between tender points and fibromyalgia symptom variables: evidence that fibromyalgia is not a discrete disorder in the clinic. Ann Rheum Dis 56:268-271, 1997.

10. Yunus MB: Fibromyalgia syndrome: new research on an old malady. BMJ 298:474-475, 1989.

11. Waylonis GW, Heck W: Fibromyalgia syndrome. New associations. Am J Phys Med Rehabil 71:343-348, 1992.

12. Fukuda K, Wilson L, Dobbins J: A community-based study of unexplained prolonged and chronic fatiguing illness in a rural area of Michigan. AACFS 1994 Proceedings, 1994.

13. Buchwald D, Umali P, Umali J, Kith P, Pearlman T, Komaroff AL: Chronic fatigue and the chronic fatigue syndrome: prevalence in a Pacific Northwest health care system. Ann Intern Med 123:81-88, 1995.

14. Fukuda K, Strauss SE, Hickie I, Sharpe MC, Dobbins JG, Komaroff A: Chronic fatigue syndrome: a comprehensive approach to its definition and study. Ann Int Med 121:953-959, 1994.

15. Komaroff AL: Clinical presentation of chronic fatigue syndrome. Ciba Found Symp 173:43-54; discussion 54-61, 1993.

16. McKenzie R, Straus SE: Chronic fatigue syndrome. Adv Intern Med 40:119-153, 1995.

17. Katon W, Lin E, von Korff M, Russo J, Lipscomb P, Bush T: Somatization: a spectrum of severity. Amer J Psychiatry 148: 34-40, 1991.

18. American Psychiatric Association: Diagnostic and Statistical Manual of Mental Disorders. American Psychiatric Press, Washington, DC, 1994.

19. Quintner JL: Somatisation disorder: a major public health issue. Med J Aust 163:558-559, 1995.

20. Bell IR: Somatization disorder: health care costs in the decade of the brain. Biol Psychiatry 35: 81-83, 1994.

21. Barsky AJ, Borus JF: Somatization and medicalization in the era of managed care. JAMA 274:1931-1934, 1995.

22. Kirmayer LJ, Robbins JM: Three forms of somatization in primary care: prevalence, co-occurence, and sociodemographic characteristics. J Nerv Ment Dis 179: 647-655, 1991.

23. Smith GR, Monson R, Ray D: Patients with multiple unexplained symptoms: their characteristics, functional health, and health care utilization. Arch Int Med 146: 69-72, 1986.

24. Buchwald D, Garrity D: Comparison of patients with chronic fatigue syndrome, fibromyalgia, and multiple chemical sensitivities. Arch Intern Med 154:2049-2053, 1994.

25. Bruno RL, Sapolsky R, Zimmerman JR, Frick NM: Pathophysiology of a central cause of post-polio fatigue. Ann NY Acad Sci 753:257-275, 1995.

26. Black DW, Doebbeling BN, Voelker MD, Clarke WR, Woolson RF, Barrett DH, Schwartz DA: Multiple chemical sensitivity syndrome: symptom prevalence and risk factors in a military population. Arch Intern Med 160:1169-1176, 2000.

27. Clauw DJ, Chrousos Gp: Chronic pain and fatigue syndromes: Overlapping clinical and neuroendocrine features and potential pathogenic mechanisms. Neuroimmunomodulation 4:134-153, 1997.

28. Unwin C, Blatchley N, Coker W, Ferry S, Hotopf M, Hull L, Ismail K, Palmer I, David A, Wessely SL: Health of UK servicemen who served in the Persian Gulf War. Lancet 353:169-178, 1999.

29. Hyams KC, Wignall FS, Roswell R: War syndromes and their evaluation: from the U.S. Civil War to Persian Gulf War. Ann Intern Med 125(5):398-405, 1996.

30. Clauw DJ: The "Gulf War Syndrome": implications for rheumatologists. J Clin Rheum 4(4):173-174, 1998.

31. Modolfsky H, Scarisbrick P, England R, Smythe H: Musculoskeletal symptoms and non-REM sleep disturbance in patients with "fibrositis syndrome" and healthy subjects. Psychosom Med 37:341-351, 1975.

32. Manu P, Lane TJ, Matthews DA, Castriotta RJ, Watson RK, Abeles M: Alpha-delta sleep in patients with a chief complaint of chronic fatigue. South Med J 87:465-470, 1994.

33. Cleveland CH, Jr., Fisher RH, Brestel EP, Esinhart JD, Metzger WJ: Chronic rhinitis: an underrecognized association with fibromyalgia. Allergy Proc 13:263-267, 1992.

34. Clauw DJ, Gaumond E, Radulovic D, Pandiri P, Ali M, Foong S, Baraniuk J: The role of true IgE mediated allergic mechanisms in the allergic symptoms of fibromyalgia. Arthritis Rheum 39 (6S):R20, 1996.

35. Mukerji B, Mukerji V, Alpert MA, Selukar R: The prevalence of rheumatologic disorders in patients with chest pain and angiographically normal coronary arteries. Angiology 46:425-430, 1995.

36. Lurie M, Caidahl K, Johansson G, Bake B: Respiratory function in chronic primary fibromyalgia. Scand J Rehabil Med 22:151-155, 1990.

37. Hiltz RE, Gupta PK, Maher KA, Blank CA, Benjamin SB, Katz P, Clauw DJ: Low threshold of visceral nociception and significant upper gastrointestinal pathology in patients with fibromyalgia syndrome. Arthritis Rheum 36(9S):C93, 1993.

38. Pellegrino MJ, Van Fossen D, Gordon C, Ryan JM, Waylonis GW: Prevalence of mitral valve prolapse in primary fibromyalgia: a pilot investigation. Arch Phys Med Rehabil 70:541-543, 1989.

39. Rowe PC, Bou-Holaigah I, Kan JS, Calkins H: Is neurally mediated hypotension an unrecognized cause of chronic fatigue? Lancet 345:623-624, 1995.

40. Wallace DJ: Genitourinary manifestations of fibrositis: an increased association with the female urethral syndrome. J Rheumatol 17:238-239, 1990.

41. Koziol JA, Clark DC, Gittes RF, Tan EM: The natural history of interstitial cystitis. J Urology 149:465-469, 1993.

42. Friedrich EG: Vulvar vestibulitis syndrome. J Reproduct Med 32(2):110-114, 1987.

43. Clauw DJ, Williams DA, Lauerman W, Dahlman M, Aslami A, Nachemson AL, Kobrine A, Wiesel SW: Pain sensitivity as a correlate of clinical status in individuals with chronic low back pain. Spine 24:2035-2041, 1999.

44. Boissevain MD, McCain GA: Toward an integrated understanding of fibromyalgia syndrome. II. Psychological and phenomenological aspects. Pain 45:239-248, 1991.

45. Hudson JI, Hudson MS, Pliner LF, Goldenberg DL, Pope HG, Jr: Fibromyalgia and major affective disorder: a controlled phenomenology and family history study. Am J Psychiatry 142(4):441-446, 1985.

46. Aaron LA, Bradley LA, Alarcon GS, Alexander RW, Triana-Alexander M, Martin MY, Alberts KR: Psychiatric diagnoses in patients with fibromyalgia are related to health care-seeking behavior rather than to illness. Arthritis Rheum 39:436-445, 1996.

47. NIH Technology Panel: Integration of behavioral and relaxation approaches into the treatment of chronic pain and insomnia. Journal of the American Medical Association 276(4):313-318, 1996.

The Hypothalamic-Pituitary-Adrenal Axis in Fibromyalgia: Where Are We in 2001?

Leslie J. Crofford

SUMMARY. Objectives: To summarize the current status of the hypothalamic pituitary adrenal [HPA] axis in the fibromyalgia syndrome [FMS].

Findings: Attention has been focused on the HPA axis in FMS because there is a perceived association of the onset of this disorder with physiologically stressful situations. The medical literature strongly supports some kind of dsyfunction in the HPA system in FMS, but when studies have compared FMS with healthy normal controls, the actual patterns of HPA axis abnormalities have been suprisingly variable. It is possible that some of this variability may relate to a variable balance between the two receptors for corticotropin-releasing hormone which exhibit opposite influences on the stress management system when activated.

Conclusions: The roles of the psychological stress response systems, including the HPA axis, remain uncertain in FMS because there has been so much variability of the findings from controlled studies. Part of the problem may be that pain is the defining symptom in the classification of

---

Leslie J. Crofford, MD, is Associate Professor of Internal Medicine, Division of Rheumatology, University of Michigan, Ann Arbor, MI 48109 USA.

Address correspondence to: Leslie J. Crofford, MD, Room 5510A, MSRB I, 1150 West Medical Center Drive, Ann Arbor, MI 48109-0680 [E-mail: crofford@umich.edu].

[Haworth co-indexing entry note]: "The Hypothalamic-Pituitary-Adrenal Axis in Fibromyalgia: Where Are We in 2001?" Crofford, Leslie J. Co-published simultaneously in *Journal of Musculoskeletal Pain* [The Haworth Medical Press, an imprint of The Haworth Press, Inc.] Vol. 10, No. 1/2, 2002, pp. 215-220; and: *The Clinical Neurobiology of Fibromyalgia and Myofascial Pain: Therapeutic Implications* [ed: Robert M. Bennett] The Haworth Medical Press, an imprint of The Haworth Press, Inc., 2002, pp. 215-220. Single or multiple copies of this article are available for a fee from The Haworth Document Delivery Service [1-800-HAWORTH, 9:00 a.m. - 5:00 p.m. [EST]. E-mail address: getinfo@haworthpressinc.com].

FMS while the HPA axis may relate more to fatigue and psychological distress. *[Article copies available for a fee from The Haworth Document Delivery Service: 1-800-HAWORTH. E-mail address: <getinfo@haworthpressinc.com> Website: <http://www.HaworthPress.com> © 2002 by The Haworth Press, Inc. All rights reserved.]*

KEYWORDS. Hypthalamic pituitary adrenal axis, fibromyalgia syndrome, pain, fatigue

The American College of Rheumatology has developed classification criteria for fibromyalgia [FM] that include the presence of subjective widespread chronic musculoskeletal pain and the presence of tender points, which identify an altered pressure-pain threshold (1). Clinicians, however, recognize a much broader constellation of symptoms. Fibromyalgia is commonly associated with pain syndromes involving discreet musculoskeletal areas [e.g., temporomandibular disorder, tension headache syndromes] or viscera [e.g., irritable bowel syndrome, irritable bladder]. In addition, patients complain of fatigue, cognitive and mood disturbances, and sleep disorder in the great majority of cases. Subjective symptoms are frequently accompanied by psychological distress related to their somatic symptoms and development of pain behaviors (2).

It has long been recognized that onset and exacerbation of FMS symptoms are frequently seen in response to stress. The term 'stress' should be viewed in its physiological sense as referring to a stimulus, either physical or psychological, which disturbs homeostasis and activates adaptive stress-response pathways. The principal stress-response systems are the hypothalamic-pituitary-adrenal [HPA] axis and the locus coeruleus-sympathetic nervous system (3). Physical, psychological, and behavioral symptoms have been linked to disturbances of these neurobiological pathways (3).

Corticotropin-releasing hormone [CRH] is a principal neuropeptide regulator of the HPA axis activity by virtue of its localization to the paraventricular nucleus of the hypothalamus. Corticotropin-releasing hormone receptors are, however, localized to many other brain regions and in those locations mediates other biological effects (4). In the prefrontal, cingulate, and insular cortices CRH plays a role in the affective response to stress. The behavioral and autonomic responses to stress are associated with CRH in the central nucleus of the amygdala. The interplay between the HPA axis and the sympathetic nervous system is localized to the locus coeruleus, dorsal raphe nucleus, and ventral tegmental areas. Corticotropin-releasing hormone may also play a role in the descending modulation of pain perception as coordinated in the periaqueductal gray (5). Corticotropin-releasing hormone actions are mediated by two receptors, CRHR1 and CRHR2. They share approximately 71 percent amino acid homology, and are differentially localized to different central and peripheral sites (6).

Animal studies have been important in understanding central effects of CRH. Increased CRH either by intracerebroventricular injection or transgenic overexpression results in altered food consumption, sexual behavior, sleep, locomotor activity, response to novel environment, and learning (7). Mice genetically engineered to eliminate expression of CRHR1 have an impaired stress response and reduced anxiety related behaviors (8,9). The CRHR2 knockout mice are hypersensitive to stress and have increased anxiety-related behaviors (10,11). Therefore, CRHR1 stimulates activity of the stress-response and mediates anxiogenic action, both of which are opposed by CRHR2.

It is clear that there is variability in HPA axis activity on the basis of genetic and acquired factors. Environmental factors that can alter HPA axis activity in animals include early life-stress [e.g., infection, maternal separation, aberrant maternal rearing behaviors], repeated social isolation, and chronic stress in adults (12). In humans, stress such as childhood sexual and physical abuse is associated with altered HPA axis and autonomic activity (13).

We are still unable to effectively evaluate CRH effects on specific brain regions in humans, and evaluation of HPA axis activity at the level of the hypothalamus can be achieved only indirectly, usually by providing a physiological or psychological stress. Central 'drive' to HPA axis activity, such as in melancholic depression, is determined using dexamethasone suppression testing (14). Direct evaluation of pituitary and adrenal hormones can be performed after administration of releasing hormones. However, there are many potential confounders in interpretation of HPA axis studies including time of day, since adrenal corticotropin hormone [ACTH] and cortisol are secreted with a pronounced circadian rhythm, and factors that themselves affect HPA axis activity [e.g., phase of the menstrual cycle or administered gonadal hormones, associated depression or chronic fatigue syndrome, medications, smoking, age, obesity]. All these factors make direct comparisons of the different studies somewhat problematic.

Several studies have evaluated responsiveness of the hypothalamus by providing physiologic stress including insulin-induced hypoglycemia

(15-17) and administration of interleukin-6 (18). These studies demonstrate differences in either HPA or autonomic responses compared with the control groups, but there is no consistency as to the direction of the change between studies. Dexamethasone suppression testing using the dose in melancholic depression is either normal or nonsuppression is increased (19-21). Corticotropin-releasing hormone stimulation testing evaluates the pituitary-adrenal response to exogenous hormone administration, and one can only speculate regarding the status of endogenous releasing hormones based on these studies. Studies have shown exaggerated or normal responses of ACTH with a relatively blunted cortisol after injection of supraphysiologic doses of CRH [1 μg/kg] (15,22,23). The adrenal response to exogenous ACTH has been normal (16,21) or low (17).

Basal levels of cortisol have been determined in the saliva [free], plasma [total and free], and urine [free]. Mean salivary cortisol levels were elevated (24), evening plasma cortisol levels have been reported as elevated (22,25) or normal (16), and 24 h urine cortisol levels are low (21,22,25,26) or normal (16). Circadian variation of cortisol levels is reduced (22,25), but circadian phase as compared to other biological rhythms is normal (27,28).

As can be easily seen, most studies show alterations of HPA axis activity but no consistent abnormalities have been demonstrated. This may be related, in part, to how FMS is diagnosed. The definition used to identify patients is pain, and there is no requirement as to the presence or absence of fatigue, other somatic syndromes, or psychological distress. It is likely that the influence of the HPA axis is largely manifested on these other features of FMS. Better methods to study the central components of the stress-response systems, including CRH functions unrelated to pituitary-adrenal activation, will likely allow researchers to correlate specific symptoms associated with FMS that are influenced by differences in HPA axis activity.

REFERENCES

1. Wolfe F, Smythe HA, Yunus MB, Bennett RM, Baobardier C, Goldenberg DL, Tugwell P, Campbell SM, Abeles M, Clark P, Fam AG, Farber SJ, Fiechtner JJ, Franklin CM, Gatter RA, Hamaty D, Lessard J, Lichtbroun AS, Masi AT, McCain GA, Reynolds WJ, Romano TJ, Russell IJ, Sheon RP: The American College of Rheumatology 1990 criteria for the classification of fibromyalgia. Arthritis Rheum 33: 160-172, 1990.

2. Wolfe F, Skevington SM: Measuring the epidemiology of distress: The rheumatology distress index. J Rheumatol 27: 2000-2009, 2000.

3. Chrousos GP, Gold PW: The concepts of stress and stress system disorders: Overview of physical and behavioral homeostasis. JAMA 267: 1244-1252, 1992.

4. De Souza EB, Grigoriadis DE, Webster EL: Role of brain, pituitary, and spleen corticotropin-releasing factor receptors in the stress response. Methods Achieve Exp Pathol 14: 23-44, 1991.

5. Crofford LJ, Casey KL. Central modulation of pain perception. Rheum Dis Clin NA 25: 1-13, 1999.

6. Vita N, Laurent P, Lefort S, Chalon P, Lelias J-M, Kaghad M, Le Fur G, Caput D, Ferrara P: Primary structure and functional expression of mouse pituitary and human brain corticotrophin releasing factor receptors. FEBS Let 335: 1-5, 1993.

7. Stenzel-Poore MP, Heinrichs SC, Rivest S, Koob GF, Vale WW: Overproduction of corticotropin-releasing factor in transgenic mice: A genetic model of anxiogenic behavior. J Neurosci 14: 2579-2584, 1994.

8. Smith GW, Aubry J-M, Dellu F, Contarino A, Belezikjian LM, Gold LH, Chen R, Marchuk Y, Hauser C, Bentrly CA, Sawchenko PE, Koob GF, Vale W, Lee K-F: Corticotropin releasing factor receptor 1-deficient mice display decreased anxiety, impaired stress response, and aberrant neuroendocrine development. Neuron 20: 1093-1102, 1998.

9. Timpl P, Spanagel R, Sillaber I, Kresse A, Reul JMHM, Stalla GK, Blanquet V, Steckler T, Holsboer F, Wurst W: Impaired stress response and recuded anxiety in mice lacking a functional corticotropin-releasing hormone receptor. Nature Genet 19: 162-166, 1998.

10. Bale TL, Contarino A, Smith GW, Chan R, Gold LH, Sawchenko PE, Koob GF, Vale WW, Lee K-F: Mice deficient for corticotropin-releasing hormone receptor-2 display anxiety-like behaviour and are hypersensitive to stress. Nature Genet 24: 410-414, 2000.

11. Kishimoto T, Radulovic J, Radulovic M, Lin C, Schrick C, Hooshmand F, Hermanson O, Rosenfeld M, Spiess J: Deletion of *Crhr2* reveals an anxiolytic role for corticotropin-releasing hormone receptor-2. Nature Genet 24: 415-419, 2000.

12. Crofford LJ, Demitrack MA: Evidence that abnormalities of central neurohormonal systems are key to understanding fibromylagia and chronic fatigue syndrome. Rheum Dis Clin NA 22: 267-284, 1996.

13. Heim C, Newport DJ, Heit S, Graham YP, Wilcox M, Bonsall R, Miller AH, Nereroff CB: Pituitary-adrenal and autonomic responses to stress in women after sexual and physcial abuse in childhood. JAMA 284: 592-597, 2000.

14. Carroll BJ, Feingerg M, Greden JF, Tarika J, Albala AA, Haskett RF, James NM, Kronfol Z, Lohr N, Sterner M, de Vigne JP, Young E: A specific laboratory test for the diagnosis of melancholia: Standardization, validation, and clinical utility. Arch Gen Psychiatry 38: 15-22, 1981.

15. Griep EN, Boersma JW, de Kloet EP: Altered reactivity of the hypothalamic-pituitary-adrenal axis in the primary fibromyalgia syndrome. J Rheumatol 20: 469-474, 1993.

16. Adler GK, Kinsley BT, Hurwitz S, Mossey CJ, Goldenberg DL: Reduced hypothalamic-pituitary and sympathoadrenal responses to hyoglycemia in women with fibromyalgia syndrome. Am J Med 106: 534-543, 1999.

17. Kirnap M, Colak R, Eser C, Ozsoy O, Tutus A, Kelestimur F: A comparison between low-dose (1 µg), standard-dose (250 µg) ACTH stimulation tests and insulin tolerance test in the evaluation of hypothalamo-pituitary-adrenal axis in primary fibromyalgia syndrome. Clin Endocrinol 55: 455-459, 2001.

18. Torpy DJ, Papanicolaou DA, Lotsikas AJ, Wilder RL, Chrousos GP, Pillemer SR: Responses of the sympathetic nervous system and the hypothalamic-pituitary-adrenal axis to interleukin-6. Arthritis Rheum 43: 872-880, 2000.

19. Hudson JI, Pliner LF, Hudson MS, Goldenberg DL, Melby JC: The dexamethasone suppression test in fibrositis. Biol Psych 19: 1489-1493, 1984.

20. Ferraccioli G, Cavalieri F, Salaffi F, Fontana S, Scita F, Nolli M, Maestri D: Neuroendocrinologic findings in primary fibromyalgia (soft tissue chronic pain syndrome) and in other chronic rheumatic conditions (rheumatoid arthritis, low back pain). J Rheumatol 19: 869-873, 1990.

21. Griep EN, Boersma JW, Lentjes EG, Prins AP, ven der Korst JK, de Kloet ER: Function of the hypothalamic-pituitary-adrenal axis in patients with fibromyalgia and low back pain. J Rheumatol 25: 1374-1381, 1998.

22. Crofford LJ, Pillemer SR, Kalogeras KT, Cash JM, Michelson D, Kling MA, Sternberg EM, Gold PW, Chrousos GP, Wilder RL: Hypothalamic-pituitary-adrenal axis perturbations in patients with fibromyalgia. Arthritis Rheum 37: 1583-1592, 1994.

23. Reidel W, Layka H, Neeck G: Secretory pattern of GH, TSH, thyroid hormones, ACTH, cortisol, FSH and LH in patients with fibromyalgia syndrome (FMS) following systemic injection of the relevant hypothalamic releasing-hormones. Z Rheumatol 57 (Suppl): 81-87, 1998.

24. Catley D, Kaell AT, Kirschbaum C, Stone AA: A naturalistic evaluation of cortisol secretion in persons with fibromyalgia and rheumatoid arthritis. Arthritis Care Res 13: 51-61, 2000.

25. McCain GA, Tilbe KS: Diurnal hormone variation in fibromyalgia syndrome: A comparison with rheumatoid arthritis. J Rheumatol 16 (Suppl 19): 154-157, 1989.

26. Lentjes EGWM, Griep EN, Boersma JW, Romijn FPTHM, de Kloet ER: Glucocorticoid receptors, fibromylagia and low back pain. Psychoneuroendocrinology 22: 603-614, 1997.

27. Korszun A, Sackett-Lundeen L, Papadopoulos E, Brucksch C, Masterson L, Engelberg NC, Haus E, Demitrack MA, Crofford L: Melatonin levels in women with fibromyalgia and chronic fatigue syndrome. J Rheumatol 26: 2675-2680, 1999.

28. Klerman EB, Goldenberg DL, Brown EN, Maliszewski AM, Adler GK: Circadian rhythms of women with fibromyalgia. J Clin Endocrinol Metab 86: 1034-1039, 2001.

The Autonomic Nervous System and Fibromyalgia

Manuel Martinez-Lavin

SUMMARY. Fibromyalgia [FMS] is a multisystem illness with defining features located in the musculoskeletal system. Accumulating evidence derived from heart rate variability analysis and coming from different groups of investigators demonstrates that autonomic [sympathetic] nervous system dysfunction is frequent in patients with FMS. Such dysautonomia can be characterized as relentless sympathetic *hyperactivity* with *hyporeactivity* to stress. It is proposed that this type of dysautonomia explains the multisystem manifestations of FMS. Its defining features: generalized pain and tenderness at palpation in specific anatomical points are explained through the mechanism known as "sympathetically maintained pain." *[Article copies available for a fee from The Haworth Document Delivery Service: 1-800-HAWORTH. E-mail address: <getinfo@haworthpressinc.com> Website: <http://www.HaworthPress.com> © 2002 by The Haworth Press, Inc. All rights reserved.]*

KEYWORDS. Fibromyalgia, autonomic nervous system, heart rate variability, sympathetically maintained pain, reflex sympathetic dystrophy

OBJECTIVES

This article reviews accumulating evidence showing that autonomic [sympathetic] nervous system dysfunction [ANS] is frequent in patients

Manuel Martinez-Lavin, MD, is Chief, Rheumatology Department, Instituto Nacional de Cardiologia Mexico, Mexico City, Mexico 14080.

[Haworth co-indexing entry note]: "The Autonomic Nervous System and Fibromyalgia." Martinez-Lavin, Manuel. Co-published simultaneously in *Journal of Musculoskeletal Pain* [The Haworth Medical Press, an imprint of The Haworth Press, Inc.] Vol. 10, No. 1/2, 2002, pp. 221-228; and: *The Clinical Neurobiology of Fibromyalgia and Myofascial Pain: Therapeutic Implications* [ed: Robert M. Bennett] The Haworth Medical Press, an imprint of The Haworth Press, Inc., 2002, pp. 221-228. Single or multiple copies of this article are available for a fee from The Haworth Document Delivery Service [1-800-HAWORTH, 9:00 a.m. - 5:00 p.m. (EST). E-mail address: getinfo@haworthpressinc.com].

221

with FMS, furthermore it argues that such dysautonomia is the cause of the different manifestations of this debilitating syndrome.

FINDINGS

First of all, it is important to recognize that FMS is a multisystem illness. Although its defining features [widespread pain and tenderness at palpation of specific anatomical points] are located in the musculoskeletal system, the illness has prominent manifestations in different body locations. Such distinctive features of FMS are: fatigue, sleep disorders, paresthesias, headache, anxiety, sicca symptoms, Raynaud's phenomenon, and irritable bowel. The prospective multicenter study that led to the American College of Rheumatology criteria for FMS determined that these features were more frequent in patients with FMS when compared to patients that suffered from other types of rheumatic diseases (1) [see Table 1]. So any valid theory attempting to explain the pathogenesis of FMS should first give a coherent explanation for presence of these disparate symptoms.

Our working hypothesis has been that ANS dysfunction could explain the multisystem features of FMS (2).

TABLE 1. Distinctive Features of Fibromyalgia as Defined by the Study of the Multicenter Criteria Committee of the American College of Rheumatology (1)

Defining features:

Widespread pain

Tenderness at palpation in 11 or more of 18 specific anatomic points

Distinctive features:

Fatigue

Sleep disorders

Paresthesias

Headache

Anxiety

Sicca symptoms

Raynaud's phenomenon

Irritable bowel

The ANS is the portion of the nervous system that controls the function of the different organs and systems of the body. It is "autonomic" because it works below the level of consciousness. One striking characteristic of this system is the rapidity and intensity of the onset of its action and its dissipation. The ANS is activated by centers located in the spinal cord, brain stem, and hypothalamus. These centers also receive input from the limbic system and other higher brain areas. These connections enable the ANS as the principal part of the stress response system in charge of the fight or flight reactions.

The ANS works closely with the endocrine system, particularly with the hypothalamic-pituitary-adrenal axis. The adrenal glands are rich in autonomic neurotransmitters. Another endocrine axis closely related to the ANS involves growth hormone secretion.

The peripheral autonomic system is divided into two branches; sympathetic and parasympathetic. These two branches have antagonistic actions on most bodily functions and thus their proper balance preserves homeostasis. The action of these two branches is mediated by neurotransmitters. Norepinephrine is the predominant peripheral sympathetic neurotransmitter whereas acetylcholine acts in the parasympathetic periphery (3).

The function of the ANS has been difficult to assess in clinical practice. Changes in breathing pattern, mental stress, or even posture, alter immediately and completely the sympathetic/parasympathetic balance. So, this dynamic system could not be properly studied by "static" test such as levels of circulating neurotransmitters and less so by their urinary catabolites. Clinical studies of the ANS have been based on the responses of heart rate and blood pressure to deep breathing or valsalva maneuver. Nevertheless in recent years a new powerful technique has been introduced for the study of the ANS, namely heart rate variability analysis. This method is based on the fact that the heart rate is not uniform, but it varies constantly and at random. The periodic components of this variation are dictated by the antagonistic impulses of the sympathetic and parasympathetic branches of the ANS on the sinus node. Spectral analysis of this variability is able to identify several bands. The high frequency band reflects parasympathetic influx on the sinus node. There is controversy on the significance of the low frequency band power. It appears to be modulated by both sympathetic and parasympathetic influx. Nevertheless experts agree in the notion that low frequency band/high frequency band ratio reflects sympathetic activity.

Autonomic nervous system function can be also assessed by cybernetic time domain analysis of heart rate variability. Different mathematical calculations are used to accomplish this task, such as the standard deviation of all R-R intervals, or the number of pairs of adjacent R-R intervals differing by more than 50 milliseconds, among others. Decreased heart rate variability signifies diminished vagal influx on the sinus node (4).

We used heart rate variability analysis to estimate ANS function in persons with FMS. Our first study was intended to assess the response of the ANS to the orthostatic stress. It is known that in normal circumstances there is a surge in the low frequency band power reflecting sympathetic activation as response to standing-up. We studied 19 women with FMS and 19 age matched controls. We found that women with FMS failed to increase their low frequency band power after adopting the upright posture. This response was significantly different from that of controls. We concluded that in FMS, there is an orthostatic sympathetic derangement (5). These results have been confirmed by other controlled studies using diverse types of orthostatic maneuvers (6-8) [Table 2]. As knowledge and technology of heart rate variability evolved, we undertook our second investigation. This was a long-term [24 hours] study using a Holter monitor. Thirty patients with FMS and 30 age/sex matched controls were included. One important peculiarity of this study was that during measurements, subjects were ambulatory and performing their routine activity. This is an important point when studying ANS function since bringing subjects to a clinical research center would artificially alter their autonomic behavior. Results showed that during these

TABLE 2. Controlled Studies of the Responses to Orthostatic Stress in Patients with Fibromyalgia [FMS] Using Heart Rate Variability [HRV] Analysis and/or Tilt Table Testing

Authors, year of publication (reference)	Orthostatic stress test	Results in FMS patients as compared to controls
Martinez-Lavin et al., 1997 (5)	Active orthostatic stress HRV analysis	Failure to increase low frequency band power
Bou-Holaigah et al., 1997 (6)	Passive tilt table testing	Abnormal drop in blood pressure
Kelemen et al., 1998 (7)	Active orthostatic stress HRV analysis	Failure to increase low frequency band power
Raj et al., 2000 (8)	Tilt table testing + HRV analysis during tilting	Abnormal drop in blood pressure. Blunted sympatho/vagal response to tilting

24 hours FMS patients had less heart rate variability suggesting decreased parasympathetic influx [and therefore, the converse, increased sympathetic influx] on the sinus node. Fibromyalgia patients had also an altered circadian variation of the sympathetic/parasympathetic balance. They display changes consistent with nocturnal sympathetic hyperactivity (9).

Other groups of investigators have confirmed this sympathetic hyperactivity in FMS (8,10,11) both in women and in men [Table 3].

This body of evidence derived from different groups of researchers, strongly suggest that dysautonomia is prevalent in patients with FMS. Such dysautonomia can be characterized as relentless sympathetic *hyperactivity* throughout the day [particularly at night-time] with *hyporeactivity* to stress. Sympathetic hyperactivity may explain the endocrine abnormalities that have been reported in FMS, e.g., the growth hormone axis dysfunction reported by Bennett et al. (12). They described that FMS patients have low serum levels of somatomedin-C [a growth hormone stable product]. It has been established that growth hormone secretion occurs mostly at night and that sympathetic hyperactivity impairs this secretion.

We have proposed that ANS dysfunction could explain all the multisystem features of FMS shown in Table 1, including its defining features, generalized pain and tenderness at palpation on specific anatomical points (2). So, sympathetic derangement as response to stress can explain the constant fatigue and also the morning stiffness that these patients have. This fatigue secondary to sympathetic derangement can be

TABLE 3. Controlled Studies of Heart Rate Variability [HRV] Analysis in Fibromyalgia [FMS] Patients

Authors, year of publication (reference)	Test	Results in FMS patients as compared to controls
Martinez-Lavin et al., 1998 (9)	24 hr. HRV time and frequency domain analyses. Circadian sympatho/vagal balance	Less HRV. Sympathetic hyperactivity, particularly at night
Cohen et al., 2000 (10)	20 min. HRV frequency domain analysis	Increased sympathetic activity
Raj et al., 2000 (8)	24 hr. HRV time and frequency domain analyses	Less HRV. Sympathetic hyperactivity
Cohen et al., 2001 (11)	20 min. HRV frequency domain analysis in men	Men with FMS also have sympathetic hyperactivity

compared to what happens to a constantly forced engine that becomes unable to speed-up as response to further stimulus.

Nocturnal sympathetic hyperactivity can induce the sleep disorders. It has been established that parasympathetic influx predominates during deep stages of sleep. Nocturnal sympathetic hyperactivity can irritate normal sleep patterns as suggested by our studies of concurrent heart rate variability analysis and polysomnography in patients with FMS (13).

Sympathetic hyperactivity could also explain sicca symptoms; a good example of this well known adrenergic side-effect is the dryness in the mouth of the amateur speaker. Pseudo-Raynaud's phenomenon can be easily explained on the same basis. Independent studies, also using heart rate variability analysis have proposed that dysautonomia may play a role in the pathogenesis of irritable bowel syndrome (14,15).

Special mention of the relationship of FMS with anxiety is deserved. It is clear that there is a psychological component in FMS. It could not be any other way with persons suffering from chronic intense pain. Unfortunately, the psychological component of FMS syndrome has led some physicians to diagnose these patients with pejorative labels such as hypochondriacs or hysterics. New labels have been used in recent years such as "persons with health seeking behavior" or "somatizers" (16). In our opinion these labels are totally misplaced and do not help by any means in understanding the pathogenesis of this syndrome. The fact that there is a psychological component in FMS does not diminish the validity of the diagnosis nor make patients censurable for their suffering. In our model, anxiety could be either the cause or the effect of sympathetic activity. What we believe is important for FMS research, is the net biological result of this interaction; sympathetic hyperactivity.

The two defining features of FMS [generalized pain and tenderness at palpation on defined anatomical points] and one "minor" manifestation [paresthesias], could be explained by relentless sympathetic hyperactivity that may induce pain through the mechanism known as "sympathetically maintained pain" (17).

Pain induced by sympathetic hyperactivity has experimental foundations. In a rodent model, after nerve damage sympathetic stimulation and norepinephrine are excitatory for primary skin C-fibers nociceptors. These nociceptors start to express adrenoceptors and become responsive to norepinephrine. Peripheral nerve injury also induces noradrenergic sprouting within the dorsal root ganglia. These unusual connections may give rise to both peripheral and central sensitization and may trigger the vicious cycle of sympathetic hyperactivity and pain.

In humans, one of the recognized causes of chronic pain is mediated by sympathetic hyperactivity. Reflex sympathetic dystrophy is its best known clinical expression. Pain in FMS has several features in common to the neuropathic pain of reflex sympathetic dystrophy namely: post-traumatic onset, relentless pain disproportionate to the underlying tissue damage and unresponsive to analgesic/anti-inflammatory drugs, the presence of allodynia [in FMS tender points reflect a generalized state of allodynia], paresthesias [a typical feature of neuropathic pain] and lastly, in both clinical syndromes, pain improves after sympathetic blockade (17).

CONCLUSION

Sympathetic nervous system dysfunction is frequent in FMS and may explain its multisystem manifestations. It remains to be established if this dysautonomia plays a major role in the pathogenesis of FMS. We surmise that it does. If so, new types of nonpharmacological and pharmacological therapeutic interventions intended to restore ANS homeostasis may be developed.

REFERENCES

1. Wolfe F, Smythe HA, Yunus MB Bennett RM, Bombardier C, Goldenberg DL, Tugwell P, Campbell SM, Abeles M, Clark P, Fam AG, Farber SJ, Fiechtner JJ, Franklin CM, Gatter RA, Hamaty D, Lessard J, Lichtbroun AS, Masi AT, McCain GA, Reynolds WJ, Romano TJ, Russell LJ, Sheon RP: The American College of Rheumatology 1990 criteria for the classification of fibromyalgia: Report of the Multicenter Criteria Committee. Arthritis Rheum 33; 160-71:1999.

2. Martinez-Lavin M, Hemosillo AG: Autonomic nervous system dysfunction may explain the multisystem features of FMS. Semin Arthritis Rheum 29;197-9:2000

3. Lefkowitz RJ, Hoffman BB, Taylor P. Neurotransmission. The autonomic and somatic nervous system. In Hardman JG, Limbird LE. Goodman & Gilman's The pharmacological basis of therapeutics 9th Edition 1996. McGraw-Hill, New York pp. 105-40.

4. Task force of the European Society of Cardiology and the North American Society of Pacing and Electrophysiology. Heart rate variability. Standards of measurement, physiological interpretation, and clinical use. Circulation 93; 1043-65:1996.

5. Martinez-Lavin M, Hermosillo AG, Mendoza C, Ortiz R, Cajigas JC, Pineda C, Nava A, Vallejo M: Orthostatic sympathetic derangement in subject with fibromyalgia. J Rheumatol 24;714-8:1997.

6. Bou-Holaigah I, Calkins H, Flynn JA, TuninC, Chang HC, Kan JS, Rowe PC: Provocation of hypotension and pain during upright tilt table testing in adults with fibromyalgia. Clin Exp Rheumatol 15;239-46:1997.

7. Kelemen J, Lang E, Balint G, Trocsanyi M, Muller W: Orthostatic sympathetic derangement of baroreflex in patients with fibromyalgia. J Rheumatol 25;823-5:1998.

8. Raj RR, Brouillard D, Simpsom CS, Hopman WM, Abdollah H: Dysautonomia among patients with fibromyalgia: A noninasive assessment. J Rheumatol 27; 2660-5:2000.

9. Martinez-Lavin M, Hermosillo AG, Rosas M, Soto ME: Circadian studies of autonomic nervous balance in patients with fibromyalgia. A heart rate variability analysis. Arthritis Rheum 42;1966-71:1998.

10. Cohen H, Neumann L, Shore M, Amir M, Cassuto Y, Buskila D: Autonomic dysfunction in patients with fibromyalgia: Application of power spectral analysis of heart rate variability. Semin Arthritis Rheum 29;217-27:2000.

11. Cohen H, Neumann L, Alhosshle A, Kotler M, Abu-Shakra M, Buskila D: Abnormal sympathovagal balance in men with fibromyalgia. J Rheumatol 28;581-9:2001.

12. Bennett RM, Cook DM, Clark SR, Burckhart CS, Campbell SM: Hypothalamic-pituitary-insulin-like growth factor I axis dysfunction in patients with fibromyalgia. J Rheumatol 24;1384-9:1997.

13. Martinez-Lavin M, Koo M, Meza S, Martin del Campo A, Hermosillo AG, Pineda C, Amigo MC, Nava A, Drucker-Colin R: Simultaneous studies of heart rate variability and polysomnography in patients with fibromyalgia. Arthritis Rheum 42; S344:1999.

14. Karling P, Nyhlin H, Wiklund U, Sjoberg M, Olofsson BO, Bjerle P: Spectral analysis of heart rate variability in patients with irritable bowel syndrome. Scand J Gastroenterol 33;572-6:1998.

15. Heitkemper M, Burr RL, Jarret M, Hertig V, Lustyk MK, Bond EF: Evidence of autonomic nervous system imbalance in women with irritable bowel syndrome. Dig Dis Sci 43;2093-8:1998.

16. McBeth J, MacFarlane GJ, Benjamin S, Silman AJ: Features of somatization predict the onset of chronic widespread pain; results of a large population based study. Arthritis Rheum 44;940-6:2001.

17. Martinez-Lavin M: Is fibromyalgia a generalized reflex sympathetic dystrophy? Clin Exp Rheumatol 19; 1-3:2001.

Chronic Persistent Pain
in Victims of Torture

Inge Genefke

SUMMARY. Objectives: To introduce the concept of torture, its forms, its sequele, and its treatment.

Findings: Torture involves pain and suffering intentionally inflicted upon a person for the purpose of coercing a confession, collecting information, punishing an action, or intimidation. Typically, it is perpetrated with the consent of a public official. Its aim is to destroy the person's individuality by beating, hanging, burning, and/or psychological assault. Long-term physical and psychological sequelae require treatment whose cornerstone is trust.

Conclusions: Torture is the worst violation of human rights known to man. It persists because of its political power. Research is needed to prevent torture and to help its victims. *[Article copies available for a fee from The Haworth Document Delivery Service: 1-800-HAWORTH. E-mail address: <getinfo@haworthpressinc.com> Website: <http://www.HaworthPress.com> © 2002 by The Haworth Press, Inc. All rights reserved.]*

KEYWORDS. Torture, political power, falanga, rehabilitation

Inge Genefke, MD, DMSc hc, is the Honorary Secretary-General with the International Rehabilitation Council for Torture Victims [IRCT]; and also the founder of the Rehabilitation and Research Center for Torture Victims [RCT] in Copenhagen and the International Rehabilitation Council for Torture Victims [ICRT].

Address correspondence to: Inge Genefke, MD DMSc hc, Borgergade 13, P.O. Box 9049, DK-1022 Copenhagen K, Denmark [E-mail: irct@irct.org].

[Haworth co-indexing entry note]: "Chronic Persistent Pain in Victims of Torture." Genefke, Inge. Co-published simultaneously in *Journal of Musculoskeletal Pain* [The Haworth Medical Press, an imprint of The Haworth Press, Inc.] Vol. 10, No. 1/2, 2002, pp. 229-259; and: *The Clinical Neurobiology of Fibromyalgia and Myofascial Pain: Therapeutic Implications* [ed: Robert M. Bennett] The Haworth Medical Press, an imprint of The Haworth Press, Inc., 2002, pp. 229-259. Single or multiple copies of this article are available for a fee from The Haworth Document Delivery Service [1-800-HAWORTH, 9:00 a.m. - 5:00 p.m. [EST]. E-mail address: getinfo@haworthpressinc.com].

INTRODUCTION

In the following paragraphs, I will provide the definition of torture and explain why understanding this definition is so important. When torture is the cause of pain, the level of suffering is quite unique. I will describe the different physical methods of torture, causing both acute and chronic pain. The psychological methods of torture always go hand in hand with the physical, worsening the severity of both. The sequelae of torture require active treatment but the most effective approaches are not necessarily intuitive. Future progress in this field will require integration between examinations of torture victims and research directed toward reducing the long-term effects of torture.

The official definition of torture was developed by the United Nations Convention Against Torture [Figure 1]. For an act to meet this definition of torture, four conditions must be fulfilled: 1. there must have been severe pain or suffering which had either physical and/or mental aspects; 2. the assault must have been caused intentionally; 3. there must have been a specific purpose for the assault; and 4. it must have been approved by one or more public officials.

The methods of physical torture are nearly unlimited. Figure 2 outlines a variety of methods, including those most commonly used. It

FIGURE 1. The definition of torture developed by the United Nations Convention Against Torture. Notice that there are four required components to this definition.

Definition of Torture

United Nations Convention Against Torture, Article 1:

For the purposes of this Convention, the term "torture" means any act by which severe pain or suffering, whether physical or mental
1. is intentionally
2. inflicted on a person for such purposes
3. as obtaining from him or a third person information or a confession, punishing him for an act he or a third person has committed or is suspected of having committed, or intimidating or coercing him or a third person, or for any reason based on discrimination or any kind, when such pain or suffering is inflicted by or at the investigation of or with the consent or acquiescence of a public official
4. or other person acting in an official capacity.

FIGURE 2. Physical methods commonly used in torture.

Physical Methods of Torture

- Beatings–systematic or random
- Suspension
- Falanga
- Burning
- Sexual attacks
- Electrical torture
- Water torture
- Pharmacological torture
- Mutilations
- Other methods

shall be noted from the very beginning, that psychological torture nearly always goes hand-in-hand with the physical. The conditions in torture prisons are usually quite terrible, the food is bad, the fear is immense, and there is no way to prepare for the coming pain. And again, it is done intentionally. Aid workers sometimes learn of the horrors of torture from watercolor paintings the victims produce to describe their experiences. They have illustrated beatings, hangings, including electrical torture, falanga, and burning. The pictures are not nice to look at but torture is not nice.

BEATINGS

In fact nearly 100 percent of torture victims are brutally beaten. Beating causes acute pain. It may entail hemorrhage. It can also induce permanent changes in the subcutaneous tissue. It can damage kidneys, stomachs, etc. In many cases, it will also cause chronic pain.

HANGING

The so-called Palestinian hanging involves over-stretching the nerves, tendons, and muscles, severely injuring the joints, leading to a lot of long-term sequelae. In all of these injured tissues, there is acute pain, and eventually chronic pain. Vertical hanging causes similar kinds of soft tissue damage. Commonly, the person is blindfolded and at intervals, electricity is applied to body parts. The victim cannot prepare for the electricity given, so the pain is even worse than if it were possible to prepare for it.

FALANGA

This is the term used to describe beatings on the soles of the feet. Research regarding the diagnosis and treatment of sequele from this form of torture has been presented (1). With falanga, the torturers obtain what they are trying to achieve, namely a pain which can persist for a lifetime–every step reminds the person of the torture experience.

BURNING

This form of torture is used rather often. It certainly gives immediate pain and the chronicity of discomfort from the damaged skin contributes to its chronicity.

PSYCHOLOGICAL TORTURE

The victims consider the psychological torture to be the worst. A lot of different methods are used [Figure 3]. One of these involves getting to an intended victim through the torture of beloved relatives while the intended victim is forced to watch. Can you imagine the eyes of a four-year old son being torn out, to force the father or mother to break down? That is psychological torture. In short, torturers will stop at nothing to demonstrate that they have the full power, while the victim is simply nothing.

The victims always break down if the torturer persists.

The victims do not talk about the torture later on, not even to their spouses. If inadequately treated, the suffering from the torture remains trapped inside of the victim's psyche, a pressure for the rest of his or her life.

The aim of torture is to destroy the person as an individual. In conclusion, torture is the worst violation of human rights known to man. Its power is as mighty as money.

FIGURE 3. Psychological methods commonly used in torture.

Psychological Methods of Torture

- Deprivation/Isolation
- Humiliation
- Threats of torture, invalidity
- Skin execution
- Threats against relatives/friends
- Witnessing torture
- Sexual assault
- Mental exhaustion
- Pharmacological torture
- Other methods

SEQUELAE

Torture always leaves sequelae. Unlike spontaneously acquired disorders, this condition is produced intentionally. Other conditions are caused by accidents, infectious organisms, genetic defects, or degenerative disease, but the torture is forced upon a fellow being, is man-made, and even worse, is perpetrated upon the victim for a purpose.

The sequelae from torture are manifold [Figure 4]. For the victim, the somatic sequelae can seem to be the most important issue. Essentially all torture survivors have soft tissue pain and other musculoskeletal symptoms. There is much to learn about how to care for these medical problems. But it is equally important, to recognize the psychological sequelae of torture. Failure to recognize that aspect of the torture will offset much of the benefit from treating the physical problems. This issue is made more difficult because the tortured client will very seldom admit to the therapist that an emotional symptom has anything to do with the torture. On the contrary, victims always try to cover-up that relationship by attributing the symptoms to more common conditions.

These observations help to explain why the sequelae of torture are so horrendous, why torture must be related to as a special entity among medical conditions, and why it is so clinically demanding upon the therapist to develop effective specific treatment.

FIGURE 4. The sequele of torture.

The Sequelae of Torture

Somatic

- Objective:
  - Muscular/skeleton
    - Neurological
    - Sensory organs

- Subjective:
  - Heart
  - Liver
  - "All organs"

Psychological:

- Anxiety
- Depression
- Pain
- Reduced memory/functions
- Sleep disturbance
- Sexual disturbance
- Change of identity
- Low self-esteem

TREATMENT

Several principles of treatment are outlined in Figure 5. A cornerstone in the treatment of torture victims is trust. When a torture victim enters a treatment program, he or she is likely to be distrustful and unwilling to believe in anything, lacking confidence in anyone. Gaining the victim's trust through empathy, consistency, and dependability will be critical to achieving success in a treatment program. A very close contact, preferably direct eye-contact, is of importance because it tends to instil trust and confidence.

Another important issue in the treatment of torture victims is to avoid intervention modalities that can be imagined to resemble some form of torture. With the use of some types of interventions, the victim can be jolted into a severe flash back and become nearly psychotic. For exam-

FIGURE 5. The principles of treatment.

Principles of Treatment

- Somatic: Physiotherapy
- Psychological: Psychotherapy
- Social
- Judicial
- The whole family
- Taking cultural aspects into consideration
- Avoid forms of treatment which seem similar to methods of torture

ple, if the clinician were to order an electroencephalogram on a torture victim, the procedure and its purpose must be carefully explained. The victim must be fully reassured that this test will not represent a new form of electrical torture.

Somatic treatment must always be provided hand-in-hand with psychotherapy. The torture violence was both physical and mental, so logically the treatment should integrate physiotherapy with psychotherapy. The most effective treatment program is often based on very simple methods. Attempts to use sophisticated instruments can be counterproductive.

MEDICAL EDUCATION

Finally, medical professionals need to be better prepared to work with torture victims. Rheumatologists, pain doctors, and psychiatrists who may come in contact with torture survivors should have specific training about torture, about the behavior of torture victims, and about the "pitfalls" in the treatment. In short, torture should be an item in the curriculum for education of physicians all over the world who specialize in the management of pain and related musculoskeletal conditions.

RESEARCH

Besides education, there is a big demand for further research. Much more must be learned about how to diagnosis specific torture-induced injuries and how do integrate the management of the somatic damage from torture with that of the traumatized psyche. The International Rehabilitation Council for Torture Victims and the Parker Institute in Copenhagen are cooperating regarding these matters.

In the section to follow, the reader will find additional background about torture, international efforts to eliminate it as a political tool, and to effectively treat its victims. In addition more information is provided about the history of work against torture, and the functions of the organizations which are dedicated to solving these problems.

A BRIEF HISTORY

The medical work against torture started in 1973 when Amnesty International launched a campaign against torture and asked medical doctors to take part in the work of helping and diagnosing torture victims. In the few cases where torture victims progressed to having a trial in court, they were and still often are, accused of having performed self-injury, for instance having burned themselves with cigarettes, banged their head into a wall, or thrown themselves down staircases, etc. In such cases it is very important that medical doctors be capable of performing forensic examinations to objectively document that torture has taken place.

That was why in Denmark we created the first Amnesty International medical group. It began work in 1974 and consisted of four doctors working on a voluntary basis. Soon after that, our numbers grew to 10. And after a few more years, there were about 4,000 medical doctors in 34 countries organized in Amnesty International's Medical Groups. They all worked with diagnosing victims of torture as well as developing more sophisticated diagnostic tools.

From the very beginning, we realized we had to start from scratch. At that time, no specific knowledge existed regarding torture methods or their influence on the physical and mental health of the victims. Therefore, we began by examining Chilean torture victims who had come to Denmark as refugees, and Greek victims of torture in their home country. We asked them in depth about the torture they had been exposed to and the after-effects they suffered. For us, and especially for them, it was a very difficult task and therefore we deeply appreciated their noble acceptance of being questioned and examined. I shall always remember the first meeting, when we evaluated the first 15 persons we had examined, as the most grievous one I have attended. At that time we realized that there were not only physical problems [the forensic medical evidence we were looking for], but also many mental problems in persons who had been exposed to torture–a fact, as evident as it may seem today, that no one had been aware of or had any knowledge about.

The first seminar on Violations of Human Rights Torture and the Medical Profession was held in 1978 in Athens. At that meeting about 100 medical doctors from 12 different countries were present. We created international working groups, one of which was to work with the rehabilitation of torture victims.

In 1979, we obtained permission to admit and examine torture victims at Rigshospitalet, the University Hospital in Copenhagen and were thereby able to establish the treatment principles for a rehabilitation program. The Rehabilitation and Research Center for Torture Victims [RCT] in Copenhagen was established in 1982. All along we cooperated closely with colleagues on the international level on the rehabilitation programs, especially colleagues from Latin America and Asia. In 1985 the official formation of the International Rehabilitation Council for Torture Victims [IRCT] took place, and in the years from 1992-1996 34 centers and programs were initiated with support from the IRCT. Today, we have been in contact with and worked with health professionals in far more than 100 countries. The number of centers has risen every year and all in all, there exist up to 250 centers and programs worldwide.

WHAT IS TORTURE

The torture process starts with the arrest, usually at night, with a formidable display of power and unnecessary use of violence. The "softening phase," which often follows, usually consists of a couple of days and nights of unsystematic violence including beatings, kicking, and other humiliations. Later on the real systematic torture begins when the torturers explore the weak spots of the victim to make him or her break down. And everybody breaks if that is the intention of torturers. Everybody! The final result may then be a formerly strong person, now a victim with little or no self-respect and a broken down personality, together with a false medical certificate denying any form of maltreatment. Sometimes, the final result is death. However, this is often not the intention of the torturers. Therefore, this leaves us with the sad fact that medical doctors sometimes participate in the performance of torture, voluntarily or involuntarily. The assistance of medical doctors becomes necessary for the torturers in order to make sure that the victim suffers as much as possible without crossing the line of death.

Systematic torture can be divided into physical and psychological forms, usually performed at the same time, and both intended to destroy the physical and psychological well-being of the victim for a long time to come. Torture has become a science and not only medical doctors but also psychologists in many countries are involved in developing new and even more brutal methods to break down the victims.

The following is an abbreviated summary of torture methods:

Physical Torture

- Beatings.
- Electric shocks are applied to the most sensitive areas of the body.
- The victim is suspended for hours on end by his arms or by his legs.
- The victim's head is forced under water until he or she is about to suffocate.
- The victim's skin is burned by cigarettes or red-hot iron rods.
- The victims are beaten systematically, for instance under the feet until the soles are badly damaged.
- Sexual offenses are common.
- Women in particular are attacked as sexual objects, and men are harmed in their ability to function as men. Trained dogs are used for direct attacks or for rape of both men and women.
- The situation during detention is further worsened by filthy food and drinking water.
- Freedom to move around is limited, and prisoners are packed into small cells which force them to sleep by turns.
- Sanitary conditions are extremely poor, and any request for going to the bathroom will often be turned into a pretext for torture.

Psychological Torture

- The breakdown of the personality often begins at the time of arrest, with removal of personal belongings, including life-saving drugs, glasses, etc., and replacing them with badly fitting uniforms.
- Names are replaced with numbers and the guards must be addressed with deep respect.
- Deprivation of sleep, blindfolding, lack of social contact.

- Mock executions lead the individual to transgress from reality into a nightmarish or catatonic state.
- Victims may be forced to torture each other.
- The worst of all is to witness torture of close relatives and friends [children, spouses, parents], powerless and helpless.

All these methods leave a deep sensation of helplessness, fear, and terror and can provoke hallucinations. Total isolation for months or years are common during which time the victims do not know what is going to happen, and the relatives often do not know their whereabouts. Many victims are forced into doing or saying things against their ideology or religious conviction, with the purpose of attacking fundamental parts of their identity. Political and ethical values are particularly attacked by the torturers when they force the victims to sing songs that praise everything they have been fighting against.

THE MEDICAL EFFECTS OF TORTURE

Torturers today are able to create conditions which effectively break down the victim's personality and identity as well as their ability to later on live satisfactory lives. The worst consequences of torture for the survivors are the mental sequelae. Deep feelings of guilt and shame often occur after torture. The feeling of guilt may be caused by the mere fact of survival while friends may have died under torture; or perhaps information was given that could have harmed friends. This deep feeling of guilt may also be produced by the so-called "impossible choice," when the victims have to choose between, for instance, revealing the names of their friends or seeing family members tortured.

Regardless of what the victim chooses, the end result is a disaster for which the victim feels responsible, and that is exactly what the torturer wants. Psychological studies of survivors of torture reveal especially the following symptoms:

- Emotional labiality
- Sleep disturbances
- Disturbances in ability to concentrate/remember
- Avoidance of thoughts or feelings associated with the torture
- Avoidance of activities or situations that arouse recollections of the torture
- Diminished ability to establish personal relationships

- Markedly diminished interest in several significant activities
- Sense of a foreshortened future
- Sudden acting or feeling as if the torture situation was recurring
- Feeling of change in personality
- Survivor guilt
- Anxiety
- Sexual disturbances
- Fatigue

All of these reactions we consider normal in people who have been exposed to something as abnormal and cruel as torture. The problems after torture are included in the posttraumatic stress disorder syndrome, but are worse.

Over the years we have conducted research concerning the somatic symptoms and objective findings after torture. We know that there are many complaints related to the musculoskeletal system, the neurological system, the cardiopulmonary system, the gastrointestinal system, the urological and genital systems, and we can see objective findings from all these organs. The majority of the clinical findings are in the musculoskeletal system. That is why we always recommend physiotherapy or other therapies related to this system.

TORTURE, A TRANSGENERATIONAL PROBLEM

In the past few years, we have begun to look very seriously at the effects of torture on children. Torture on children is performed in a number of countries, sometimes for the purpose of affecting pressure on the parents, who are often forced to witness. In some countries, homeless kids are tortured in order to force them off the streets. But even more often, children become victims of torture in a more indirect way. If a parent is tortured, it brings great disturbance to the entire family. Children are often left without the necessary explanations and the parents' silence creates fearful fantasies and guilt in the child. Some parents become overly protective; others cannot care for their children in an emotionally satisfactory way. Thus, torture is a transgenerational problem and should be treated as such. Moreover, it expands the effects of torture onto entire families. This spill-over effect magnifies the devastating results of torture.

THE MAGNITUDE OF THE TORTURE PROBLEM

Several human rights organizations are trying to assess the magnitude of the torture problem. Many researchers, including scholars in the Danish rehabilitation movement at the Rehabilitation Council for Torture Victims in Copenhagen have performed studies on refugee populations in European countries. The picture is bleak and sometimes difficult to discern.

However, I will mention a few studies which at least can be indicative of what we are dealing with.

- A very recent study of 462 refugees living in Norway shows that 25 percent of the men and five percent of the women had been exposed to torture (2).
- Of the refugee population world-wide, between five and 35 percent, or 1.6 to five million people, have been tortured (3).
- In the United States, approximately 400,000 former torture victims reside (4).
- In Denmark, there are approximately 78,000 refugees [Danish Department of Interior]. A survey among 10,000 asylum seekers entering Denmark in the late 1980's show that 18.5 percent of the men and 3.8 percent of the women had been exposed to torture or other violent abuse. Approximately 10 percent of the Asian refugees and up to 50 percent of the African refugees had been tortured (5). The results of a close-up study of refugees from the Middle East from 1994, 30 percent of all refugees from this area had been exposed to torture; 55 percent of the males and 12 percent of the females (6).
- The Chilean government has admitted to the United Nations Committee Against Torture [CAT] that the former government was responsible for 100,000 victims of torture. This must be considered a minimum number (Genefke, unpublished).

The numbers vary a great deal from study to study. Noting our research and thousands of interviews with torture victims, I have no doubt that the figures are in fact even much higher than survey research has indicated. We know that many victims are so traumatized by the shame they are feeling, that they cannot make themselves reveal they are torture victims, especially when questioned by government officials or other authority figures. Thus, we don't have a precise number and we never will. But we do know that victims of torture can be counted in the millions.

REHABILITATION MODELS

Today we know how to rehabilitate the torture victims. We have developed different rehabilitation models, which are used at many centers and programs world-wide.

One of them is the holistic approach, where all aspects of life are taken into consideration; the psychological, somatic, social, legal, spiritual, familial, and cultural aspects. A point of conceptual importance is that we are not considering torture survivors to be sick, but simply to have normal reactions to a very abnormal event.

The main treatment principles are:

- To treat physical and psychological symptoms at the same time,
- To secure the patient's trust and confidence,
- To respect the individual,
- To avoid situations which remind the patients of torture,
- To inform carefully about examinations.

Psychological insight therapy. This form of therapy consists of the following phases–the meeting, the initial setting, the emotional phase, reiteration, and end of therapy.

Psychological supportive therapy. We use this where we are dealing with practical matters like bodily dysfunctions, etc., social matters, like housing and language, and integrational matters, for refugees to get a basic understanding of the new country, so it is a balance between insight and supportive psychotherapy.

Special programs for children and families. Couple therapy, family therapy, individual child therapy, group therapy, and network meetings are important.

Out-reach method for screening and rehabilitation of torture victims. This model has four points of importance: availability, accessibility, adaptability, and appropriateness. Availability refers to the services being available to meet the health needs, both general and special. Accessibility means that the services must not be too distant or culturally insensitive. Adaptability refers to the likelihood of the project being acceptable to the refugees/nationals and therapeutically effective at the same time. Appropriateness is related to the question of whether a project is appropriate to the groups of torture victims covered by it.

Psychosocial support and treatment to dislocated war victims and torture victims. The aim is to facilitate the social functioning of the person by: Strengthening adaptive coping mechanisms, discouraging nonadaptive processes, and facilitating access to social opportunities. Furthermore, to facilitate the psychological working of traumatic experiences, loss and bereavement people have had by: Consoling, comforting and protecting them, sharing their experiences and feelings, recognizing their suffering and pain, and supporting them to express grief when the first survival needs are satisfied. Finally, to treat the persons who have developed a psychic disturbance.

Counselling. It is defined as a method that, to some degree, takes into account a deeper understanding of the individual's experiences, giving relief and understanding, and helping the person to solve problems and to make choices. The counsellor must respect the confidentiality of information given and must be capable of handling situations which are loaded with painful feelings without getting lost, and use them for the benefit of the client. He must also be skilled in analyzing problems and give advice and know how to help the client make his own decisions. The counselling program is designed to be accomplished by persons who are not health professionals such as doctors, psychologists, etc. We created this program because in many countries there are not a sufficient number of health professionals, but other very good professionals, like for instance teachers, even journalists or monks and nuns, etc., can learn the program and perform very effectively, not as deeply as a psychotherapist of course, but they can really help victims.

The aim of counselling is to increase awareness of experienced traumas and the reactions to these. Furthermore, to give relief from the psychological suffering to reduce after effects of traumatic experience and to help the person regain control of life situations in order to become a full-blown member of society again. The counsellor must therefore always respect the confidentiality of information given and must be capable of handling situations which are loaded with painful feelings without getting lost himself and use them for the benefit of the client. The counsellor must also be skilled in analysing problems and give advice and know-how to help the client make his or her own decisions.

THE ROLE OF THE RHEUMATOLOGIST
AND PHYSIOTHERAPIST

The premises, the appearance, and the attitude of the therapists. Everything that can remind the torture survivors of imprisonment and situations of torture should be avoided. As far as possible we avoid waiting time for the client before an appointment. Treatment rooms should have no clinical appearance, but are cozy and decorated with ornaments and pleasant colors. During treatment, private clothes are used instead of uniforms. The treatment should not inflict pain, especially during initiation of treatment where the client is in a physical and psychological condition of stress and therefore hypersensitive. It is of utmost importance to create a good and confident atmosphere. During imprisonment and torture the client has lost his self-respect and confidence in himself and in others. Accordingly the building up of mutual confidence is the presupposition for treatment.

Common clinical symptoms in victims of torture. There is a fine consistency between the symptoms and the signs within the locomotor system, as opposed to the signs and symptoms from the vital organs. Actually, it is often found that the reason for the organic complaints is bound to the malfunctions in the locomotor system. Some of the most common symptoms are lack of concentration and of memory, headache, either due to nightmares and lack of sleep or due to disinformation from the proprioceptors together with dysfunction of the masticatory system and dysfunctions in the genuine joints of the cervical spine.

There is a high incidence of pain due to dysfunctions in the rest of the spine and the peripheral joints and muscles in particular. These are typical sequels after beating, suspension or fixation in awkward body positions, etc.

Late effects of falanga [beating on the soles of the feet with iron bars, whips, etc.] are pain in the calves and the feet together with an abnormal spatial orientation [clients from the Middle-East]. This kind of torture provokes in the acute phase huge swelling which causes destruction of the tissue structures in the feet and the calves.

Cooperation with rheumatologist and physiotherapist. Cooperation with a rheumatologist is recommended, if possible. The client is offered individual physiotherapy lasting one hour twice a week, and according to need, training in a hot water pool, swimming and fitness training.

RHEUMATOLOGICAL TREATMENT APPROACH
TO TORTURE VICTIMS

The first meeting between the client and the therapist. The first meeting should have the form of a dialogue in order to avoid a situation of interrogation. The therapist should be calm and empathetic and express knowledge about torture and its sequels. This is being done in order to relieve the feeling of isolation, guilt, and shame which is always present in our clients.

Special attention during treatment. There are always lots of individual considerations to be taken during treatment of a victim of torture. Among other things it is most important to situate oneself in front of the client, to avoid going behind the client without explaining why, to avoid placing the client in strong light, etc. At all times one should pay attention to the reactions of the client both verbal and nonverbal. Many clients are very shy and do not want to undress, since they have been undressed during torture as a part of the humiliation. In each case we evaluate whether the client should be treated fully dressed or partly undressed. For the same reason, the treatment should always start at a neutral part of the body, and areas such as the pelvic area will not be treated until late in the treatment course, in case sexual torture has taken place.

Considerations on the choice of instruments for the treatment. Careful introduction is needed to the use of treatment tables and mirrors. Treatment with ultrasound or laser is often postponed until late during the course, since many clients have been submitted to electrical torture and therefore may not accept electrotherapy. In case of electrical torture treatment with electrodes such as transcutaneous nerve stimulation and short-wave treatment for which fixation is required such as mechanical traction will not be used because of the reminding of torture.

The course of individual treatment. A variety of physiotherapy methods should be applied to relieve pain and improve function, all in accordance with the findings on the physiotherapy examination. Soft tissue treatment plays a major role in the overall treatment of torture survivors, since they have large amounts of adhesive connective tissue within and between the musculoskeletal structures. This scar tissue gives rise to dysfunction due to tightness and pain. As a preliminary treatment gentle effleurage is given to painful areas. The purpose is to help the client to accept being touched, to reduce pain and to relax the muscles. When possible, other methods are introduced such as pain-relieving massage, softening of tight fibrous tissues, stretching of tight muscles and connective tissue, proprioceptive stimulation, and mobilization of stiff joints. Most clients have a changed posture [e.g., they have developed a stooping posture] which can be corrected over time when the client starts improving physically as well as psychologically.

Special attention should be directed to the respiratory patterns which are sensitive to a person's psychological state of mind. Respiratory relaxation and reeducation techniques are applied either alone or combined with other physiotherapy methods.

The treatment of falanga-symptoms consists primarily of softening massage to the maltreated tissues of the soles of feet, mobilization of fixated joints of the foot, loosening of the fascia and stabilization of the unstable joints in the feet and the calves. Parallel to this treatment the muscle balance is reestablished.

It is very important to stress that the methods used for survivors of torture are no different from all physiotherapeutic modalities–only they are adapted to this very special group of patients. Thus, a deep knowledge of a broad variety of treatment techniques combined with experience, pragmatism, imagination, and flexibility is required.

Interrelationship between physical and psychological symptoms. During treatment it should be pointed out to the client the interrelationship between different kinds of torture, the clinical signs and some of the psychological signs and symptoms. If for instance the client experiences respiratory problems and heart symptoms, it may be a physical manifestation of his fear. In this way his perception of the body can be approached. This is a very important part of the treatment since many clients have an altered perception of parts of the body during and after the torture. Sometimes the clients have a very modest knowledge of human anatomy and therefore benefit from information based on anatomical illustrations and books.

Flash-back. Sometimes it happens that a client is experiencing a flash-back [a short reactive psychosis where the client imagines himself outside of time and place]. He often relives a situation, e.g., from a prison, because something [for example a noise, a gesture, a color, or a light] provoked his memory. This may also happen during physiotherapy. When this happens it can be difficult to get in contact with the client who will be in his own world of thoughts and imagine himself back in prison. The therapist will then stay by the client and make sure that he is not hurt, but should not touch him. Usually it will be possible to "call him back" fairly quickly by telling him in a calm voice where he really is.

Ordering of aiding devices. Many clients need different kinds of auxiliary devices, such as angora-underwear, special shoes, foot supports, braces, mattresses, chairs, etc. Sometimes, it is necessary to make a home visit in order to evaluate the need for devices.

Physical activation of the client apart from individual treatment sessions. The client is asked to do specific exercises at home in order to give him a better muscle balance and a better understanding of the body.

Duration of physiotherapy treatment. The duration of the treatment course is being adjusted to the symptoms of the individual client and may last as long as six months or sometimes more. It is being followed by a final examination by the physiotherapist and possibly by a rheumatologist. Most of the clients experience a considerable relief of pain in joints and muscles, less headache, less fatigue, better physical fitness, and a better understanding and acceptance of the body. They will also gain a better posture, a better body balance, and a freer way of walking. Many torture victims complain of chronic pain from the musculoskeletal system, often with neurogenic pain, hyperalgesia, and allodynia. With this in mind, it is not the task of the physiotherapist to make the patient free of pain, but to guide him to a better understanding of the nature of the pain, and the pain influence on physical functions. During the course of treatment they have been given instructions as to how they through a variety of exercises and suitable rest- and working-positions can prevent relapses.

Two international seminars for physiotherapy educators were held in Copenhagen in 1995 and 1997. The seminars were joint ventures between World Confederation for Physical Therapy and IRCT. Physiotherapy educators from all five regions were gathered in Copenhagen to discuss how physiotherapy for torture survivors should be implemented in the curriculum for physiotherapists. A curriculum has been developed and can be delivered if requested from IRCT.

Conclusion. In a number of countries the word torture is difficult to use. It may be dangerous to mention or many create apprehension and fear. It was suggested that words like organized violence and abuse were appropriate in describing the same atrocities. It became obvious for the participants how extensive torture is and the magnitude of the psychological and physical sequelae. As a consequence all agreed that the subject should be implemented in the curriculum to create awareness of the problem.

INTERNATIONAL CONVENTIONS AND DECLARATIONS

Before 1974, when the medical work against torture started, the only relevant conventions and declarations against torture were the Hippocratic Oath and United Nations Universal Declaration of Human Rights. Since the work started, there has been a true explosion of relevant conventions and declarations, not only from international and regional bodies like United Nations and the Council of Europe but also ethical codes and declarations specifically for the health professions: doctors, nurses, and physical therapists.

The definition of torture we use today is the definition from the United Nations Convention Against Torture and Other Cruel, Inhuman or Degrading Treatment or Punishment, of December 10, 1984, which entered into force in June, 1987. In this Convention, torture is defined as:

> Any act by which severe pain or suffering, whether physical or mental, is intentionally inflicted on a person for such purposes as obtaining from him or a third person information or a confession, punishing him for an act he or a third person has committed or is suspected of having committed, or intimidating or coercing him or a third person, or for any reason based on discrimination of any kind, when such pain or suffering is inflicted by or at the instigation of or with the consent or acquiescence of a public official or other person acting in an official capacity. It does not include pain or suffering arising only from, inherent in or incidental to lawful sanctions.

It is very important that the United Nations–our World Society–has a standpoint and has established a definition.

In the United Nations Convention Against Torture, I want specifically to underline what we consider the most important Articles: Article 2, 4, 6, 10 and 14.

Article 2: Paragraphs 2 and 3 of this Article say:

> 2. No exceptional circumstances whatsoever, whether a state of war or a threat of war, internal political instability or any other public emergency, may be invoked as a justification of torture.

> 3. An order from a superior officer or a public authority may not be invoked as a justification of torture.

There are thus three very important points in Article 2:

a. No torture allowed,
b. No excuse–whatsoever,
c. An order: No excuse.

Article 4: Paragraph 1 of this Article says:

Each State Party shall ensure that all acts of torture are offences under its criminal law. The same shall apply to an attempt to commit torture and to an act by person which constitutes complicity or participation in torture.

Article 6 concerns impunity: Paragraph 1 of this Article says:

Upon being satisfied, after an examination of information available to it, that the circumstances so warrant, any State Party in whose territory a person alleged to have committed any offence referred to in article 4 is present shall take him into custody or take other legal measures to ensure his presence.

Article 10 concerns education

Each State Party shall ensure that education and information regarding the prohibition against torture are fully included in the training of law enforcement personnel, civil or military, medical personnel, public officials and other persons who may be involved in the custody, interrogation or treatment of any individual subjected to any form of arrest, detention or imprisonment.

This concept can thus be seen not only as a moral obligation of the world society, but also as the legal obligation of a State Party.

Article 14 concerns assistance to victims of torture

Each State Party shall ensure in its legal system that the victim of an act of torture obtains redress and has an enforceable right to fair and adequate compensation, including the means for as full rehabilitation as possible. In the event of death of the victim as a result of an act of torture, his dependents shall be entitled to compensation.

We are here talking about the three famous M's:

* Moral rehabilitation–Obtain redress
* Money rehabilitation–Fair and adequate compensation
* Medical rehabilitation–Means for as full rehabilitation as possible–physical, mental and social, including the family

In order to control the implementation of the United Nations Convention Against Torture in the countries who have ratified it, the CAT has been set up, composed of 10 experts. The Committee meets in Geneva twice a year. The States parties to the Convention are obliged to report to the Committee how the Convention is implemented in domestic law and in practice.

Today, 110 countries out of 186 have ratified the United Nations Convention. We are constantly urging all relevant international organisations to put pressure on the remaining 76 countries.

The Vienna Declaration. An important United Nations Declaration is the Vienna Declaration and Program of Action, adopted at the World Conference on Human Rights in June 1993. All 185 United Nations member states adopted it by consensus. In this document, a whole page concerns torture and the work against torture. The specific page on torture contains eight paragraphs, all worded in a very strong, clear and efficient language. In this manuscript, only the most important paragraph in my opinion, namely paragraph 57, will be quoted:

> The World Conference on Human Rights therefore urges all States to put an immediate end to the practice of torture and eradicate this evil forever through full implementation of the Universal Declaration of Human Rights as well as the relevant conventions, and, where necessary, strengthening of existing mechanisms. The World Conference on Human Rights calls on all States to cooperate fully with the Special Rapporteur on the question of torture in the fulfilment of this mandate.

Furthermore, since 1984 the United Nations–again the World Society–has had a Special Rapporteur on Torture, and the United Nations Voluntary Fund for Victims of Torture was created in 1981.

Following the World Conference on Human Rights in Vienna in 1993, a United Nations High Commissioner for Human Rights was appointed in April 1994. One of his most essential tasks is to work against torture. In June 1994 he visited the RCT from where he launched an appeal against torture, which he named the Copenhagen-Appeal. In this appeal he emphasises the importance of all States working against torture, and furthermore implementing fully the Convention Against Torture, especially with a view to the rehabilitation of torture victims and their families.

The United Nation's document entitled "Principles of Medical Ethics relevant to the role of health personnel particularly physicians, in the protection of prisoners and detainees against torture and other cruel, in-human or degrading treatment or punishment" [1982], clearly states in Principles 2 and 4 that doctors under no circumstances may participate in torture. However, it is not only the United Nations who by legal inter-ventions works against torture.

The Council of Europe's "Convention for the Prevention of Torture and Inhuman or Degrading Treatment or Punishment" went into force in 1989. A Committee for the Prevention of Torture controls the imple-mentation of the Convention. The members of this Committee visit prisons and other places where people are detained, in order to reveal whether torture and/or ill treatment takes place. It reports back confi-dentially to the country visited and suggests recommendations based on the findings of the Committee. This preventive work has proved to be very efficient.

The World Medical Association has also made a strong statement against torture, i.e., the so-called "Declaration of Tokyo" from 1975. This declaration contains a medical professional definition of torture, which resembles the definition in the United Nations Convention Against Torture. However, the United Nations definition only refers to govern-ment-sanctioned torture, which is the level on which the World Society can have influence. The Tokyo-Declaration says quite clearly that: "the doctor shall not countenance, condone or participate in the practice of torture." World Medical Association has further made a Resolution on Human Rights from 1995. Also the International Council of Nurses and World Confederation for Physical Therapy have made strong position statements and guidelines concerning torture.

TORTURE, THE STRONGEST WEAPON AGAINST DEMOCRACY

As I have already mentioned earlier, torture creates enormous amounts of fear in the victims and in the victims' environment. This is also the intention of the torturers. Because frightened people do not fight, you create a very effective means of subduing any opposition in a dictator-ship. Torture is used by governments to stay in power, governments which would otherwise have been removed. The spill-over effect tor-ture has from the individual victim to the family–and from the family onto the entire community–is an effective weapon against opposition and change. This is also why torturers oftentimes have no intention of killing their victims. They want them to stay alive and to go back to their community–broken and changed. Others in the community are going to think twice and thrice before they take up a fight. The scariness of watching what torture does to your friends and role models causes passivity as well as well-founded fear for your own life. Democracy and participation are two of the same kind. Passivity is only beneficial for dictators. So, one of the most important preconditions for the foundation for a stable democracy is freedom from torture and treatment and counselling of those who have been tortured.

Not only is torture a profound obstacle for democracy, it is also a hindrance for development. I would like to refer to the Vienna Declaration which in article 5 refers to the close connection between development and human rights. It says that:
All human rights are:

- Universal,
- Indivisible,
- Interdependent, and
- Interrelated.

This is both the case for civil rights, socioeconomic rights and rights to development. Thus, we cannot talk about development without specifically examining the situation regarding torture in a given country or region. The right to development is only possible if the civil rights and the socioeconomic rights are included in all development planning.

The Vienna Declaration also states in article 8: "Democracy, development and respect for human rights and fundamental freedoms are interdependent and mutually reinforcing. Democracy is based on the freely expressed will of the people to determine their own political, economic, social, and cultural systems and their full participation in all aspects of their lives." It cannot, I believe, be stated more clearly than that.

INTERNATIONAL WORK OF THE INTERNATIONAL REHABILITATION COUNCIL FOR TORTURE VICTIMS

The international work of IRCT has increased tremendously over the past years. Lobbying for victims of torture has become increasingly important and we work intensely with international bodies such as the United Nations, the European Union and national parliaments, including the United States Congress. We also work on group levels and individual levels, especially do we organize international seminars for health professionals and now also journalists in all parts of the world: Latin and Central America, Asia, Africa, and Western and Eastern Europe—each year about 15-20 international seminars. All together, we have established educational programs for health professionals such as medical doctors, nurses, physiotherapists, judges, and documentarists in more than 100 countries. The IRCT specifically works with many medical, nurses and physiotherapist organizations in order to enhance the general knowledge level of torture rehabilitation and to put the spotlight on the issue amongst all health professionals around the globe. These organizations include the World Medical Association, World Confederation for Physical Therapy, International Council of Nurses, World Psychiatric Association, and several international medical associations such as the Indian Medical Association, Nepal Medical Association, Malaysian Medical Association, and Pakistan Medical Association.

The International Rehabilitation Council for Torture Victims network program. Another major pillar in our work is the provision of assistance to establish programs and centers for victims of torture all over the world. We give advice and support to existing centers, including financial support, not only for rehabilitation, but also for research and documentation. The strong increase in new center and program establishments has made grounds for the formation of a more regionalized structure of the IRCT. In the future, we will emphasise the position of region centers in Asia and Latin America in order to support them into functioning as both clearinghouses and strongholds in general for the rehabilitation movement in those regions.

The IRCT will support the establishment of information-documentation centers in those particular regions. These clearinghouses will become knowledge centers for all aspects of torture and related research. This will make it much easier for local and national health organizations, health professionals, and media to access crucial new and valid information on torture.

Documentation. From the documentation center in Copenhagen, we distributed information and educational material on torture and related issues since 1987. Knowledge is influence, and we are proud of our documentation center which contains more than 38,000 records, including a vast amount of research and other documentation on torture and its effects. Close to 10,000 loans and requests were processed during 2,000, 40-50 percent of these going to foreign users from all over the world. The IRCT is presently initiating a major international documentation project, the Global Torture Victims Information System, which will contain information on instances of torture, as well as the ensuing treatment processes, supplied by rehabilitation centers from all over the world. Through the communication of such data, gathered from rehabilitation centers world-wide, a reliable, international base of information on the occurrence of torture, the methods used by perpetrators, as well as on the work to rehabilitate survivors, will become available for the first time. In addition, we publish our own quarterly journal, "Torture." Information activities have been established, for instance, we are on the Internet with an informative web site. Furthermore, we have produced a number of books in many different languages such as Arabic, Albanic, Chinese, Russian, Ukrainian, Spanish, French, English, etc., as well as articles and films. Within the last four years we have informed and educated 29,300 persons.

Press work. We also try as much as possible to keep the international press informed of all important news related to torture victims and rehabilitation. We have developed media strategies for approaching the press in order to make the message effective and heard.

Funding. We have established general funding opportunities for centers world-wide by: Lobbying activities aimed at governments to pledge [higher] contributions to United Nations Voluntary fund for Victims of Torture, making reports on estimated "Need for funding of rehabilitation services world-wide" [United Nations paper 1996], working for the creation of a special budget line for rehabilitation of torture victims in the European Union, working for funding via development aid agencies such as Danish Agency for Development Assistance, Swedish International Development Cooperation Agency, Norwegian Agency for Development Cooperation, etc., and by working for private funding, i.e., the Oak Foundation which is our most important private donor.

The 26 June Campaign. The 26 June Campaign is one of the IRCT's most effective international advocacy tools. Since the inauguration of the United Nations International Day in Support of Victims of Torture in 1997 the occasion has achieved a relatively high international profile, and a large number of international media outlets carried stories on the subject of torture on 26 June this year. The year 2001 was the fourth consecutive year in which the IRCT co-ordinated the 26 June campaign on behalf of Coalition of International Non-Governmental Organizations against Torture [including: Amnesty International, the Association for the Prevention of Torture, the International Federation of Action by Christians for the Abolition of Torture, the International Rehabilitation Council for Torture Victims, Seeking Reparation for Torture Survivors, and the World Organization against Torture]. This year, 26 June was commemorated by 252 rehabilitation centers and human rights organizations in 95 countries in all parts of the world.

The 2001 campaign was reported in the national media of a large number of countries, as well as global coverage on British Broadcasting Corporation World Service, Radio Netherlands [broadcasting in Spanish into Latin America] and United Nations World Radio, to name just three agencies with which the IRCT dealt directly, and we hope next year's campaign will have as much publicity as this year.

This year, the global campaign was launched by UNHCHR Mary Robinson, who presented the global ratification campaign, which the IRCT is conducting on behalf of CINAT. Letters were sent to all States, which have not ratified the United Nations Convention against Torture or which have reservations–either general or to the competence of the Committee against Torture.

Prevention. Lastly, but not less important, I want to stress the area of prevention. Here, we have strengthened our efforts considerably in recent years. Prevention and advocacy are sometimes interrelated, for example, our lobbying efforts are closely related to the ultimate goal of preventing torture from happening in the first place.

In addition, prevention obviously has to go hand in hand with rehabilitation. Even though it sounds simple, it is of course a very difficult task. However, the prevention program at the IRCT has had great success, even with limited staff and funding, it has been able to initiate changes of attitudes and accommodate new and critical thinking about torture around the globe. Let me spend a few minutes introducing you to the concepts of prevention as we distinguish them as medical doctors. In the prevention of torture, you can use the exact same concepts of prevention as you do with any medical illness.

Within the medical world, primary prevention of disease means the prevention of the occurrence of the disease in the first place. Secondary prevention means reducing the number of outbreaks of the disease and tertiary prevention stands for the treatment and relief of the disease but not necessarily its cure.

If we translate that into the prevention of torture, we get the following distinctions:

- *Primary prevention*, tries to prevent the practice of torture before it even occurs and is aimed at society in general.
- *Secondary prevention* deals with the reduction of the number of tortured and is aimed at groups that have been or may be involved in torture, e.g., the police, the prison department, judges, civil ser-

vants, etc. They should be influenced not to practice torture in their work.

- *Tertiary prevention* deals with reducing the results of torture. It is person-related and aims to give help, rehabilitation, and treatment to the torture victim in order to lessen the effects of torture.

On the primary level, the IRCT attempts to involve many different professional groups as well as the political level. The organization has participated actively in the United Nations work group drafting an Optional Protocol for the Convention against Torture. Other international and highly renowned institutions with which IRCT has had contacts include the Raoul Wallenberg Institute in Lund, Sweden, and the Organization for Security and Co-Operation in Europe. Here, it is important to note that tertiary prevention is the foundation for primary prevention. The treatment of an individual constitutes a value beyond treating him or her. It also creates the necessary knowledge for doctors, so they can initiate prevention on the primary as well as secondary levels. What I mean is: we need the medically based knowledge of torture before we can address decision makers and law enforcement personnel. The IRCT has worked to disseminate knowledge of torture amongst health professionals, including the magnitude of the problem, the methods of torture, the effects of various torture methods, the victims' coping mechanisms, etc. Only when we have this knowledge, can we affect relevant groups in society.

On the secondary level, I would like to mention a few educational programs in which IRCT has been involved. Police officers from Bosnia Herzegovina, South Africa, Ukraine, Palestine, and China have visited Denmark, and IRCT has met with more than 500 international law enforcement personnel in more than 60 countries, exploring new and more humane ways of conducting police work and the underlying devastating long lasting effect of torture in the victims' body and mind. We have also discussed that torture is degrading–not only to the victims–but to the torturers themselves. Abroad, IRCT has been conducting seminars for law enforcement personnel, including prison officials, on several continents, including Africa, Latin America, and Asia. The IRCT personal takes part in prison visits in co-operation with members of international human rights bodies, to several countries.

On the tertiary level, seminars are held to train health personnel in the various treatment methods, to create a forum for the participants from the various countries to exchange experiences, and to stimulate the creation of treatment centers.

CONCLUSION

Twenty-five years of professional medical and psychological work against torture has proved the following: Today we have sufficient knowledge. We know now how torture affects the individual. We know about torture methods, after-effects–short- and long-term–and we know how to diagnose, which is of course extremely important. We know how to rehabilitate the victims and how to rehabilitate them according to different models. We work very hard to help establishing new treatment centers because without rehabilitation of victims of torture, development and democracy will be at stake. Not only do we as a world community owe it to the victims, but it is necessary to heal the wounds of torture in a country in order to have peace and tranquillity.

We have enough experience to be able to speak about torture and its effects in a more substantial and assured way. Together we have sufficient basic knowledge [i.e., social analysis on a medical and psychological basis] allowing us to make very strong statements–also to politicians and decision makers–against the practice of torture, and to disclose torture even when performed in its most "sophisticated" ways. The fact that our knowledge is founded on social analysis and with a medical and psychological basis is, in our opinion, the reason why politicians and decision makers listen to us.

We have a unique knowledge because our organization and network is founded on a professional basis [as doctors, psychologists, nurses, physical therapists, social workers, etc.]. We have a specific professional knowledge about torture. The analysis and documentation we, as health professionals, have made concerning torture is our strength. It reveals torture as a power instrument "playing" with the physical and psychological health of human beings. This, I think, is why torture is disgusting and offending to most people. The fact that totally healthy people are tortured with the acceptance and knowledge of their own government is despicable. Our research has proved that torturers who work for governments are aiming at breaking down the victims, and we know that they are always capable of doing so if that is their intention.

Our research has proven that all over the world torture methods [there are cultural differences] are basically the same, because the aim of torture is the same. Our research has proved that torture is used as a power instrument often used against people who are working for better and more democratic conditions in their own country, primarily people like student leaders, union leaders, honest politicians, journalists, leaders of ethnic minorities, etc.

Our research has revealed that torture is used in one third of the countries in the world today because governments want to stay in power, and that is why they use torture as their means. Our research and the research of the IRCT network have revealed this pattern. We should use all our strength and energy to spread this horrible knowledge. The people in power, i.e., the people responsible for torture, have of course always known these facts. The new thing is that we, who want to help the victims, now understand how horrible and long-lasting the effects of torture really are. Now we are as clever as the torturers and they cannot fool us anymore.

When we started talking about torture some 25 years ago, there was silence about what really happened under torture. At that time, we were not aware that the torture victims could not break this silence because of the torture-induced shame, guilt, personality changes, low self-esteem, anxiety, depression, etc. Because the torture victims were suffering so much psychologically, they could not explain. This knowledge, and the fact that we can explain it as professionals, is a weapon in our hands—thereby we can break the silence.

But who will listen? How do you reach the public? How do you reach the most important decision makers? One of the answers is targeted advocacy work, including press work. Advocacy has become increasingly important for IRCT and we dedicate many man-hours to that particular work area. We believe that we, as an international organization, have a moral obligation to advocate on behalf of the millions of victims. Exhibits, the IRCT homepage, research for television-documentaries, participation in hearings, dissemination of press releases, participation in urgent actions, lobbying on national and international levels—everything is aimed at calling attention to the need for rehabilitation of torture victims and the abolition of torture. In fact, it is our democratic world which we defend, no matter where on the globe the torture is taking place.

In order to help, we need to speak out and expose the countries using government sanctioned torture. We need to support organizations working against torture and we should always treat torture victims with respect. Only this way we can show our disgust for torture. Each and every one of us has a choice between doing something or staying passive. As Edmund Burke said: "The only thing necessary for the triumph of evil is for good men to do nothing."

REFERENCES

1. Amris K, Torp-Pedersen S, Prip K, Qvistgaard E, Danneskiold-Samsoe B, Bliddal H: Changes in the plantar fascia after falanga torture diagnosed by ultrasound [us]: preliminary results. J Musculoske Pain 9 (suppl#5):11, 2001.

2. Lie B: Psykosociale problemer blant nylig ankomne flyktninger i Norge: Rapport Fra Undersøkelsen. Psykososialt Senter for Flyktninger, Oslo, 1998.

3. Baker R: Psychological Problems of Refugees. British Refugee Council: European Consultation on Refugees Exiles, London, 1985, pp. 1-141.

4. Anonymous: Torture victims in the United States. The Center for Victims of Torture, Minneapolis, MN, USA 2001.

5. Kjersem HJ: Migrationsmedicin i Danmark: Vurdering Af Nogle Migrationsmedicinske Problemstillinger Blandt Asylansøgere Og Flygtninge. Dansk Røde Kors Asylafdelingen, 1996, pp.1-78.

6. Montgomery E, Foldspang A: Criterion-related validity of screening for exposure to torture. Torture 4(4):115-118, 1994.

The Development
of Widespread Pain After Injuries

Dan Buskila
Lily Neumann

SUMMARY. Objective: To evaluate the evidence suggesting the development of widespread pain and fibromyalgia [FMS] after musculoskeletal injuries.

Findings: Few studies have determined the frequency of a precipitating event occurring prior to the onset of widespread pain and FMS. Evidence comes mostly from case series or case reports. The strongest evidence supporting the development of widespread pain and FMS comes from an Israeli study in which adults with neck injuries had a 10-fold increased risk of developing FMS within one year of their injury, compared with adults with lower extremity fractures. Although widespread pain and FMS may be associated with trauma, the present data from the literature are insufficient to indicate whether causal relationships exist between injuries and widespread pain. It was suggested that precipitating triggers such as injuries might interact with genetic factors, and together cause the development of FMS, which is the result of central nervous system dysfunction. The outcome of post-injury widespread pain/FMS was found in most of the reports to be worse than that of idiopathic FMS. So-

Dan Buskila, MD, is Professor of Medicine, Soroka Medical Center and Faculty of Health Sciences, Ben-Gurion University of the Negev, Beer-Sheva, Israel.

Lily Neumann, PhD, is Professor in Biostatistics, Epidemiology Department, Faculty of Health Sciences, Ben-Gurion University of the Negev, Beer Sheva, Israel.

Address correspondence to: Dan Buskila, MD, Department of Medicine B, Soroka Medical Center, P.O. Box 151, Beer Sheva 84101, Israel [E-mail: lily@bgumail. bgu.ac.il].

[Haworth co-indexing entry note]: "The Development of Widespread Pain After Injuries." Buskila, Dan, and Lily Neumann. Co-published simultaneously in *Journal of Musculoskeletal Pain* [The Haworth Medical Press, an imprint of The Haworth Press, Inc.] Vol. 10, No. 1/2, 2002, pp. 261-267; and: *The Clinical Neurobiology of Fibromyalgia and Myofascial Pain: Therapeutic Implications* [ed: Robert M. Bennett] The Haworth Medical Press, an imprint of The Haworth Press, Inc., 2002, pp. 261-267. Single or multiple copies of this article are available for a fee from The Haworth Document Delivery Service [1-800-HAWORTH, 9:00 a.m. - 5:00 p.m. (EST). E-mail address: getinfo@haworthpressinc.com].

261

cial systems and social acceptability of work disability play a strong role in determining the outcome of post-injury FMS.

Conclusions: Widespread pain and FMS are obviously associated with injury. However, overall data are insufficient to indicate whether causal relationships exist between injury and FMS.

Future studies should prospectively document the chronology of symptoms from the onset of the injury and repeatedly evaluate the patients for disability, quality of life, change in occupation, and litigation status. *[Article copies available for a fee from The Haworth Document Delivery Service: 1-800-HAWORTH. E-mail address: <getinfo@haworthpressinc.com> Website: <http://www.HaworthPress.com> © 2002 by The Haworth Press, Inc. All rights reserved.]*

KEYWORDS. Widespread pain, fibromyalgia, injuries, posttraumatic fibromyalgia

INTRODUCTION

Fibromyalgia [FMS] syndrome is a chronic painful musculoskeletal disorder of unknown cause. Despite extensive research, the etiology and pathophysiology of FMS are still unclear. Physical and emotional trauma have been reported anecdotally to be precipitating factors in FMS, and it is not uncommon for patients with FMS to report the onset in relation to an accident or an injury (1,2). The issue of injuries triggering the development of widespread pain and FMS has generated much controversy, since it has not only medical but also considerable medicolegal implications (3).

Indeed, evidence that musculoskeletal injury or trauma can cause widespread pain comes mostly from a few case series or case reports and it is often insufficient to establish causal relationships. The possible association between injury and widespread pain/FMS has recently been systematically reviewed (4,5).

The aim of this article is to evaluate the evidence that injury can initiate widespread pain/FMS and its medicolegal implications.

INJURY AND WIDESPREAD PAIN/FIBROMYALGIA SYNDROME: IS IT ASSOCIATED?

Few studies have attempted to determine the frequency of a precipitating event occurring prior to the onset of FMS, or the prevalence of FMS following a specific musculoskeletal trauma. Several authors have recently characterized posttraumatic or reactive FMS (1,2,6,7). A retrospective chart review found that 29 of 127 FMS patients [23 percent] identified a specific precipitating event prior to the onset of symptoms (1). These events were usually traumatic, such as a motor vehicle accident [MVA], an injury, or surgery. In a study of patients with posttraumatic FMS (2) a total of 60.7 percent noted the onset of symptoms after an MVA, and 12.5 percent noted symptom onset after a work injury, 7.1 percent after surgery, 5.4 percent after a sports-related injury, and 14.3 percent after other various traumatic events. Twenty-three of 24 patients with chronic postaccident pain had FMS (8) and 10.5 percent of 38 patients after whiplash trauma fulfilled the criteria for diagnosing FMS (9). The strongest evidence supporting an association between injury and FMS is an Israeli study in which 22 [21.6 percent] of 102 adults with neck injuries developed FMS within one year of their trauma, compared with only one of 59 adults with lower extremity fractures [P = 0.001] (10). All subjects were recruited at an occupational medicine clinic. Almost all FMS-related symptoms were more common and more severe in the neck injury group. Fibromyalgia syndrome was noted at a mean of 3.2 months [±1.1] after the trauma. Neck injury subjects with FMS [N = 22] had more tenderness, had more severe and more prevalent FMS related symptoms, and reported lower quality of life and more impaired physical functioning than did those without FMS [N = 80]. This study suggests that some areas of the body are more susceptible than others to a traumatic incident thus, trauma to the neck is associated with a higher incidence of FMS, whereas even major trauma to the legs, such as fracture, has no similar impact. Interestingly, Radanov et al. (11) have shown that two years after whiplash injury of the neck, 18 percent of the patients still had injury-related symptoms, including fatigue, headaches, anxiety, sleep disturbances, and muscle tenderness. It is possible that some of the symptomatic patients would have satisfied the criteria for FMS, but this disorder was not studied in the report by Radonov et al. (11).

INJURY AND WIDESPREAD PAIN/ FIBROMYALGIA SYNDROME: CAUSATION AND MEDICOLEGAL ASPECTS

Many patients with FMS report that their condition started with a physical or emotional trauma, infection, or surgery (12). Overall data from the literature are insufficient to indicate whether causal relationships exist between injury and widespread pain/FMS. The absence of evidence, however, does not mean that causality does not exist; rather it implies that appropriate studies have not been performed. A study of the clinical course of 104 randomly selected workers who had not returned to work in three months following soft tissue injury showed that the greatest negative effect for return to work was associated with psychological distress and functional disability (13). In this study the presence of fibromyalgic tender points was one of the valid predictors of delay in return to work.

It was suggested that the questions of whether injury can cause FMS or whether other psychosocial factors are more important are worthy of further examination in the medicolegal context (14). The issue of causality in FMS has been addressed by Wolfe and the Vancouver Fibromyalgia Consensus Group (15). They concluded that the cause[s] of FMS is [are] incompletely understood and that there may be events reported by the patient as precipitating and/or aggravating, including physical trauma. It was suggested that in determining the relationship between FMS and antecedent events, the physician should consider the patient's opinion, and review the events and pertinent collateral information, including current and past medical and psychosocial history. The chronology of symptoms should be documented (15). Our study on the association between neck injury and FMS suggests that soft tissue injury to the neck can result in an increased incidence of FMS compared with other injuries (10).

Trauma in the form of an accident or work injury is often a focus in determination of medicolegal disability in subjects developing chronic widespread pain/FMS. Although FMS obviously may be associated with injury, the question is whether trauma can cause FMS or whether other factors, such as pain behavior, societal enhancement, or psychosocial factors, are the overwhelming causes (16). Furthermore, even though trauma may cause FMS in selected cases, is it necessarily associated with work disability? Gordon (14) has proposed that in determining the relationship between the antecedent injury and the development of FMS, the physician should assess underlying pre-existing medical and psychological conditions, along with details of the severity of the accident and documentation of the patient's activities and pain symptoms before and since the accident. He states that from his experience, frank malingering is unusual in this patient population. However, the patient's post behavior and psychological state are a key to understanding this possibility (14). This diagnostic approach may help the assessor to determine whether the accident was a risk factor in the cause of FMS, an aggravating one that advanced pre-existing FMS or only a component in the development of FMS but not the sole cause of a condition that was going to develop anyway (14).

Moldofsky et al. (8) reported on 24 patients with postaccident pain, all had FMS with one exception. The eight patients who had their litigation resolved were compared with the 16 who had pending medicolegal claims. No significant differences between the two groups, in terms of FMS symptoms, current disability, and sleep patterns, were found. Seven of the eight patients with resolved litigation were unemployed due to impairment or disability. Patients with unresolved litigation remained employed with modification requirements, such as part-time work, alteration of work place, or the provisions of special aids. The successful resolution of litigation in this small group of patients with FMS did not lead to an improvement in their symptomatology, their psychophysiologic dysfunction, or their overall economic well being.

Buskila et al. (10) reported from Israel that 20 of 102 patients with neck injuries filed an insurance claim. There was no difference in the prevalence of FMS, tender point count, quality of life, and pain and fatigue symptoms between those that filed and did not file a claim. All of the Israeli patients with postaccident FMS continued to be employed. This is in contrast to other reports (15). The Israeli experience suggests that the social system and the social acceptability of work disability play a strong role in determining the outcome of trauma and FMS. Wolfe (16) has suggested that limiting the payments for patients with FMS will decrease claims and encourage them to consider themselves as less disabled.

PROGNOSIS

Although the majority of patients with FMS have chronic symptoms and despite the presence of disability risk factors, most patients with FMS maintain a good range of normal daily activities and continue working (14). Few studies have addressed the issue of outcome in postinjurious FMS. Turk et al. (17) demonstrated that patients with posttraumatic FMS present quite different pictures than patients with idiopathic FMS. Specifically, posttraumatic patients with FMS reported significantly higher degrees of pain, disability, life interference and affective distress, as well as lower levels of activity than did the idiopathic patients with FMS.

Similarly, Greenfield et al. (1), in a study of 127 patients with FMS, reported that reactive patients with FMS were more disabled and had less physical activity, greater loss of employment, and greater disability compensation than the rest of the patients with FMS. Waylonis and Perkins (2) have reported in contrast that the outcome of posttraumatic FMS was not different from that of spontaneous FMS. However, this study had some methodologic weaknesses, since the authors were able to contact only 23 percent of 773 patients with posttraumatic FMS eligible to be included in the study. We have recently assessed the outcome of patients with neck injuries originally examined in 1996 (10) [three years later, in 1999]. We were able to recruit 78 of 102 subjects [76 percent]. Fifty percent of the subjects having postneck injury FMS in 1996 still had FMS in 1999. All of them were females and all the subjects continued to be employed [unpublished data].

FUTURE DIRECTIONS

Although FMS may be associated with antecedent injury, the current literature reveals that data are insufficient to indicate whether causal relationships exist between trauma and FMS. The strongest evidence supporting an association between trauma and FMS, the Israeli neck injury study (10), should be corroborated by further studies.

Future epidemiologic studies of trauma and widespread pain/FMS are needed to address potential or predictive causality. These studies should document the chronology of symptoms following an injury, both prospectively and longitudinally. The patient should be assessed for symptoms and tenderness immediately after the accident and then be repeatedly evaluated using both subjective [questionnaires assessing physical functioning and quality of life, visual analog-scales for self-rating] and objective [point count and dolorimetry threshold] measures. Such a design will enable the clarification of the relationship between injury [trauma] and widespread pain/FMS.

REFERENCES

1. Greenfield S, Fitzcharles M, Esdaile JM: Reactive fibromyalgia syndrome. Arthritis Rheum 35:678-681, 1992.

2. Waylonis GW, Perkins RH: Post-traumatic fibromyalgia. A long-term follow-up. Am J Phys Med Rehabil 73:403-409, 1994.

3. White KP, Harth M, Teasell RW: Work disability evaluation and the fibromyalgia syndrome. Semin Arthritis Rheum 24:371-381, 1995.

4. White KP, Carette S, Harth M, Teasell RW: Trauma and fibromyalgia: Is there an association and what does it mean? Semin Arthritis Rheum 29:200-216, 2000.

5. Buskila D, Neumann L: Musculoskeletal injury as a trigger for fibromyalgia/posttraumatic fibromyalgia. Curr Rheumatol Reports 2:104-108, 2000.

6. Bennett RM: Disabling fibromyalgia: Appearance versus reality. J Rheumatol 20:1821-1824, 1993.

7. Romano T: Valid complaints or malingering? Clinical experiences with posttraumatic fibromyalgia syndrome. West Virg Med J 86:198-202, 1990.

8. Moldofsky H, Wong MTH, Lue FA: Litigation, sleep symptoms and disabilities in postaccident pain (fibromyalgia). J Rheumatol 20:1935-1940, 1993.

9. Magnusson T: Extracervical symptoms after whiplash trauma. Cephalgia 14: 223-227, 1994.

10. Buskila D, Neumann L, Vaisberg G, Alkalay D, Wolfe F: Increased rates of fibromyalgia following cervical spine injury: A controlled study of 161 cases of traumatic injury. Arthritis Rheum 40:446-452, 1997.

11. Radanov BP, Sturzenegger M, Di Stefano G: Long-term outcome after whiplash injury: A 2-year follow up considering features of injury mechanism and somatic, radiologic, and psychosocial findings. Medicine (Baltimore) 74:281-297, 1995.

12. Aaron LA, Bradely LA, Alarcon GS, Triana-Alexander M, Alexander RW, Martin MY, Alberts KR: Perceived physical and emotional trauma as precipitating events in fibromyalgia. Arthritis Rheum 40:453-460, 1997.

13. Crook J, Moldofsky H: The clinical cause of musculoskeletal pain in empirically derived groupings of injured workers. Pain 67:427-433, 1996.

14. Gordon DA: Chronic widespread pain as a medicolegal issue. Bailliere's Clin Rheumatol 13:531-543, 1999.

15. Wolfe F: The fibromyalgia syndrome: A consensus report of fibromyalgia and disability. J Rheumatol 23:534-539, 1996.

16. Wolfe F: The fibromyalgia problem. J Rheumatol 24:1247-1249, 1997.

17. Turk DC, Okifuji A, Starz TW, Sinclair JD: Effects of type of symptom onset on psychological distress and disability in fibromyalgia syndrome patients. Pain 68: 423-430, 1996.

Index

MPI. *See* Multidimensional Pain
    Inventory (MPI)
MPSs. *See* Myofascial pain syndromes
    (MPSs)
MSK. *See* Medullary sponge kidney
    (MSK)
Multidimensional Pain Inventory
    (MPI)
  in fibromyalgia, 92-93
    validity of, 92-93
    profiles of, differential treatment
        repsonses as function of, 94
Multiple chemical sensitivity,
    described, 204f
Muscle(s), skeletal, aging effects on,
    12-14
Muscle contraction, isometric, pain
    modulation during, 49-50
Muscle fiber type I, injury to,
    141-142,142t
Muscle pain
  aging and, 5-22
    chronic fatigue syndrome, 17
    effects on skeletal muscle, 12-14
    introduction to, 6
    muscle oxidative damage, 14-16
    pathologic conditions, 18
    perception of, physiologic
        changes in, 11-17
  assessment of, 99-102
  in the elderly, 11-18
    aging and, 18
    chronic fatigue syndrome, 17
    effects on skeletal muscle, 12-14
    muscle oxidative damage, 14-16
    pathologic conditions, 10-11
    perception of, physiologic
        changes in, 11-17
  findings related to, 126-128,127f
  inflammatory, pathophysiology of,
    121-129. *See also*
    Inflammatory myopathies
  study of, objectives of,
    122-126,123f-125f,126t

Myofascial pain syndromes (MPSs),
    165-175
  gender predilection for, 168
  histology of, 167-168
  hypersensitivity and, 167
  introduction to, 166
Myofascial release, for fibromyalgia
    with myofascial trigger
    points, 183-184
Myofascial trigger points
  fibromyalgia with, physical therapy
    approach to, case example,
    177-190. *See also*
    Fibromyalgia, with
    myofascial trigger points,
    physical therapy approach to,
    case example
  identified, 182t
MYOPAIN 2001, xv-xviii
  attendance at, 1
  introduction to, 1-3
MYOPAIN meetings
  clinical and scientific objectives of,
    xv
  history of, xv-xvi
Myopathy(ies), inflammatory,
    pathophysiology of, 121-129.
    See also Muscle pain,
    inflammatory,
    pathophysiology of

Nepal Medical Association, 253
Neumann, L., 261
NEURIGEN Project, 12,14
Neurodynamic testing, in assessment
    of fibromyalgia with
    myofascial trigger points, 182
Neuroendocrinological aberrations,
    fibromyalgia due to, 51-52
Neuroimaging, of persistent pain
    conditions, 76-81
Nitric oxide, 41
Nitric oxide synthase, 41